Rehabilitation of Paralysis Due to Apoplexy

Written by Pan Chang
Translated by Li Zhaoguo and Xu Qilong
Illustrated by Xu Lin

FOREIGN LANGUAGES PRESS BEIJING

First Edition 2004

Home Page:
http://www.flp.com.cn
E-mail addresses:
info@flp.com.cn
sale@flp.com.cn

ISBN 7-119-03192-9

Published by Foreign Languages Press
24 Baiwanzhuang Road, Beijing 100037, China

Distributed by China International Book Trading Corporation
35 Chegongzhuang Xilu, Beijing 100044, China
P.O. Box 399, Beijing, China

Printed in the People's Republic of China

FOREWORD

Apoplexy, known as wind stroke in traditional Chinese medicine (TCM), is usually seen in hypertension, cerebral hemorrhage and cerebral infarction as defined in modern medicine. At present, about a third of the provinces and municipalities in China have entered the era of an ageing society. There are about two million aged people who suffer from wind stroke each year in China, among whom about 70% have various sequelae. With the increase of the ageing population and the development of medical science, the morbidity and survival rate of apoplexy and the rate of its resultant after paralysis occurs have also increased.

Paralysis due to wind stroke usually means that patients are unable to manage their own life. Though various factors are responsible for patient debility, such as constitutional factors and pathological conditions, correct nursing and rehabilitative treatment are the key factors involved in handling it. It is evident that correct nursing and rehabilitative treatment can greatly reduce the sequelae rate, prevent spasms and rigidity of the joints, increase the rehabilitative rate of bodily functions and improve the quality of survival.

It is certain that to provide correct nursing methods and knowledge of rehabilitative treatment for patients with paralysis due to wind stroke is the duty of every medical and nursing worker. For this purpose, the author has written this book based on over ten years of clinical treatment and research into paralysis due to wind stroke. Since medical terms and the body positions are difficult for general readers to understand, this book is illustrated in detail with necessary explanations for readers' convenience. In order to make it easy for readers to understand the directions and range of the physiological movement of the main joints, so as to correctly do functional exercises, Chapter 2 is devoted to the illustration and explanation of the movement of each main joint in the human body.

The book introduces different nursing and rehabilitative therapeutic methods according to the acute stage, convalescence and sequelae, making it more convenient for readers to study and manipulate.

The rehabilitative treatment usually begins three to seven days after the pathological conditions become stable. Clinical practice shows that correct relaxation and slow separation of each joint and independent active functional exercises when the patient is conscious and free from remarkable inhibition will not aggravate the pathological conditions. Even cerebral hemorrhage will not recur. For patients with hypertension and general vascular sclerosis (including coronary heart disease), critical conditions also will not appear if the patients do not withhold the breath and make great efforts in functional exercises.

Clinical practice finds that correct rehabilitative treatment is a course lasting up to three months. It is generally believed that the restoration of neural function terminates within six months and it is difficult to restore after half a year. So, early rehabilitative treatment can promote blood circulation, propel venous recovery, promote metabolism, and reduce local damage in the brain. Besides, the formation of collateral circulation in the brain will improve cerebral ischemia and promote the rehabilitation of the limbs.

To restore the functions of the affected limbs earlier, patients must correctly understand and perform the rehabilitative therapeutic methods. The following points should be borne in mind.

1. Correctly understand the terms used in this book, such as bending the shoulder joint, extending the elbow joint, dorsal bending of the wrist joint, palmar bending of the wrist joint, dorsal bending of the ankle joint, metatarsal bending of the ankle joint, etc. Besides, upward (anterior, lateral) turning of the palm means a supine position of the forearm and vice versa.
2. Familiarity with the muscle groups. Appendix 1 in this book covers the muscle groups involved in the movement of the main joints. Readers, and medical and nursing workers engaging in rehabilitative medicine, should become familiar with them, especially the starting and ending points of each skeletal muscle. Such a familiarity is helpful for correct and systematic functional training or selection of sites for performing treatment.
3. Moderate exertion in doing exercise: no matter if the exercise is done by the patient actively, or passively with the help of doctors or relatives, the effort used and the range selected should be moderate, avoiding making efforts to enable each joint to reach the normal physiological movement range; otherwise, the joint pains can easily occur. Besides, patients with paralysis due to wind stroke usually experience sensory disturbance and bradyesthesia, so that any exercise involving great exertion will cause subcutaneous ecchymoma. In the early stages, patients are forbidden to do exercises with heavy loads, because it is easy to cause dislocation of the joints.
4. Correct location of the acupoints. This is a key to the curative effect of rehabilitative treatment. The correct location of each acupoint is expounded in the book. If readers are still unclear, please refer to the commonly used bone measurement and simple ways to locate acupoints in Appendix 2 in this book or other specialized works.

On the whole, the rehabilitation process of the patients with paralysis due to wind stroke is a process of substitute functional training and the restoration of the injured nerves. This means that the patients study to develop new functions to substitute for the lost ones, and restore the formal functions of their body through restoration and reconstruction of the functions of the nerves.

In writing this book, I am indebted to Mr. Xu Lin, who has drawn all the illustrations, and Mr. Li Yuqin, who has supported and cooperated with me.

I would also like to acknowledge my relatives, who have helped me heart and soul in my study of medicine.

There must be errors in this book due to my limited knowledge. Criticism and advice are welcome and will be adopted in the next edition.

Pan Chang

CONTENTS

Chapter 1
GENERAL INTRODUCTION

Wind stroke, a term used in traditional Chinese medicine (TCM), is a kind of acute cerebrovascular disease marked by sudden coma accompanied by hemiplegia, distortion of the face, dysphasia or sudden hemiplegia without fainting. Since its occurrence is sudden, involving rapid changes, and violent in development, similar to the way the wind blows in nature, so it is called wind stroke in TCM.

Wind stroke is a disease due to disturbance of the blood circulation in the brain. Usually wind stroke is divided into two categories according to the cause, pathogenesis and manifestations. The first category is called hemorrhagic wind stroke or hemorrhagic cerebrovascular disease, including cerebral hemorrhage and subarachnoid hemorrhage. The second category is called ischemic wind stroke or ischemic cerebrovascular disease, including temporal cerebral ischemic seizure and cerebral infarction (including cerebral thrombosis and cerebral embolism).

1. DIFFERENTIATION OF DISEASE

Under normal conditions, the blood is transported to the brain through the cerebral vessels to provide necessary nutrients for the brain tissues (nerve cells) to maintain the physiological activities of the brain. If there is cerebral arteriosclerosis that makes the vascular wall brittle and narrow, or leads to dissecting aneurysm, it may cause the breaking or stagnation of the vessels due to various factors such as excitation, anxiety, overexertion and hypotension (or hypertension), consequently leading to disturbance in blood circulation, ischemia in part of the cerebral tissues and edema, which further result in dysfunction of the cerebral nerves and various manifestations of wind stroke.

(1)Cerebral hemorrhage

Cerebral hemorrhage refers to the breaking of the vessels in the cortex of the brain and extravasation of the blood. There are symptoms of headache, vomiting, coma and hemiplegia in most patients. Cerebral hemorrhage is the most serious type of wind stroke. The clinical manifestations vary due to differences in the regions subject to the hemorrhage.

① Capsuloganglionic hemorrhage

It is usually marked by paralysis of the opposite side limb, sensory disturbance in half of the body and hemianopsia.

② Thalamus hemorrhage

Scanty thalamus hemorrhage on one side may produce symptoms of light paralysis of the limbs, sensory disturbance of one side of the body and obvious disturbance of proprioceptive sense due to a topoanesthesia-like inability to tell which finger is touched. Profuse thalamus hemorrhage on both sides is usually marked by frequent spurting vomiting of a coffee-like substance, polyuria, glucose in the urine, paralysis of the four limbs, and both eyes staring toward the tip of the nose. The prognosis is usually unfavorable.

③ Cerebrolobar hemorrhage

The usual manifestations are headache and vomiting. Frontal lobar hemorrhage is usually accompanied with restlessness, anxiety, paralysis of the opposite side limbs and anandia. Parietal lobar hemorrhage is usually accompanied with sensory disturbance of the opposite side. Temporal lobar hemorrhage is usually accompanied with restlessness, anxiety and sensory aphasia. Occipital lobar hemorrhage is usually accompanied with hemianopsia. The prognosis is usually favorable.

④ Pontine hemorrhage

The brain stem is a region susceptible to hemorrhage. The usual manifestations are paralysis of one side of the face and limbs on the opposite side. Profuse hemorrhage usually causes paralysis of the four limbs, miosis, high fever, coma, even convulsion and irregular breathing. The prognosis is usually unfavorable.

⑤ Cerebellar hemorrhage

Scanty hemorrhage is often marked by dizziness, sharp headache, frequent vomiting, unclear speech and unstable walking. Profuse hemorrhage usually leads to sudden death.

⑥ Ventricular hemorrhage

Primary ventricular hemorrhage is seldom seen. Secondary ventricular hemorrhage is usually marked by vomiting, polyhydrosis, cyanotic coloration or paleness of the skin. One or two hours after the onset, unconsciousness occurs along with high fever, paralysis of the four limbs or stiff convulsions, unstable blood pressure and irregular breathing. The prognosis is unfavorable.

(2) **Subarachnoid hemorrhage**

This is an independent disease of hemorrhagic wind stroke. Primary subarachnoid hemorrhage is caused by the direct flow of blood into the subarachnoid cavity from the surface of the brain and the broken vessels in the bottom of the brain. Secondary subarachnoid hemorrhage is cerebral hemorrhage caused by the flow of blood into the subarachnoid cavity or ventricles of the brain through the cerebral tissues. Generally speaking, an occurrence before the age of 30 is usually caused by deformity of the vessels; occurrence after 40 is usually due to dissecting aneurysm; occurrence after 50 often results from hypertension and breaking of the vessels due to arteriosclerosis. The usual clinical manifestations are acute headache, vomiting, and stiffness of the neck, which may be accompanied by anxiety, delirium and hallucination, or convulsions and coma. This disease tends to recur and care must be taken to prevent relapse.

(3) **Temporary cerebral ischemia**

Temporary cerebral ischemia of the arterial system in the neck is usually marked by flaccidity of one limb or half of the body, sensory disturbance in half of the body, aphasia or vision disorder of one eye. Temporary cerebral ischemia due to vertebral-basal arterial system is usually marked by dizziness, blurred vision, ambiopia, nausea and vomiting, dysphagia and ataxia. The symptoms normally last only a matter of minutes, with the longest duration being no more than 24 hours, hence the name temporary cerebral ischemia.

(4) Cerebral thrombosis

Cerebral thrombosis, the most common type of wind stroke, is caused by ischemia, softening and necrosis of local cerebral tissues due to obstruction of the narrowed cerebral vessels with blood coagulation. The usual symptoms are hemiplegia, aphasia and sensory disturbance. Clinically, it is often seen among people ranging in age from 55 to 60. It occurs more frequently in males than females. It is marked by an attack in quiet conditions, slow onset and gradual aggravation; continuing consciousness and no sensory disturbance; temporary cerebral ischemia, hypertension, cerebral arteriosclerosis, hyperlipemia and diabetes history.

① Thrombosis in the cervical arterial system usually causes paralysis of the opposite side, sensory disturbance or aphasia.

② Thrombosis in the vertebral-basal arterial system often leads to dizziness, nausea, vomiting, ambiopia, crossed dyscinesia and sensory disturbance, dyslalia, dysphagia and choking in drinking water.

(5) Cerebral embolism

Embolism (including cardiogenic embolism, bacterial embolism, arteriosclerosis embolism, fat embolism and air embolism) in the blood is due to various factors flowing into the cerebral arteries whereby the blood blocks the cerebral arteries and causes a series of cerebral neural symptoms similar to cerebral thrombosis. Clinically, it often occurs among people aged 20 to 40. It frequently occurs suddenly due to overexertion and excitation. It often causes headache, vomiting and sensory disturbance accompanied by rheumatic heart disease and atrial fibrillation history.

2. DIFFERENTIATION OF SYNDROME

TCM believes that wind stroke is related to the heart, liver, spleen and kidney, caused by wind, phlegm, dampness and stagnation in the vessels that prevent Qi (vital energy) and blood from circulating or blocking the upper orifices, leading to endogenous miscellaneous disease characterized by deficiency in the "root" and excess in the "branch," as well as predominance in the upper and deficiency in the lower.

(1)Syndrome due to invasion of pathogenic factors into the meridians and vessels.

This syndrome is shallow in location, light in nature; or, it is caused by invasion of pathogenic factors into the viscera. Usually, there is no lapse in consciousness, only dyscinesia and sensory disturbance. Invasion of pathogenic factors into the collaterals usually causes numbness of the skin and distortion of the face. However, invasion of pathogenic factors into the meridians often leads to paralysis, dysphasia, numbness of the limbs and a distorted face. These two conditions are collectively termed an attack of the meridians. Clinically, there are five types of wind stroke syndrome.

① Wind-phlegm blocking the collaterals. The symptoms accompanying it are dizziness, grayish and light-colored tongue with a thin, white or white and greasy coating, taut and slippery pulse.

② Extreme hyperactivity of the liver-Yang. The symptoms are dizziness, headache (involving the vertex and both sides of the head), reddish complexion and eyes, bitter taste in the mouth and dry throat, restlessness and susceptibility to rage, constipation and yellowish urine, reddish or deep-colored tongue with yellowish or dry coating, taut and powerful pulse.

③ Phlegm-heat and Fu-excess. The symptoms are vomiting of phlegm and saliva, reddish complexion and restless fever in the afternoon, abdominal distension and constipation, reddish tongue with yellowish greasy or grayish black tongue, taut-slippery and large pulse.

④ Qi-deficiency and blood stasis. The symptoms are a light white complexion, swelling and distension of the hand and foot, shortness of breath and fatigue, palpitation and spontaneous sweating, grayish light-colored tongue or tongue with ecchymoses and petechia, thin and slow or thin and ragged pulse.

⑤ Yin-deficiency and wind-disturbance. The symptoms are dizziness, tinnitus or deafness, tremor of the hands and feet, dysphoria and sleeplessness, reddish or deep-red tongue with scanty or no coating, thin and taut or rapid pulse.

(2)Syndrome due to invasion of pathogenic factors into the viscera

This syndrome is deep in location and serious in nature, with unconsciousness and sensory disturbance and dyscinesia. An attack of the Fu-organs usually causes trance and mental confusion, while an attack of the Zang-organs frequently leads to unconsciousness. Clinically, it is divided into blockage syndrome (including Yang-blockage and Yin-blockage) and collapse syndrome, both of which are marked by sudden fainting and unconsciousness.

① Blockage syndrome

This syndrome is accompanied by lockjaw, clenched hands, anuria and constipation, and stiff limbs. Furthermore, the syndrome due to blockage of the orifices by wind-fire is characterized by hemiplegia, reddish complexion and eyes, clenched and spasming hands, even convulsions and opisthotonus, reddish or deep-red tongue with yellow and dry or burned black coating, taut and rapid pulse; the syndrome due to blockage of orifices by phlegm-fire is marked by hemiplegia, stiffness of limbs, restlessness, profuse sputum and rapid breath, red eyes, stertor (abnormal snoring) and feverish body, constipation, reddish tongue with yellowish thick and greasy coating, slippery, rapid and powerful pulse; the syndrome due to confusion of the orifices by phlegm-dampness is characterized by hemiplegia, flaccidity and coldness of the limbs, profuse sputum and drooling, grayish and dirty complexion, light-colored tongue with white and greasy coating, sunken and slippery or slow pulse.

② Collapse syndrome

This syndrome is marked by exhaustion of the primordial Qi, mental derangement, flaccidity of the four limbs, pale complexion, closed eyes and open mouth, miosis, stertor with weak breath, flaccidity of hands and cold limbs, profuse and continuous sweating, even cold dampness all over the body, incontinence, contracted tongue with light purplish and whitish slippery coating, scattered or indistinct pulse.

3. DYSFUNCTION

Statistical analysis shows that about 70% of those who survive wind stroke suffer from dysfunction to varying degrees.

(1) **Dyscinesia**: Symptoms of hemiplegia (the major dysfunction and seen in about 40% of the cases) and even paralysis of the four limbs are seen in the vertebral system; the symptoms beyond the vertebral system are varied involuntary movements such as tremor, athetosis, non-coordination and unstable walking.

(2) **Sensory disturbance**: Including anesthesia or hypoesthesia on the opposite side, and sensitive or abnormal sensation such as sharp pain.

(3) **Psychical dysfunction**: Manifestation of true personality due to loss of reasoning, usually seen in depression, fantasy, anxiety, delusion and mania.

(4) **Aphasia**: Anandia is marked by unclear and infrequent speech, and stuttering; sensory aphasia is characterized by smooth speech with disordered words.

(5) **Dysfunction of the vegetative nerve**: Abnormal sweating over the affected side.

(6) **Neuro-paralysis of the cerebral nerves**: Central facial paralysis (such as distorted mouth, shallowness of the nasolabial groove with normal condition of the wrinkles over the forehead), strabismus on the same side and dysphagia.

(7) **Special dysfunction**: Agnosia—the patient is unable to distinguish things with the eyes, but can differentiate by hearing and smell. Apraxia: the patient can walk involuntarily, but cannot walk in a selected direction; the hands can move, but cannot imitate the actions of others.

(8)**Dysfunction in urination and defecation**: Retention of urine and constipation or incontinence.

Among the dysfunctions mentioned above, hemiplegia is the one that most frequently leads to disability (over 40%). So, the rehabilitation of hemiplegia is an important task for medical workers to undertake.

4. REHABILITATION OF HEMIPLEGIA

The rehabilitation of hemiplegia depends on the degree of the damage to the cerebral neural cells and the pathological changes of the cerebral vessels on the one hand, and rehabilitative treatment on the other. Delayed rehabilitative treatment or incorrect functional exercises will affect the rehabilitation of limb functions, and even lead to disability, such as transverse walking, swinging the hip and drooping foot.

The rehabilitation of hemiplegia usually goes through the following stages:

(1) **Complete paralysis stage (stage I):** Two weeks from the occurrence, 0 degree of the myodynamia, inability of the affected limbs to contract. At this stage passive functional exercise can be done.

(2) **Combined reaction and involuntary contraction stage (stage II):** The myodynamia is 1-2 degrees, the function of the affected limbs begins to return, with slight voluntary movement, spasm of the muscles and some low degree of involuntary movement. Passive functional exercise can be done with the help of doctors and nurses. The patient also can do passive functional exercise, unaided, or self massage.

① Combined reaction: At the early stage of hemiplegia, when the affected limbs are unable to contract, strong exercise of the muscles on the healthy side may cause atrophy of the muscles on the affected side, such as contraction of the greater pectoral muscle, sternocleidomastoid muscle and adductive muscle groups on the hip joint. It aggravates, with an increase in the muscular spasms on the affected side and attenuates, with the improvement of the pathological conditions. Thus, it is not physiological activity, but a kind of primitive moving model in the rehabilitative course of the affected limbs.

② Voluntary contraction: It can produce the smallest voluntary movement but cannot stimulate the movement of the joints.

(3) **Common movement stage (stage III):** The myodynamia is 3 degrees and there is obvious contraction of the muscles on the affected limbs that propels the movement of the joints. But this is a kind of fixed movement. For example, the contraction of the flexors on the upper

limbs is certainly the combined contraction of the muscles on the shoulder, elbow, wrist and finger, that is, common movement. And the spasm of the muscles gradually aggravates. Incorrect treatment at this stage will easily cause spasms and stiffness of the joints. So, doctors and nurses should help the patients correctly perform functional exercise with Tuina (massage) therapy so as to enable each joint to separate from the combined movement and reduce the spasms. Proper sitting exercise is also applicable at this stage.

(4) **Separated movement stage (stages IV and V):** The myodynamia is 3-4 degrees. The affected limbs are bent and extended to move the muscles on the joints separately, such as simple bending and extending the elbow and wrist joints. The muscular spasms will be alleviated and the patient can sit or stand. Sitting and standing exercises can be done actively at this stage with the combined use of Tuina therapy for smoothing the joints and strengthening the myodynamia.

(5) **Voluntary movement stage (stage VI):** The myodynamia is 4-5 degrees. The affected limbs can stand and walk freely with high speed. The coordination and acrobatic movement are obviously improved, and the symptoms of muscle spasm have basically disappeared. The functional exercises of standing, walking forwards and backwards, and going up and down stairs can be done with the combined use of Tuina therapy. The patients may do some other exercises, such as writing and picking up small glass beads.

Chapter 2

ILLUSTRATED EXPLANATION OF THE MOVEMENTS OF THE MAIN JOINTS IN THE HUMAN BODY

To get familiar with the movement of the main joints in the human body is beneficial for understanding the following chapters. For this purpose, this chapter is devoted to a concise and simple explanation of the joints in the order of head and neck, waist and back, shoulder, elbow, wrist, finger, hip joint, knee, ankle and toe.

1. HEAD AND NECK

(1) Bending of the atlantooccipital articulation (anterior bending of the head): The head is bent till the jaw gets near the chest in a range of 30°-35° (fig. 2-1).

(2) Extension of the atlantooccipital articulation (posterior bending of the head): The head is raised backward till the jaw is away from the chest in a range of 30°-35° (fig. 2-2).

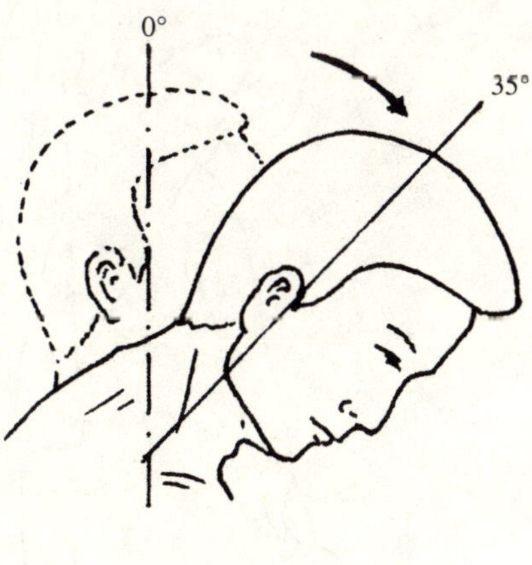

Fig. 2-1 Bending of the atlantooccipital articulation (anterior bending of the head)

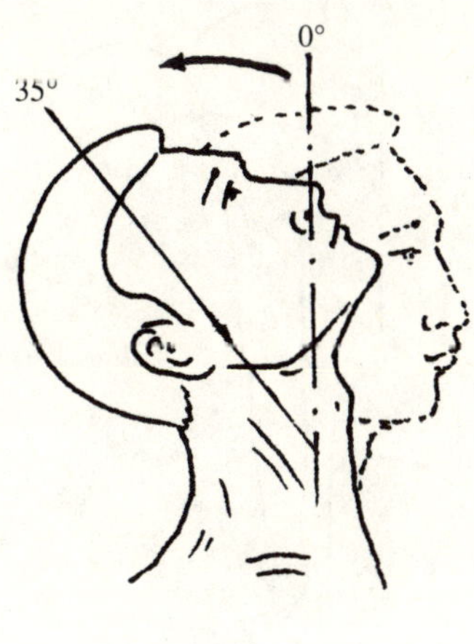

Fig. 2-2 Extension of the atlantooccipital articulation (posterior bending of the head)

(3) Lateral bending of the atlantooccipital articulation (lateral bending of the head): The head is bent laterally to the left or right with the ear getting near the shoulder of the same lateral side (the shoulder should not be raised) in a range of 45° (fig. 2-3).

(4) Rotation of the atlantooccipital articulation (rotation of the head): The head is rotated from the left to the right or from the right to the left in a range of 30° (fig. 2-4).

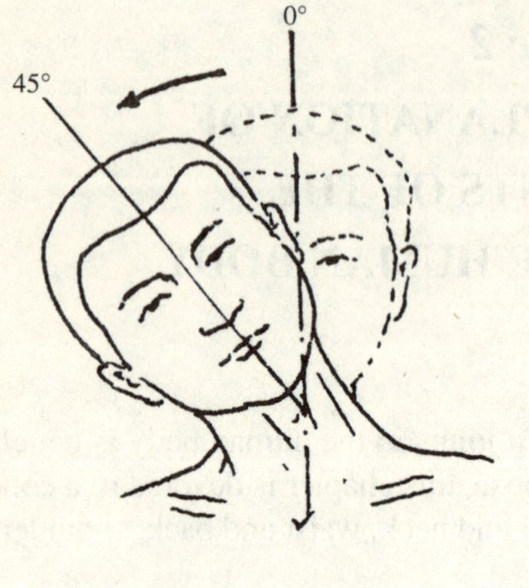

Fig. 2-3 Lateral bending of the atlantooccipital articulation (lateral bending of the head)

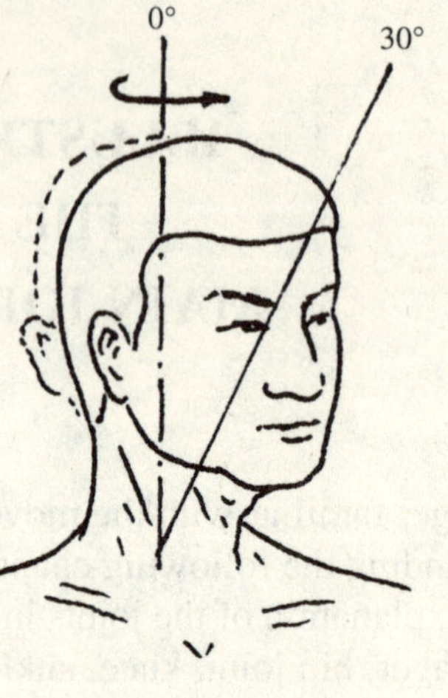

Fig. 2-4 Rotation of the atlantooccipital articulation (rotation of the head)

2. WAIST AND BACK

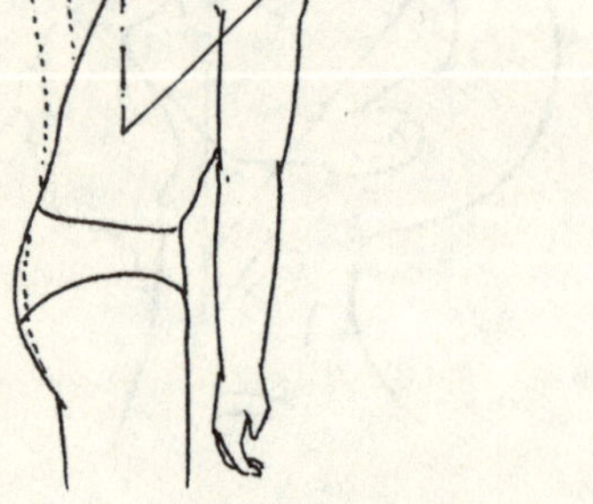

Fig. 2-5 Bending of the spine (anterior bending of the waist)

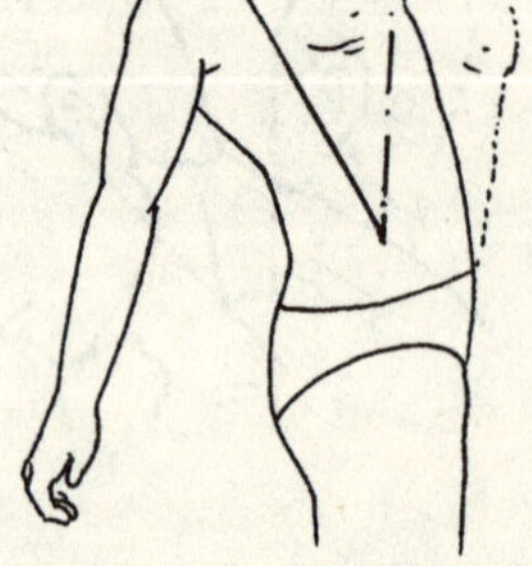

Fig. 2-6 Extension of the spine (posterior bending of the waist)

(1) Bending of the spine (anterior bending of the waist): The upper part of the body is bent to the chest and abdomen in a range of about 45° (fig. 2-5).

(2) Extension of the spine (posterior bending of the waist): The upper part of the body is bent backward in a range of about 30° (fig. 2-6).

(3) Lateral bending of the spine (lateral bending of the waist): The upper part of the body is bent to the right or left in a range of about 30° (fig. 2-7).

(4) Rotation of the spine (rotation of the waist): The upper part of the body is rotated from the right to the left or from the left to the right without moving the lower part of the body, in a range of about 45° (fig. 2-8).

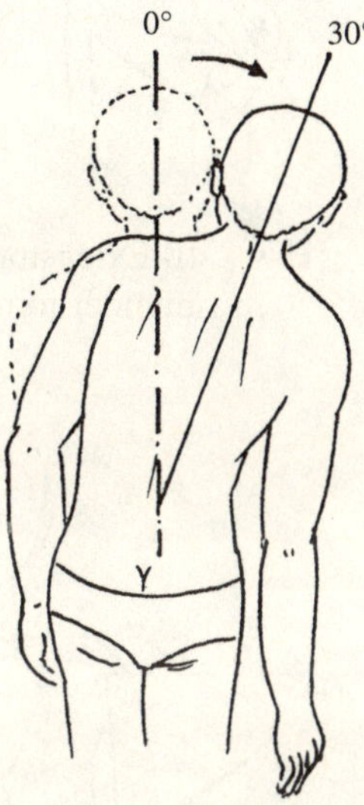

Fig. 2-7 Lateral bending of the spine (lateral bending of the waist)

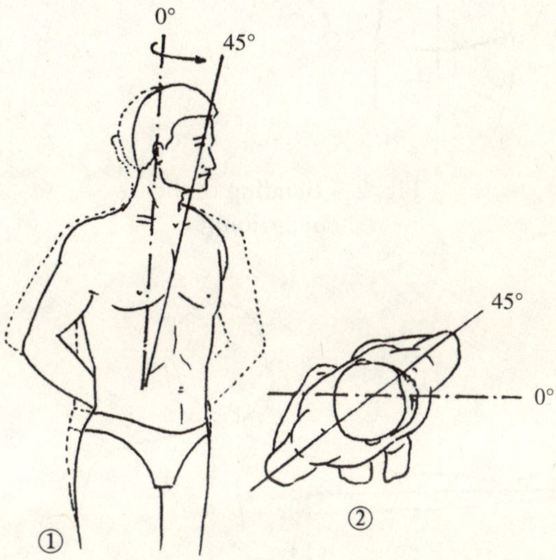

Fig. 2-8 Rotation of the spine (rotation of the waist)

3. UPPER LIMBS

(1) Bending of the shoulder joint: The upper limbs are extended straight forward horizontally without raising the trunk in a posterior direction, in a range of about 90° (fig. 2-9).

(2) Extension of the shoulder joint: The upper limbs are bent straight backward in a range of about 35° (fig. 2-10).

(3) Abduction of the shoulder joint: The upper limbs are raised horizontally from the same lateral side and away from the body in a range of about 90° (fig. 2-11).

(4) Adduction of the shoulder joint: The upper limb is turned back to the same side from lateral upward position or the elbow is turned to the midline in a range of about 90°+30° (fig. 2-12).

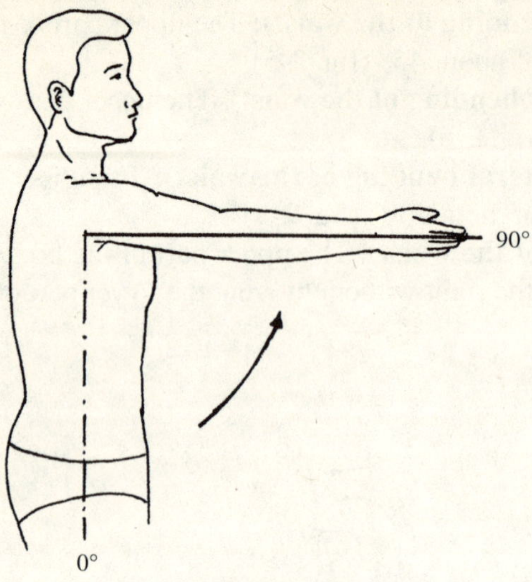

Fig. 2-9 Bending of the shoulder joint

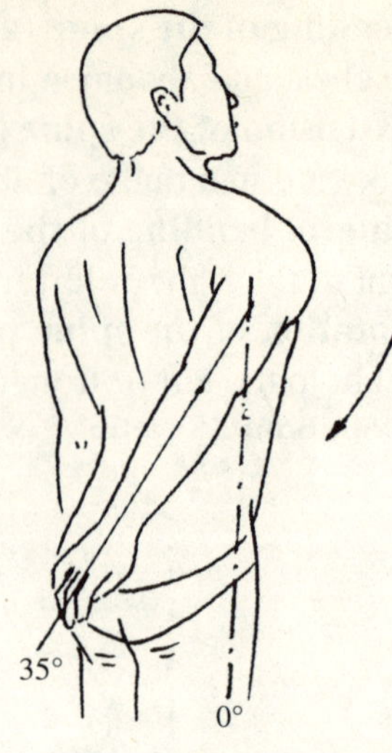

Fig. 2-10 Extension of the shoulder joint

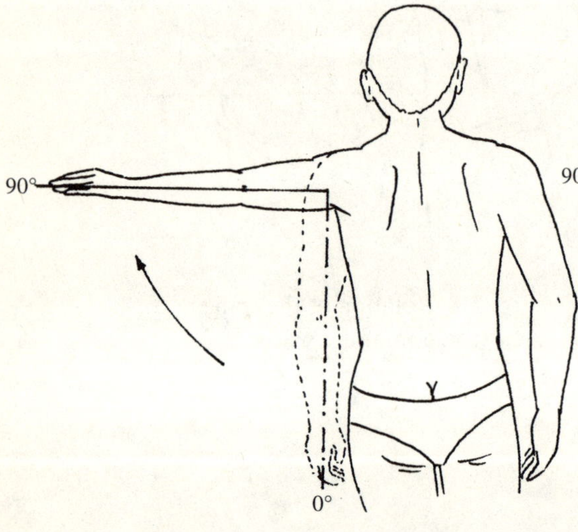

Fig. 2-11 Abduction of the shoulder joint

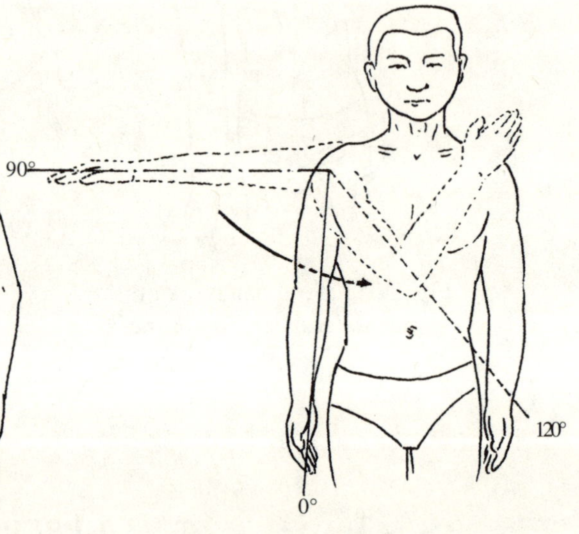

Fig. 2-12 Adduction of the shoulder joint

(5) Eversion of the shoulder joint: The upper arm is rotated laterally in a range of about 45° (fig. 2-13).

(6) Intorsion of the shoulder joint: The upper arm is rotated medially in a range of about 80° (fig. 2-14).

(7) Bending of the elbow joint: The forearm is bent toward the upper arm in a range of 135°-150° (fig. 2-15).

(8) Extension of the elbow joint: The elbow is bent and the forearm is extended in a range of 0° or extended backward in a range within 10° (fig. 2-16).

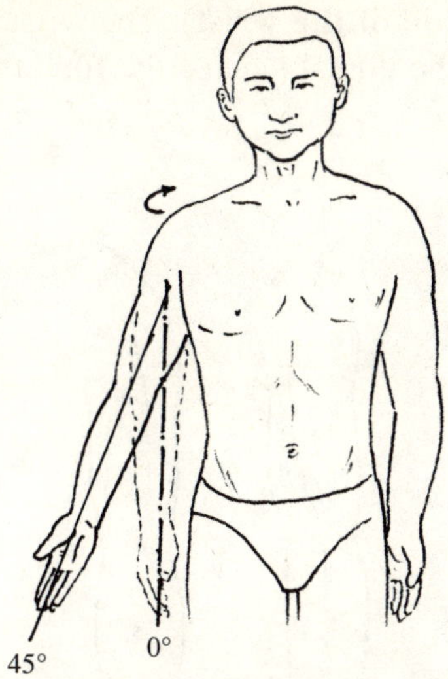

Fig. 2-13 Eversion of the shoulder joint

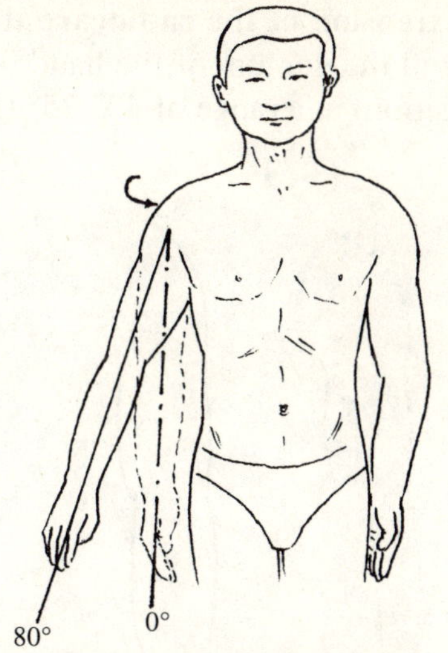

Fig. 2-14 Intorsion of the shoulder joint

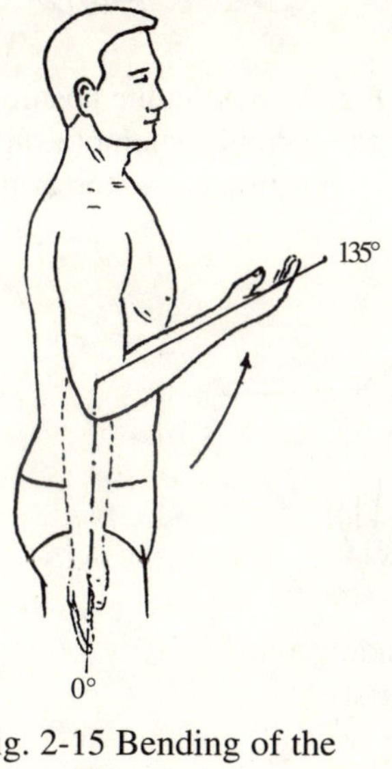

Fig. 2-15 Bending of the elbow joint

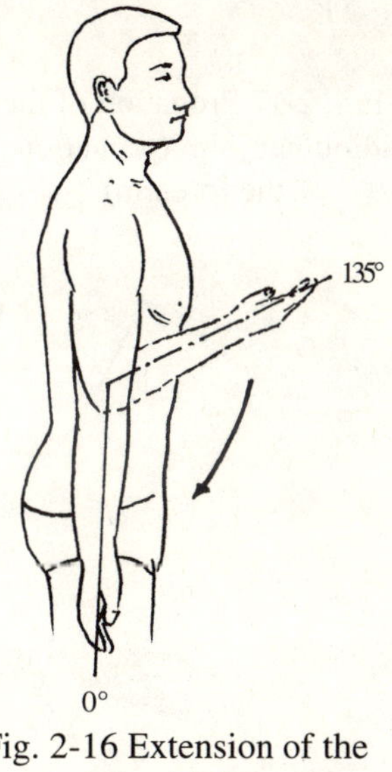

Fig. 2-16 Extension of the elbow joint

(9) Pronation of the radioulnar joint (pronation of the forearm): The palm is turned from medial position to posterior position in a range of about 90° (fig. 2-17).

(10) A supine position of the radioulnar joint (a supine position of the forearm): The palm is turned from medial position to anterior position in a range of about 90° (fig. 2-18).

(11) Bending of the radiocarpal joint (bending the wrist): The wrist is bent and the palm is turned near the palmar side of the forearm (bending the palm) in a range of about 60° (fig. 2-19).

(12) Extension of the radiocarpal joint (extension of the wrist): The wrist is turned backward and the dorsum of the hand is turned near the dorsal side of the forearm (dorsal bending position) in a range of 40°-75° (fig. 2-20).

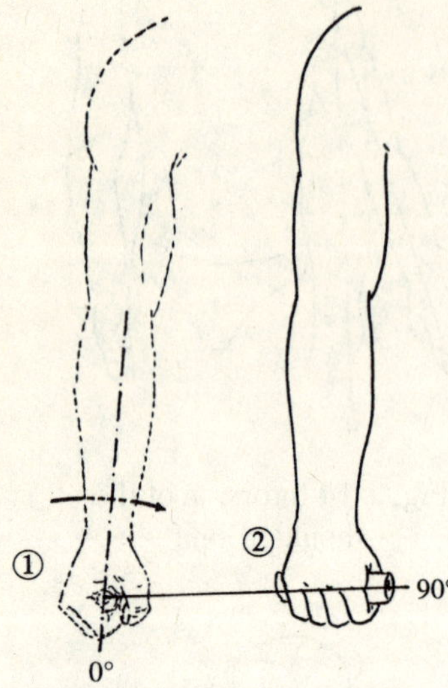

Fig. 2-17 Pronation of the radioulnar joint (pronation of the forearm)

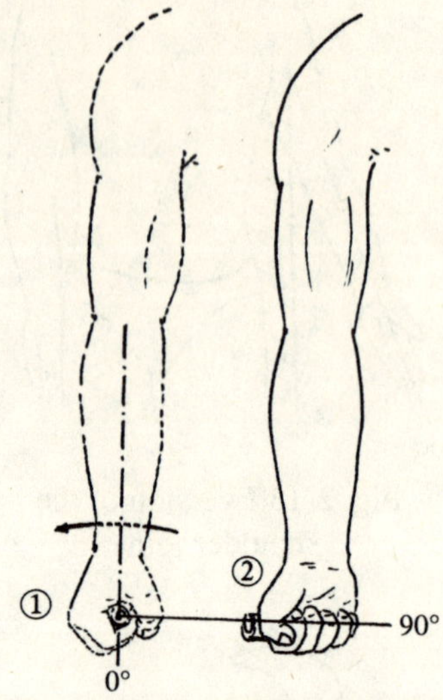

Fig. 2-18 A supine position of the radioulnar joint (a supine position of the forearm)

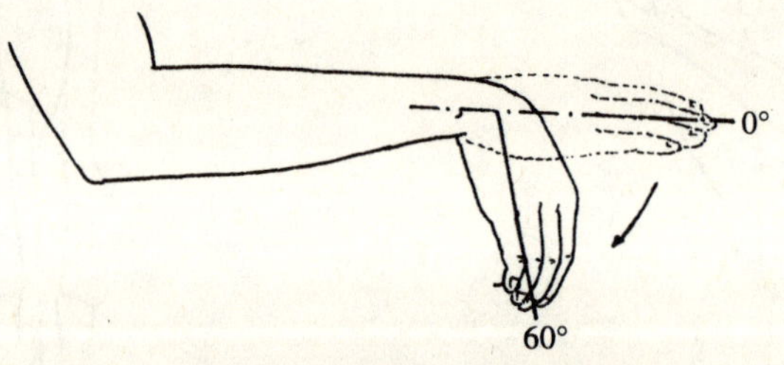

Fig. 2-19 Bending of the radiocarpal joint (bending the wrist)

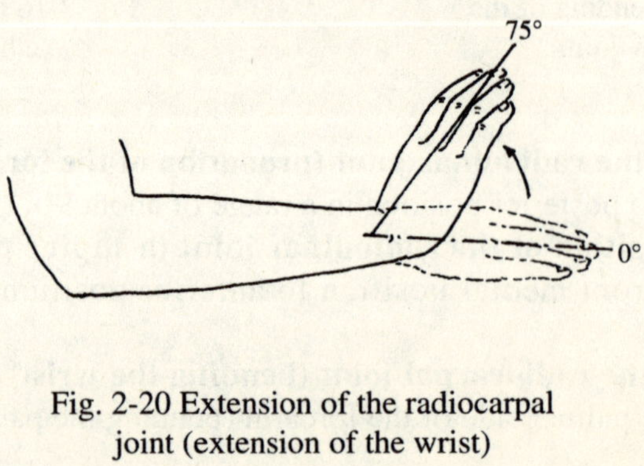

Fig. 2-20 Extension of the radiocarpal joint (extension of the wrist)

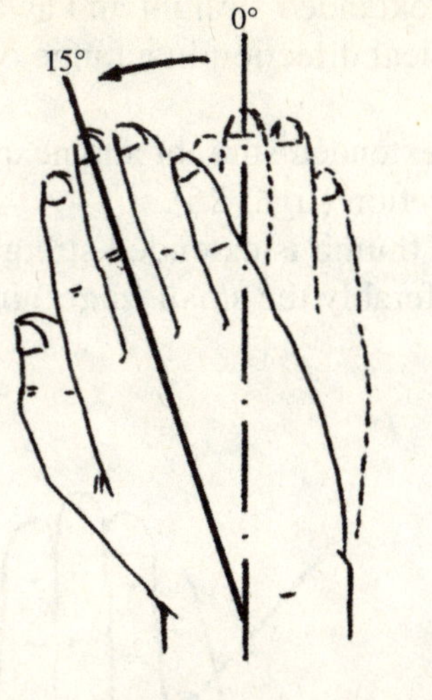

Fig. 2-21 Abduction of the radiocarpal joint

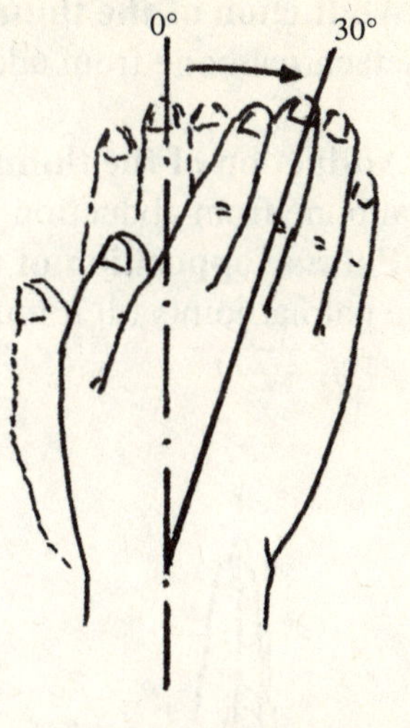

Fig. 2-22 Adduction of the radiocarpal joint

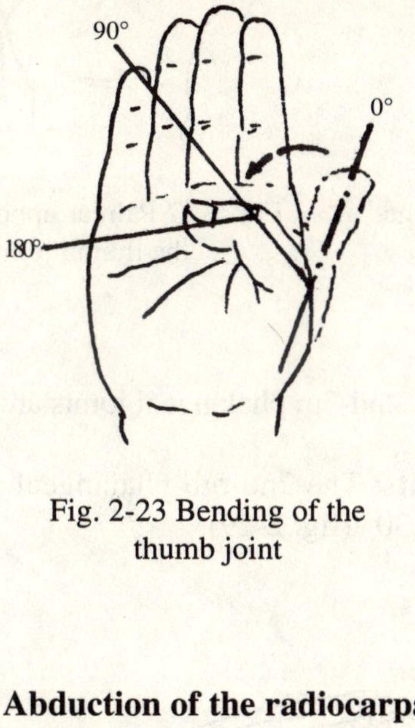

Fig. 2-23 Bending of the thumb joint

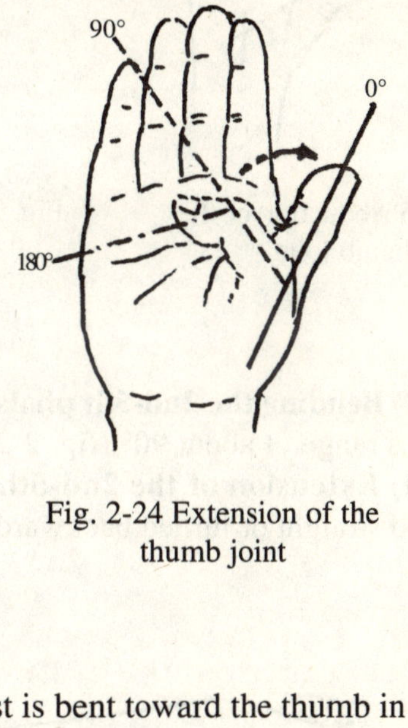

Fig. 2-24 Extension of the thumb joint

(13) Abduction of the radiocarpal joint: The wrist is bent toward the thumb in a range of about 15° (fig. 2-21).

(14) Adduction of the radiocarpal joint: The wrist is turned toward the small finger in a range of about 30° (fig. 2-22).

(15) Bending of the thumb joint: The thumb is bent toward the major thenar eminence. The metacarpophalangeal and phalangeal articulations are bent in a range of about 90° (fig. 2-23).

(16) Extension of the thumb joint: The thumb is extended straight and parallel to the second metacarpal bone (fig. 2-24).

(17) Abduction of the thumb joint: The thumb is extended straight and away from the second metacarpal bone from adduction position to vertical direction in a range of about 45° (fig. 2-25).

(18) Adduction of the thumb joint: The thumb is extended straight and near the second metacarpal bone from abduction position to vertical direction (fig.2-26).

(19) Palmar opposition of the thumb joints: The thumb is extended straight and bent toward the palmar joints till it touches other fingers (preferably the small finger) in a range of about 45° (fig. 2-27).

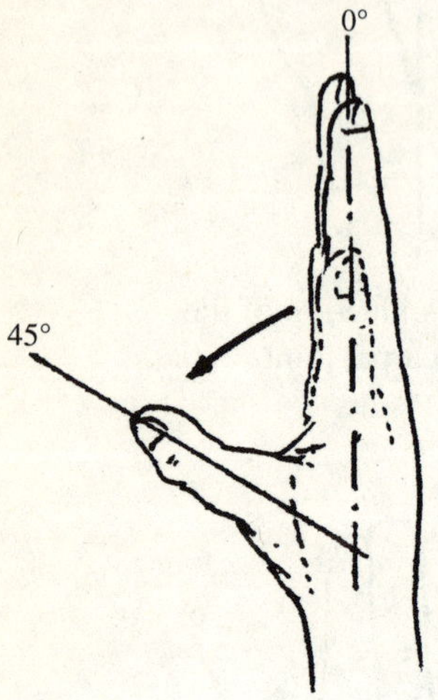

Fig. 2-25 Abduction of the thumb joint

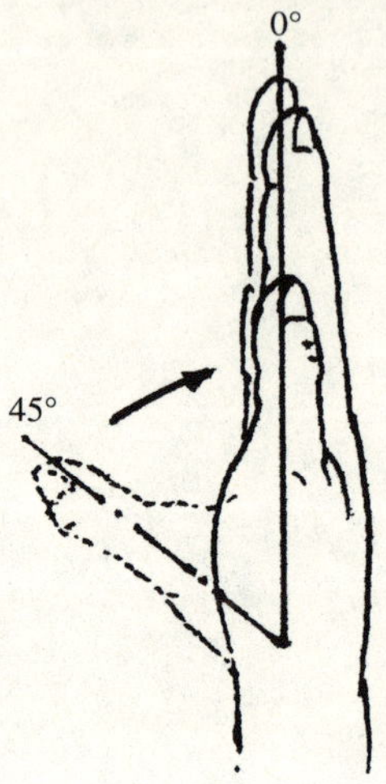

Fig. 2-26 Adduction of the thumb joint

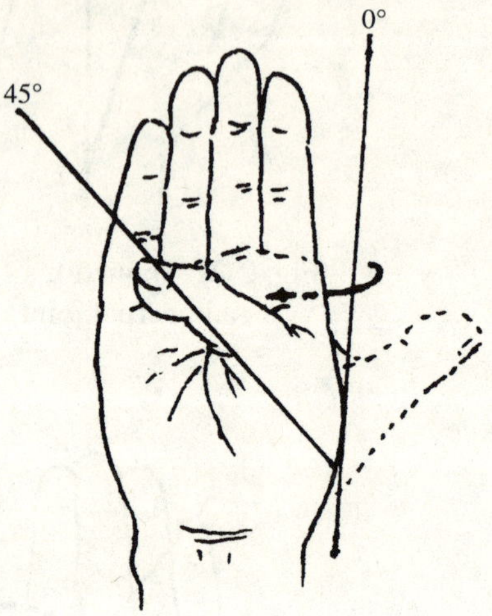

Fig. 2-27 Palmar opposition of the thumb joints

(20) Bending the 2nd-5th phalangeal joints: The 2nd-5th phalangeal joints are bent into a fist in a range of about 90° (fig. 2-28).

(21) Extension of the 2nd-5th phalangeal joints: The 2nd-5th phalangeal joints are extended straight or turned backward in a range about 30° (fig. 2-29).

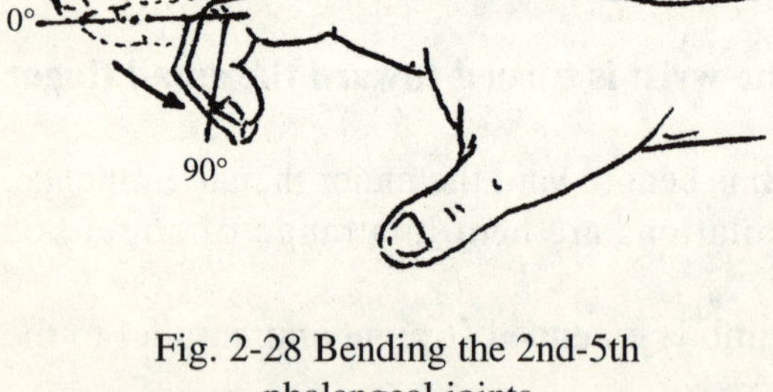

Fig. 2-28 Bending the 2nd-5th phalangeal joints

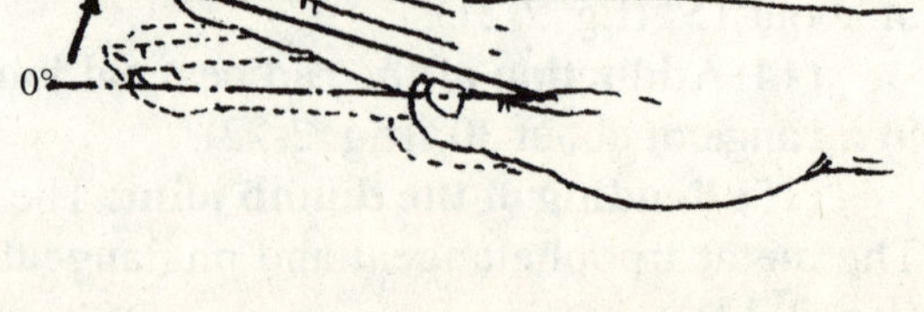

Fig. 2-29 Extension of the 2nd-5th phalangeal joints

(22) Abduction of the 2nd-5th phalangeal joints: The 2nd-5th phalangeal joints are extended straight, with the middle finger as the center, and forked toward both sides in a range of about 30° (fig. 2-30).

(23) Adduction of the 2nd-5th phalangeal joints: The 2nd-5th phalangeal joints are extended straight, with the middle finger as the center, and ranked together (fig. 2-31).

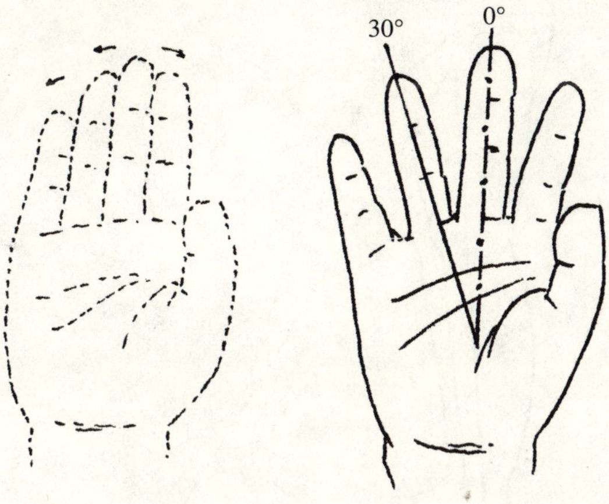

Fig. 2-30 Abduction of the 2nd-5th phalangeal joints

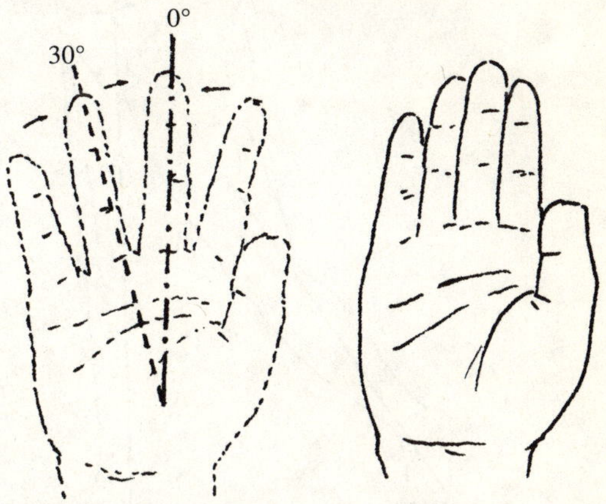

Fig. 2-31 Adduction of the 2nd-5th phalangeal joints

4. LOWER LIMBS

(1) Bending the hip joint: The lower limbs are bent in an anterior direction. When bending the knee, the thigh may touch the abdomen. The maximum range is about 125° (fig. 2-32).

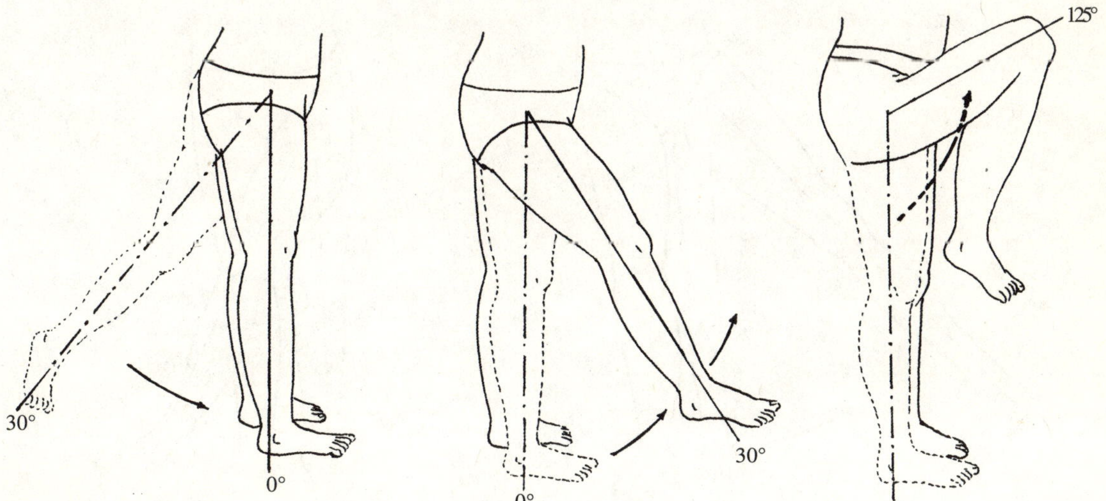

Fig. 2-32 Bending the hip joint

(2) Extending the hip joint: The lower limbs are bent in a posterior direction, surpassing the vertical position of the body about 30° (the waist should not be bent backward) (fig. 2-33).

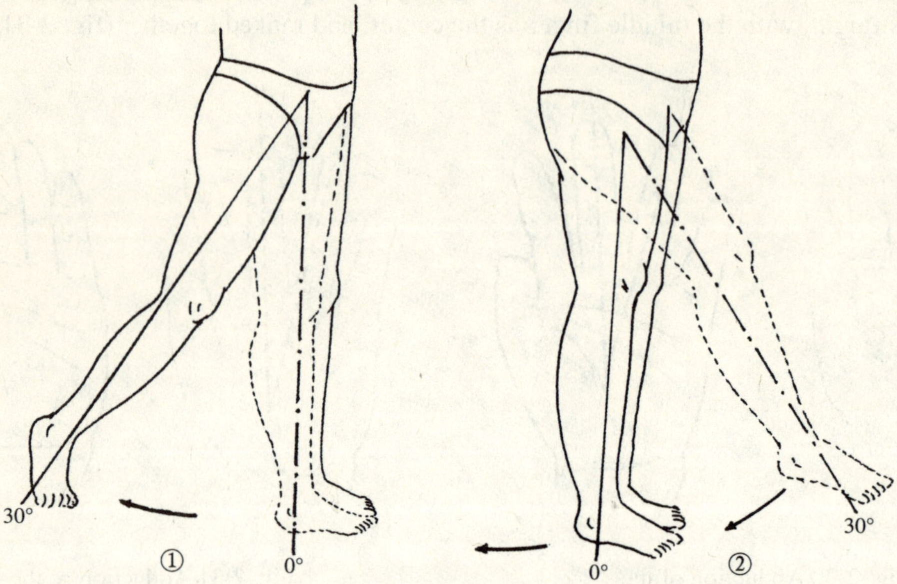

Fig. 2-33 Extending the hip joint

(3) Abducting the hip joint: One of the lower limbs swings away from the other lower limb in a range of about 60° (fig. 2-34).

(4) Adducting the hip joint: One of the lower limbs gets close to or over the other lower limb in a range of about 30° (fig. 2-35).

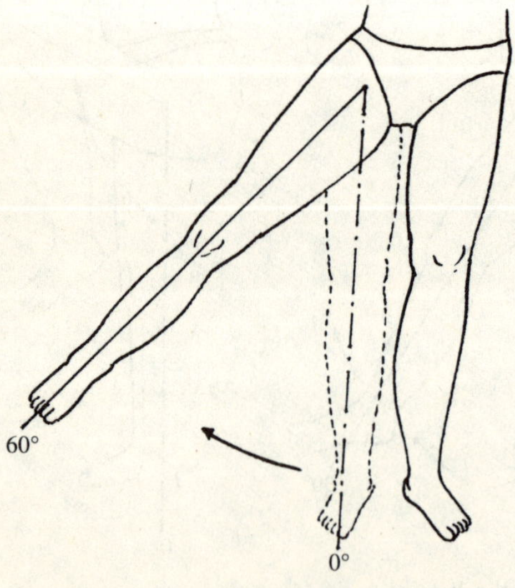

Fig. 2-34 Abducting the hip joint

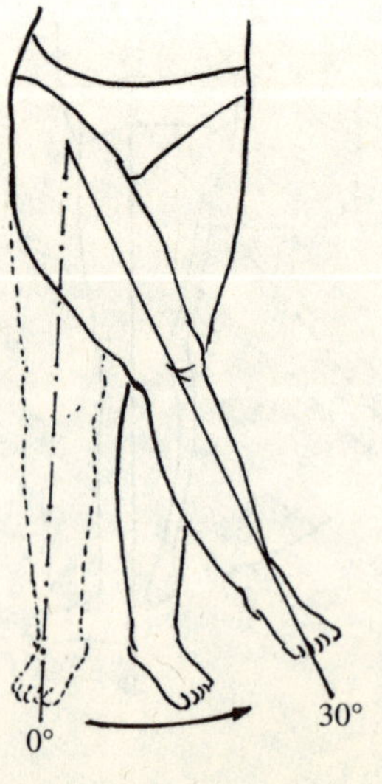

Fig. 2-35 Adducting the hip joint

(5) Eversion of the hip joint: The thigh is turned laterally in a range of 30°-45° (fig. 2-36).

(6) Intorsion of the hip joint: The thigh is turned medially in a range of about 40°-50° (fig. 2-37).

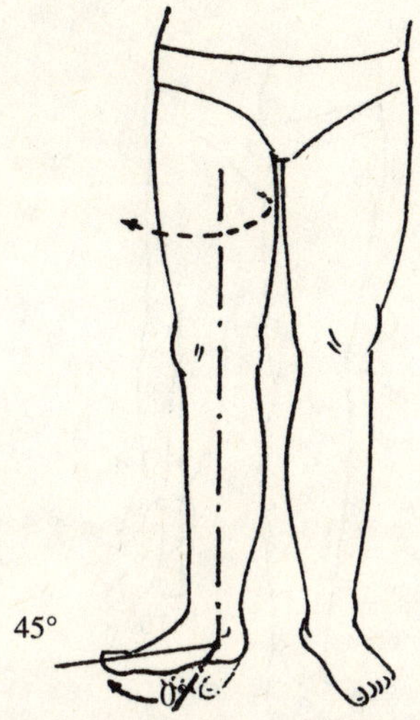

Fig. 2-36 Eversion of the hip joint

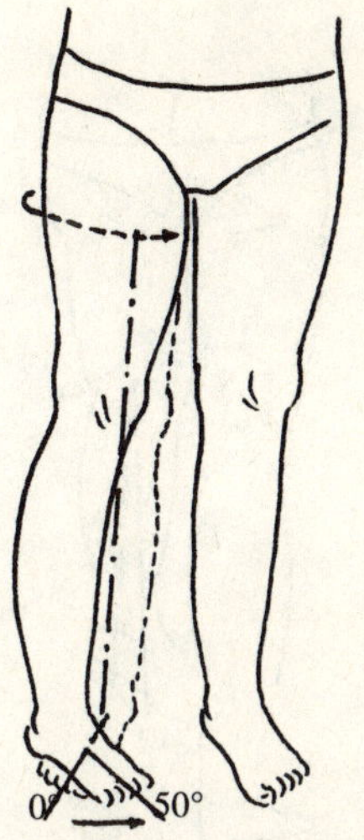

Fig. 2-37 Intorsion of the hip joint

(7) Bending the knee joint: The shank is bent backward to get near to the thigh in a range of about 90°. The maximum range is 120°- 150° (fig. 2-38).

(8) Extending the knee joint: The knee is bent and the shank is turned away from the thigh in a standing position. The maximum range is 5° (fig. 2-39).

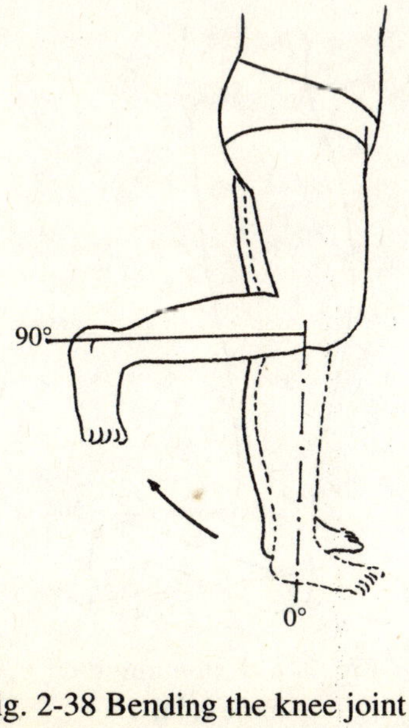

Fig. 2-38 Bending the knee joint

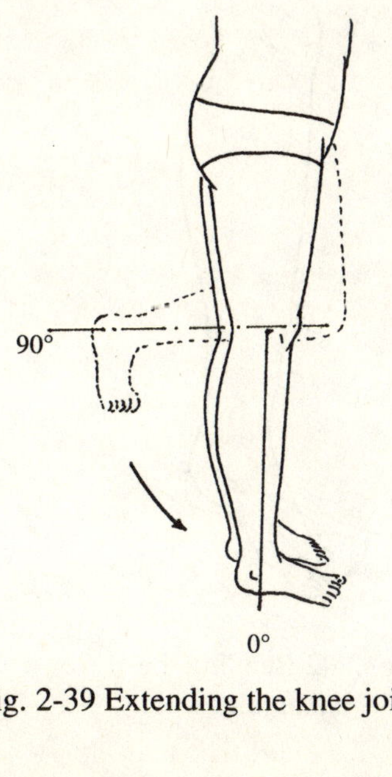

Fig. 2-39 Extending the knee joint

(9) Eversion of the knee joint: The shank and knee are respectively turned medially and laterally in a range of about 10° (fig. 2-40).

(10) Intorsion of the knee joint: The shank and the knee joint are respectively turned laterally and medially in a range of about 10° (fig. 2-41).

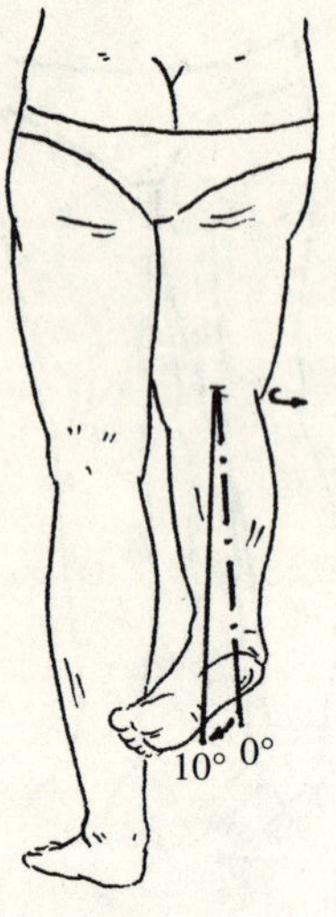

Fig. 2-40 Eversion of the knee joint

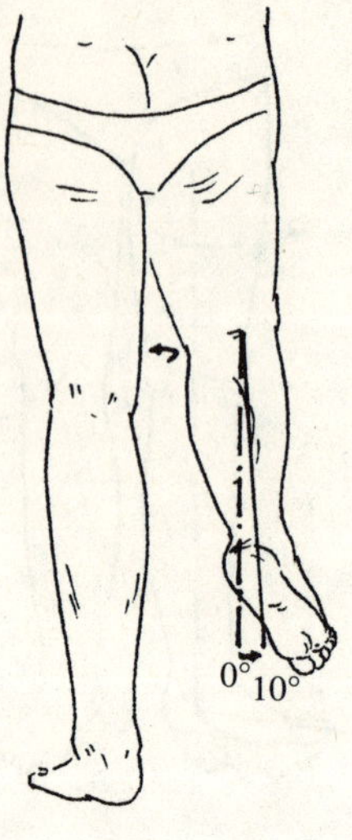

Fig. 2-41 Intorsion of the knee joint

(11) Bending the ankle joint: The dorsum of the foot and the shank are bent in an anterior direction downward from a vertical position in a range of 20°-30° (fig. 2-42).

(12) Extending the ankle joint: The dorsum of the foot and the shank are turned upward from vertical position to a straight anterior position in a range of 40°-45° (fig. 2-43).

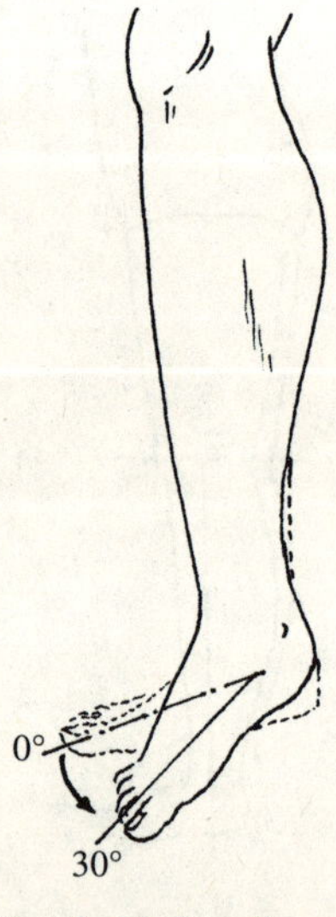

Fig. 2-42 Bending the ankle joint

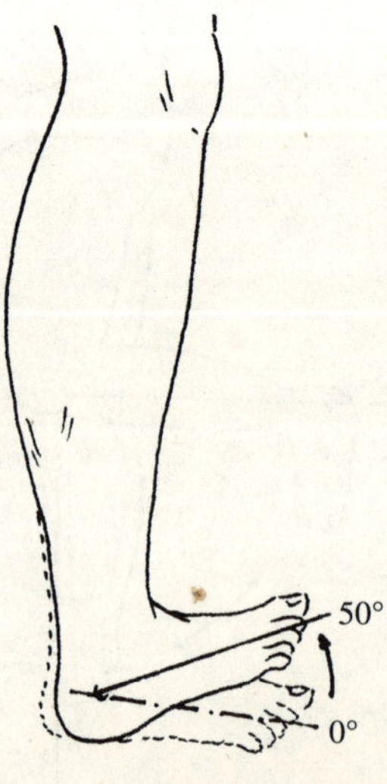

Fig. 2-43 Extending the ankle joint

(13) Eversion of the ankle joint: The foot turns laterally and the sole faces the external side in a range of about 35° (fig. 2-44).

(14) Intorsion of the ankle joint: The foot is bent medially and the sole faces the internal side in a range of about 60° (fig. 2-45).

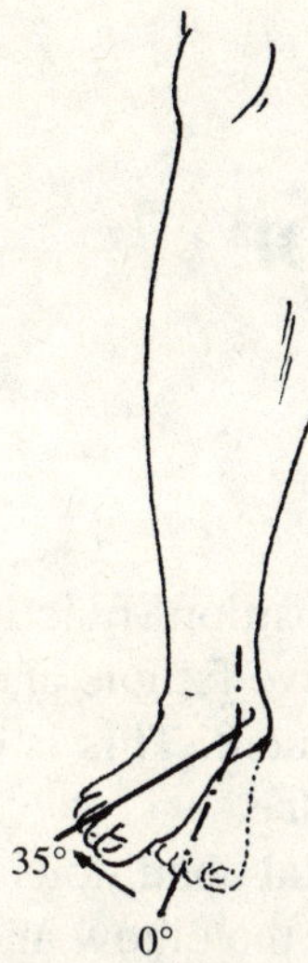

Fig. 2-44 Eversion of the ankle joint

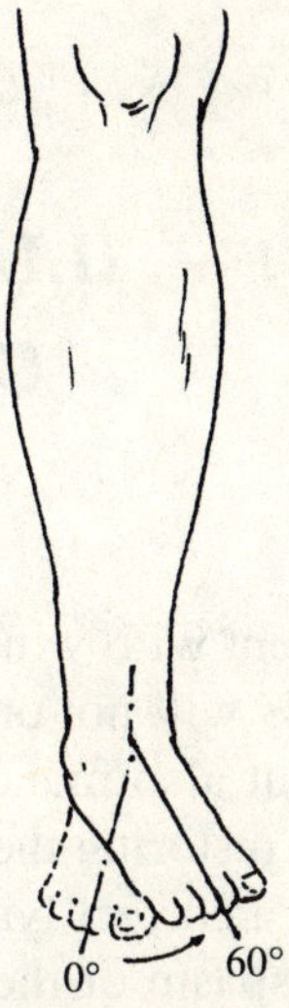

Fig. 2-45 Intorsion of the ankle joint

(15) Bending the toe joint: The toes are bent downward in a range of about 45° (fig. 2-46).

(16) Extending the toe joint: The toes are turned upward in a range of 60°-90° (fig. 2-47).

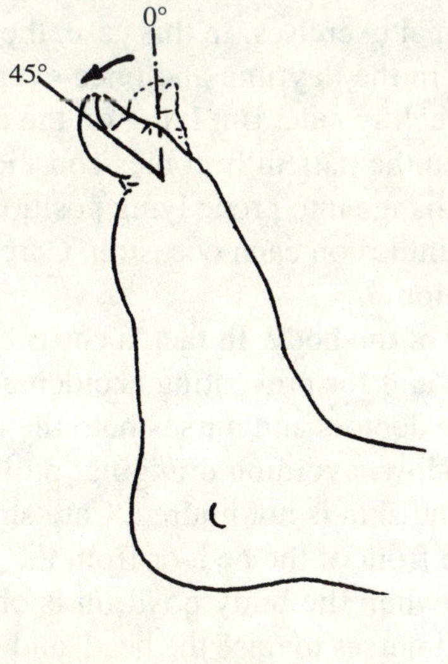

Fig. 2-46 Bending the toe joint

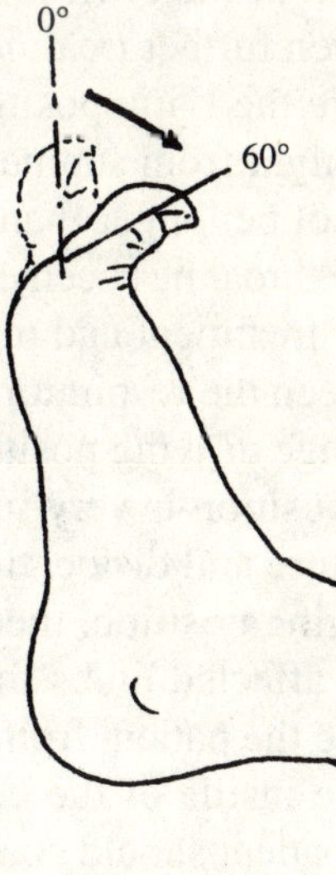

Fig. 2-47 Extending the toe joint

Chapter 3

ILLUSTRATED EXPLANATION OF CORRECT LYING POSITIONS

The patient with wind stroke should maintain a correct lying position (functional lying position). This will not only make the patient feel comfortable, relieve fatigue and alleviate symptoms, but also make it convenient for examination and treatment. This is especially important for restoring the functions of the limbs and reducing sequelae.

Keeping a correct lying position can prevent specific pathological conditions caused by flaccidity or spasm of the muscles (such as lifting the hip, bending the elbow and walking obliquely; leaning the trunk forward when standing; etc.) and secondary dysfunctions due to static lying (such as semi-dislocation of the shoulder joint and stiffness of the knee joint) as well as keep the activity range of the joints as much as possible.

It is clinically observed that the main lying position selected by the patient is supine. However, prolonged maintenance of any kind of position will inevitably lead to necrosis of the soft tissues due to disturbance of local tissue, neural nutrition and blood circulation. At the early part of the acute stage, the patient may change the lying position once every two hours under the condition that it will not affect the treatment and blood pressure. When the patient has moved out of the critical stage and the life signs have become stable, the affected limbs should be given further treatment and exposed to functional exercises. In this case, the patient should change the lying position once every two hours in the daytime and once every three hours in the night from supine position to lying on the healthy side. But lying on the affected side should not be longer than one hour each time. When the patient becomes conscious and sputum in the throat has been eliminated, he or she may change into prone lying position if it is necessary for treatment and nursing, no more than 30 minutes on each occasion. Care should be taken to keep the respiratory tract smooth in the position.

The change of lying position is not simply a turning of the body. In fact, a correct change of the lying position is very important for rehabilitation and for preventing accidental injury (such as fracture and dislocation of joints). So, when the doctors and nurses help the patients change the lying position, the action must be mild and slow, avoiding dragging, pulling and pushing. The affected limbs should be slightly lifted so the skin is not injured. Care should be taken to move the patient from the back of the bed to the front of the bed, or from the edge of the bed to the inside of the bed, so as to avoid falling when the body position is changed. Besides, the patient should cooperate with the doctors and nurses to raise the head, and turn the shoulder, waist and hip. Before the patient changes the body position, he or she should take several deep breaths in order to calm down.

In order to enable the patient to keep a correct lying position, this chapter introduces five supine positions, two lateral lying positions and two prone positions with illustrations. These nine positions are provided for the patients to choose. Besides, four methods for changing body positions are illustrated for doctors and nurses to follow.

1. BASIC BODY POSITION FOR SUPINE LYING

(Fig. 3-1)

[Method] The patient lies in a supine position with the head and neck cushioned 15cm (for the patient with hemorrhagic wind stroke, the head and neck can be cushioned slightly higher) and kept vertical with the trunk. The shoulder and arm of the affected limb is kept in a salute posture (about 50°abduction, 15° intorsion and 40°bending of the shoulder, and about 90° bending of the elbow) with a pillow cushioned beneath. The wrist is extended about 50°. The fingers are slightly bent with a roll of gauze 5cm in diameter held in the fingers. The inferior and lateral sides of the knee on the affected side are coshioned with soft pillows. The knee is bent about 30° and the ankle joint is kept at 0°. The foot is cushioned with a plate or a sandbag. The healthy limb extends naturally.

[Effect] To prevent shoulder joint adhesion, semiluxation, stiffness and spasm of the elbow, finger and knee joints, flexing and cramps of the wrist joints, drooping and intorsion of the foot, eversion and deviation of the hip joint.

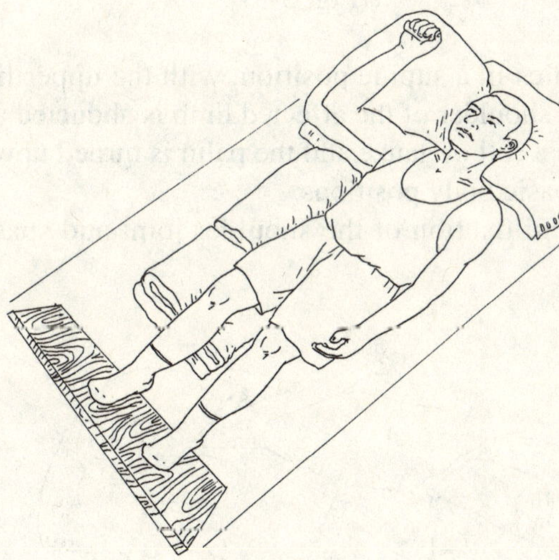

Fig. 3-1 Basic body position for supine lying

2. ABDUCTING THE SHOULDER IN A SUPINE POSITION

(Fig. 3-2)

[Method] The patient lies supine with the upper limb on the healthy side placed beside the body. The shoulder on the affected side is abducted about 60° and the elbow is slightly bent. The shoulder, elbow and hand are cushioned with pillows, and the palm faces upward. The other methods are the same as that of the basic body positions.

[Effect] To prevent shoulder joint adhesion and semiluxation as well as spasm of the elbow joint due to prolonged bending.

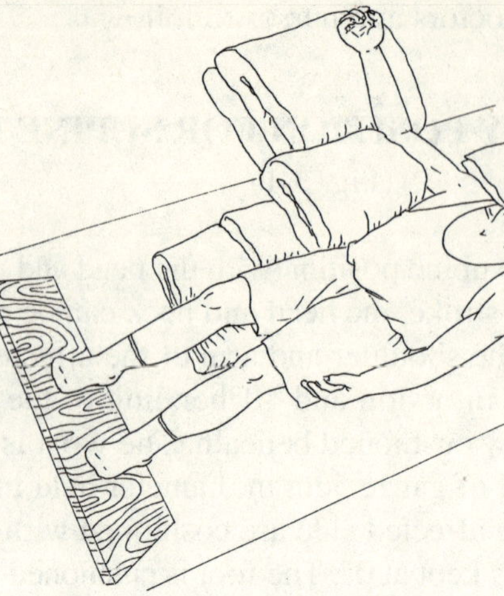

Fig. 3-2 Abducting the shoulder in a supine position

3. EXTENDING THE ELBOW IN A SUPINE POSITION

(Fig. 3-3)

[Method] The patient lies in a supine position, with the upper limb on the healthy side placed beside the body. The shoulder of the affected limb is abducted about 30° and the elbow is extended. The hand holds a roll of gauze and the palm is turned upward. The other methods are the same as that of the basic body positions.

[Effect] To prevent semiluxation of the shoulder joint and spasm of the elbow due to prolonged bending.

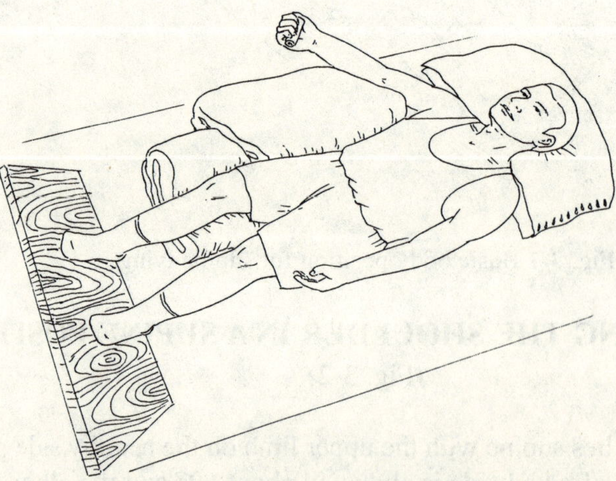

Fig. 3-3 Extending the elbow in a supine position

4. BENDING THE ELBOW IN A SUPINE POSITION

(Fig. 3-4)

[Method] The patient lies in a supine position with the upper limb on the healthy side placed alongside the body. The shoulder on the affected limb is slightly abducted, the wrist slightly extended and the fingers are slightly bent. The hand is put on the chest and the palm is turned upward. The elbow joint is bent. The other methods are the same as that of the basic body positions.

[Effect] To prevent pain and adhesion of the shoulder due to prolonged abduction affecting blood circulation as well as stiffness of the elbow joint.

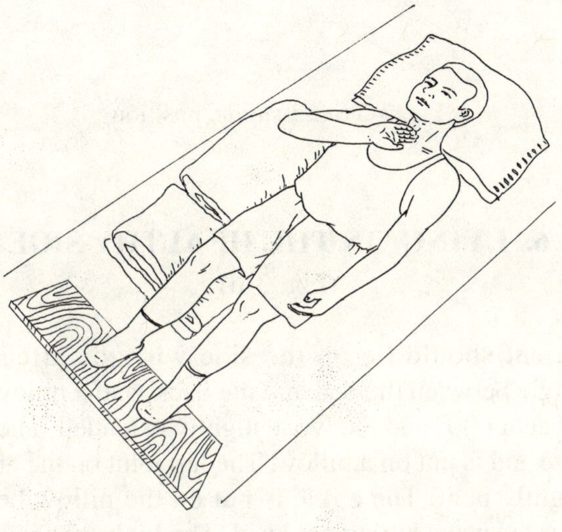

Fig. 3-4 Bending the eldow in a supine position

5. SEMI-SUPINE POSITION

(Fig. 3-5)

[Method] The patient is in a semi-supine position with the affected side on the upper, with approximately a 30° angle between the bed and the back, and a pillow below. The shoulder on the affected side is extended about 30° and abducted about 50°. The elbow is extended and the fingers are slightly bent, the hand resting on the pillow with the palm downward. The hip on the affected side is extended and the knee is slightly bent. The ankle is put on the pillow or before a plate at 0°. The upper and lower limbs on the healthy side are arranged naturally in a comfortable position.

[Effect] To prevent bedsores and great fluctuation in blood pressure, and make it convenient for discharging sputum and relieving spasm of the elbow joints. The other methods are the same as that of the basic body positions.

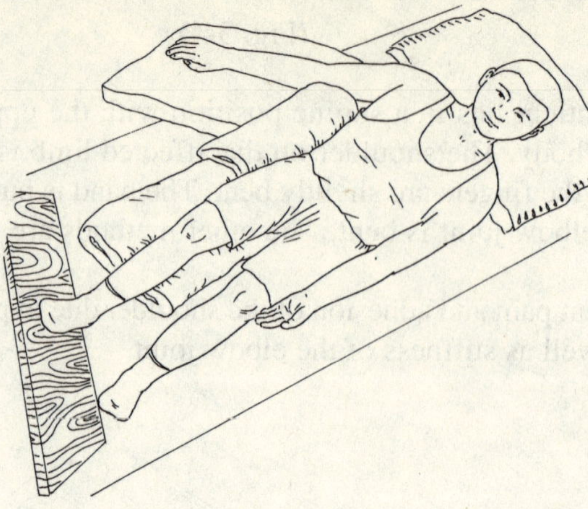

Fig. 3-5 Semi-supine position

6. LYING ON THE HEALTHY SIDE
(Fig. 3-6)

[Method] The patient should lie on the side with the affected side upward, with approximately a 100° angle between the bed and the back, and a pillow beneath the armpit and chest. The elbow is bent about 90° and the wrist slightly extended. The fingers are bent and the hand holds a roll of gauze and is put on a pillow. The hip joint on the affected side is bent about 30° and the knee is slightly bent. The ankle is put on the pillow beneath the shank on the healthy side at 0° in order to keep a horizontal level. The limbs on the healthy side are arranged naturally in a comfortable position.

[Effect] To prevent bedsores, semiluxation of the shoulder joint and stiffness of the hip and knee joints. The other methods are the same as that of the basic body positions.

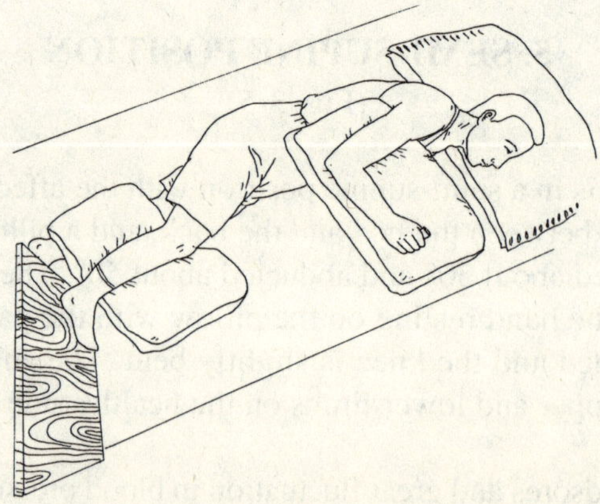

Fig. 3-6 Lying on the healthy side

7. LYING ON THE AFFECTED SIDE

(Fig. 3-7)

[Method] The patient should lie with the affected side below, with approximately a 120° angle between the back and the bed. The shoulder and elbow on the affected side are slightly bent; the hand holds a roll of gauze and rests on the pillow with the palm upward. The hip and knee joints are slightly bent and the ankle is put before a plate at 0°. The shoulder on the healthy side is bent about 45°, the elbow is bent and the hand is put on the pillow with the palm downward to support the body. The hip and knee joints are bent about 90° with a pillow beneath to support the body.

[Effect] To strengthen the myodynamia of the muscle groups at the neck, shoulder, chest, waist, back, buttock and lower limbs on the affected side so as to prevent bedsores that may result on the healthy side from prolonged lying.

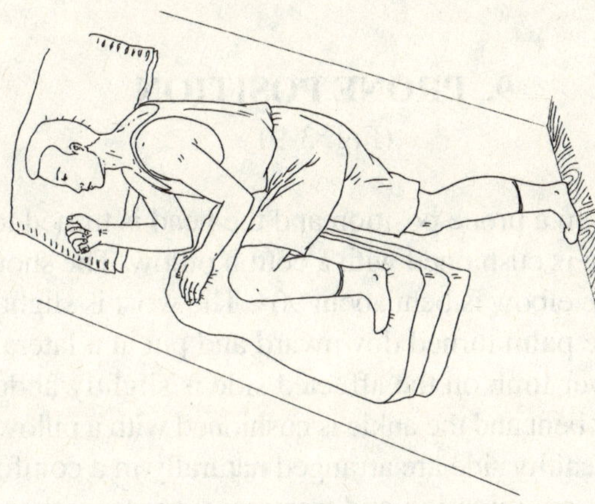

Fig. 3-7 Lying on the affected side

8. SEMI-PRONE POSITION

(Fig. 3-8)

[Mcthod] Thc paticnt is in a scmi-pronc position with the affected side uppermost, the head turned to the affected side with a pillow beneath. There should approximately be an 150° angle between bed and back, and the chest and abdomen are cushioned with a pillow. The shoulder on the affected side is abducted and the elbow is bent, both about 90°. The wrist is slightly extended and the hand holds a roll of gauze with the palm turned downward and put in a lateral and upward position in relation to the head. The hip and knee joints on the affected side are slightly bent. The ankle is cushioned with a pillow at 0°. The limbs on the healthy side are arranged naturally in a comfortable position.

[Effect] To strengthen the myodynamia of the muscles on the chest and abdomen on the affected side as well as the functions of the heart and lungs, so as to prevent bedsores.

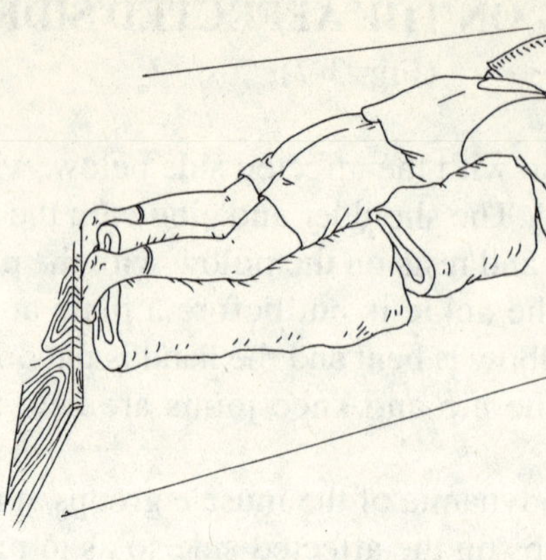

Fig. 3-8 Semi-prone position

9. PRONE POSITION
(Fig. 3-9)

[Method] The patient is in a prone position and the head is turned to the affected side with a pillow beneath. The abdomen is cushioned with a cotton pillow. The shoulder on the affected side is abducted about 45°, and the elbow is bent about 90°. The wrist is slightly extended and the hand holds a roll of gauze with the palm turned downward and put at a lateral and upward position in relation to the head. The lower limb on the affected side is slightly abducted and the hip joint is adducted. The knee is slightly bent and the ankle is cushioned with a pillow or put on the edge of the bed at 0°. The limbs on the healthy side are arranged naturally in a comfortable position.

[Effect] To facilitate for examination and treatment; to strengthen the myodynamia of the muscles on the chest and abdomen and the functions of the heart and lungs; and to prevent bedsores on the back, waist and sacral region and semiluxation of the shoulder joint.

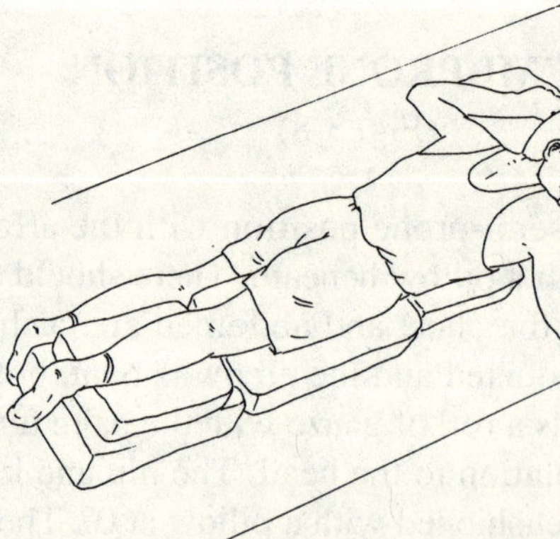

Fig. 3-9 Prone position

10. PASSIVE CHANGE FROM A SUPINE TO A PRONE POSITION
(Fig. 3-10)

[Method] The patient lies in a supine position and the hand on the healthy side grasps the hand on the affected side and is placed on the abdomen. The foot on the healthy side is crossed under the foot on the affected side. The doctor or nurse stands on the affected side, holding the shoulder on the affected side with one hand and supporting the lower part of the knee on the affected side with the other, to help the patient turn the body slowly to the healthy side, slightly raising the lower limb on the affected side and moving the shoulder on the affected side to a lying position on the healthy side. Then, the upper limb on the affected side is placed in an upward position in relation to the head and the body is turned to a prone position. The patient is helped to move the hand on the healthy side away from the lower part of the abdomen and adjusted into a functional pronation.

[Effect] To improve the functional state of the heart and cerebral vessels and promote the restoration of the coordinating function of both the healthy and affected sides; to strengthen the passive movement of the patient; and to promote the restoration of the myodynamia of the muscles on the affected side.

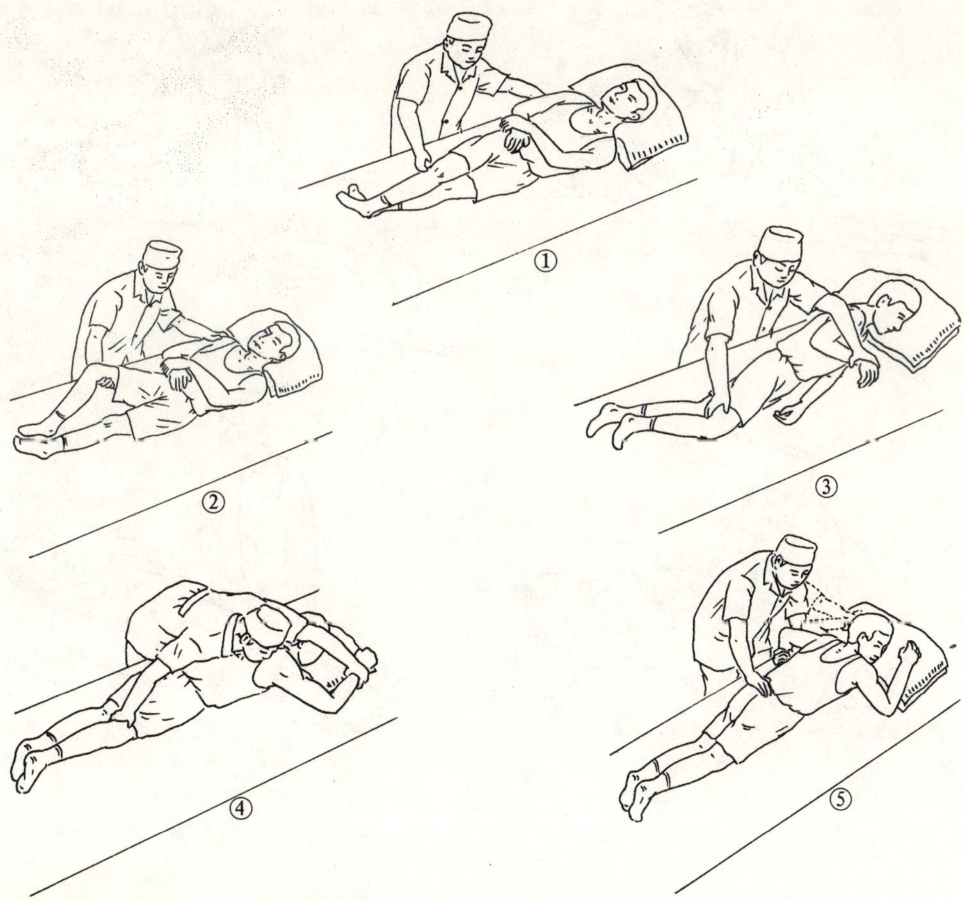

Fig. 3-10 Passive change from a supine to a prone position

11. PASSIVE CHANGE FROM A PRONE TO A SUPINE POSITION
(Fig. 3-11)

[Method] The patient is in a prone position and the hand on the healthy side holds the hand on the affected side and raises it over the head. The doctor or nurse stands on the healthy side and holds the shoulder and hip on the affected side respectively to enable the patient to raise the head, turn the body slowly to the healthy side and raise the hand on the affected side as much as possible. When the body is being turned, the doctor or nurse slowly bends the shoulder and hip on the affected side to help the lower limb on the affected side turn to a lying position on the healthy side. Then, the doctor or nurse turns the patient's body to a supine position and adjusts it to a functional supine position.

[Effect] To improve the functional state of heart and brain vessels; promote the restoration of the functions of both the healthy and affected sides; to strengthen the passive movement of the patient; and to enlarge the moving range of all the joints and reinforce the myodynamia of the muscles on the affected side.

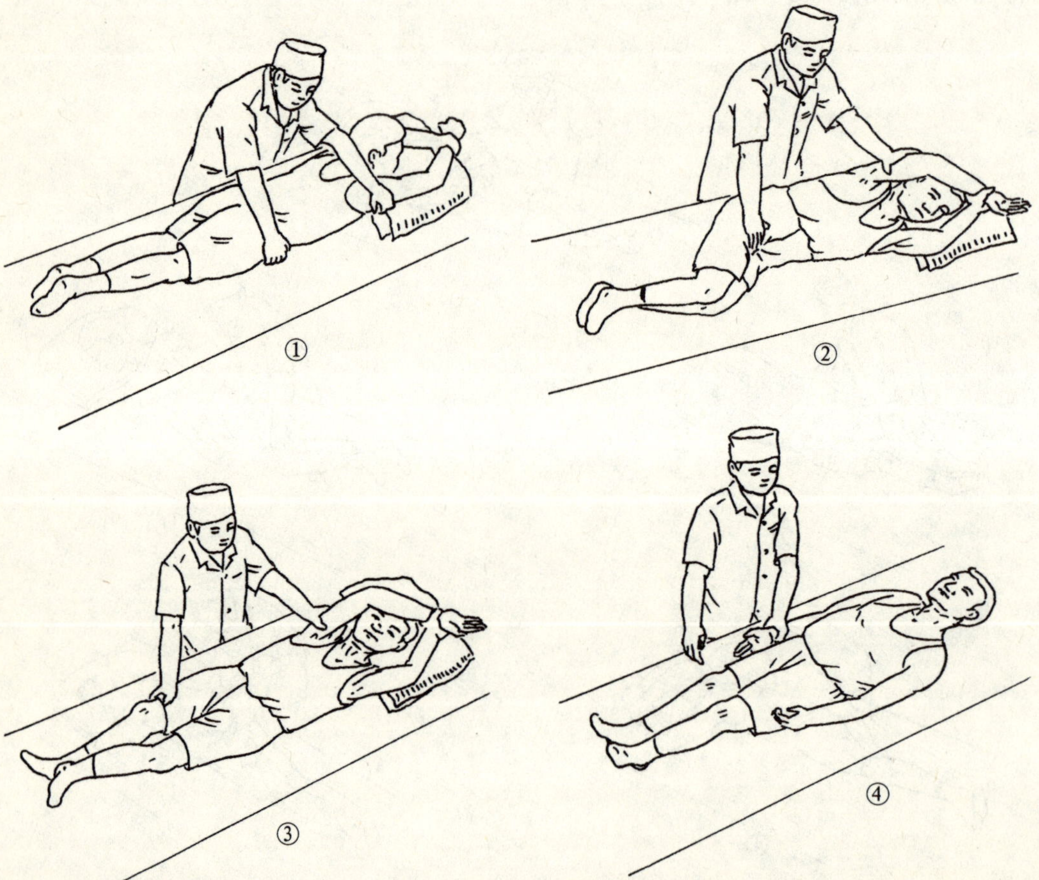

Fig. 3-11 Passive change from a prone to a supine position

12. ACTIVE CHANGE FROM A SUPINE TO A PRONE POSITION (Fig. 3-12)

[Method] The patient is in a supine position. The hand on the healthy side holds the hand on the affected side to raise it over the head, while the foot on the healthy side is placed under the foot on the affected side. The patient raises the head to tûrn to the healthy side, breathes in, and raises the hand on the affected side with the help of the hand on the healthy side. The foot on the healthy side supports the foot on the affected side to help the waist turn to a lying position on the healthy side. Then, the patient breathes out and continues to turn the body to a prone position. The doctor or nurse helps the patient adjust to a functional prone position.

[Effect] To strengthen the functions of the heart and lungs and promote metabolism; and to improve the quality of active movement so as to prevent stiffness and spasms of all the joints.

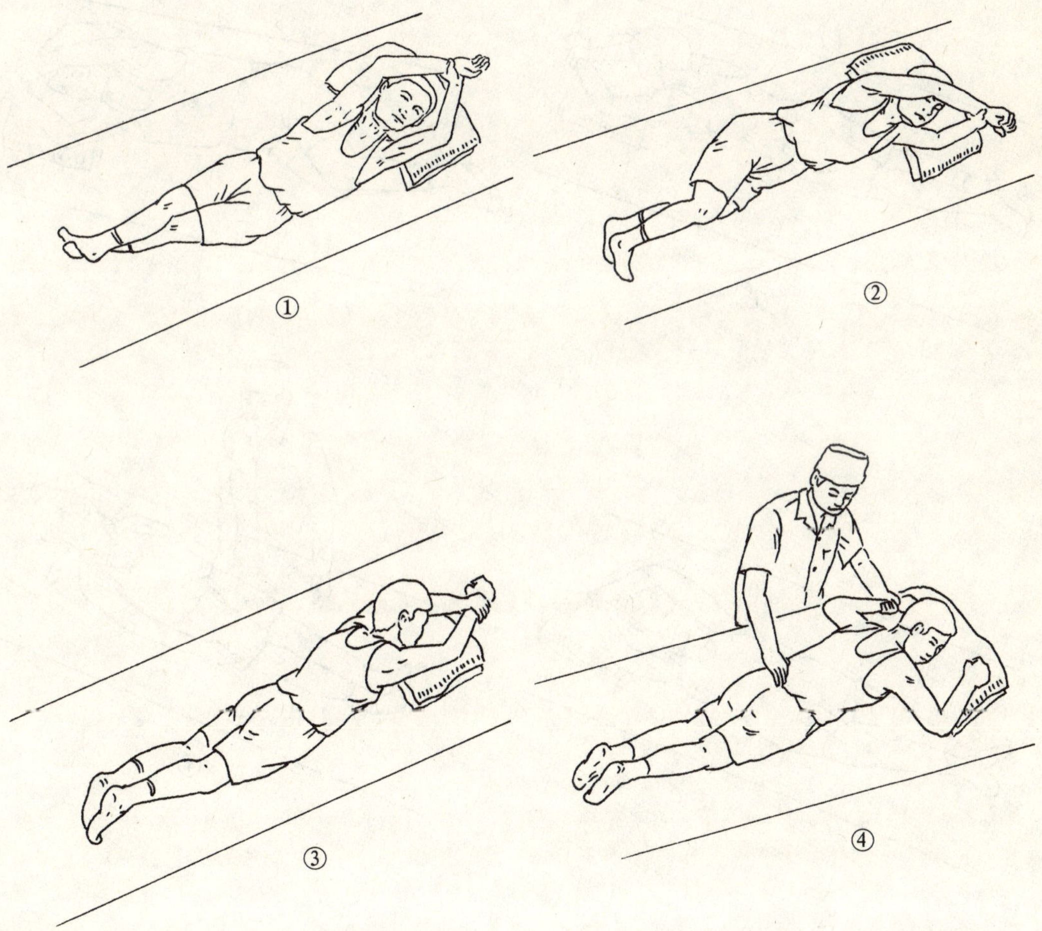

Fig. 3-12 Active change from a supine to a prone position

13. ACTIVE CHANGE FROM A PRONE TO A SUPINE POSITION (Fig. 3-13)

[Method] The patient is in a prone position and the hand on the healthy side holds the hand on the affected side to raise it over the head. The head is raised and turned to the affected side. Then, the patient breathes in and the hand on the healthy side raises the hand on the affected side. At the same time, the waist turns with the trunk to a lying position on the healthy side. The patient breathes out and continues to turn the body into a supine position. The doctor or nurse helps the patient adjust his or her body to a functional supine position.

[Effect] To strengthen the functions of the heart and lungs and promote metabolism for the benefit of rehabilitation; to enlarge the moving range of the shoulder, back and waist; and to prevent deformity of the shoulder, elbow and spine joints.

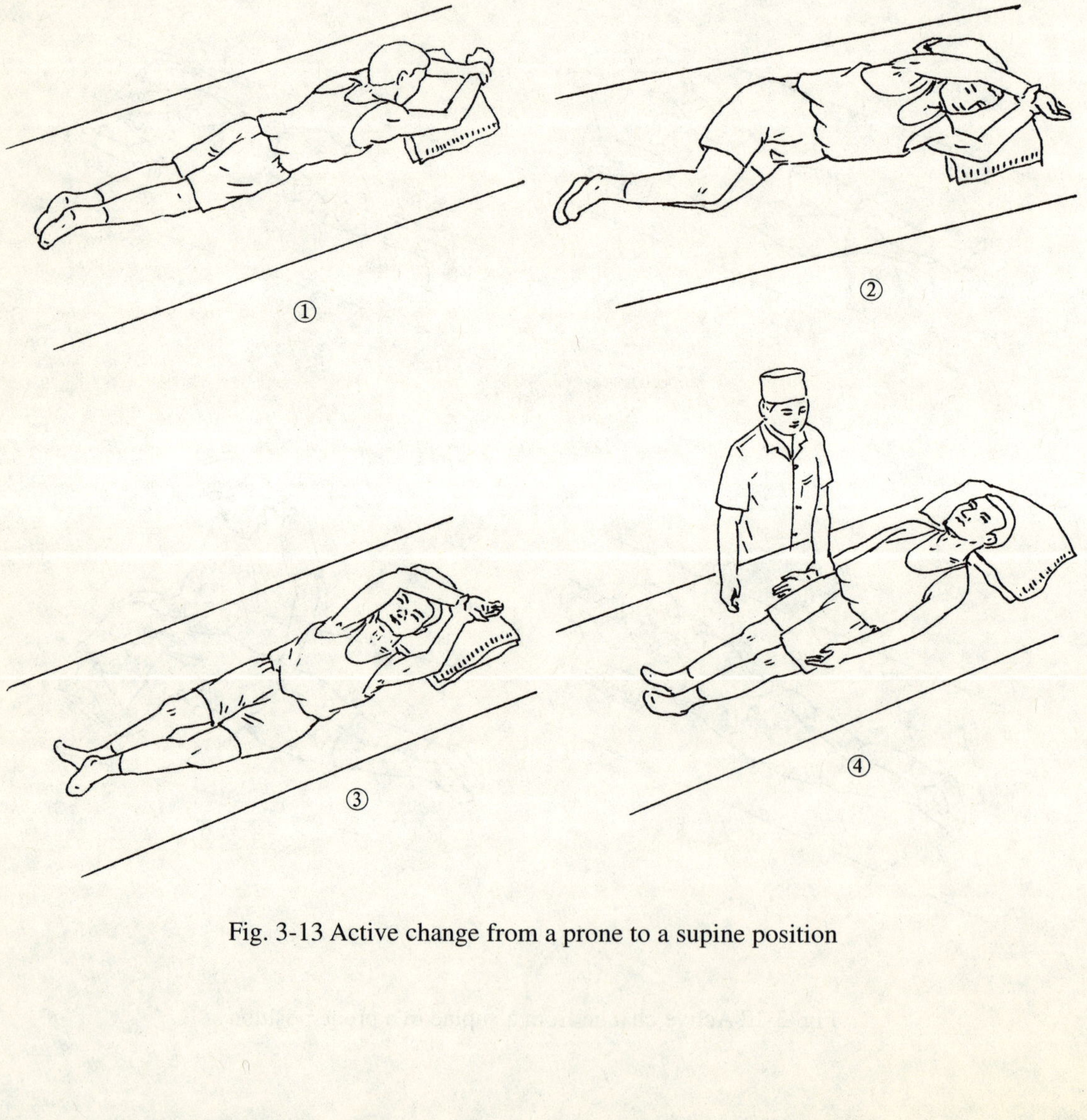

Fig. 3-13 Active change from a prone to a supine position

Chapter 4

ILLUSTRATED PASSIVE FUNCTIONAL EXERCISES AT THE ACUTE STAGE

After the improvement of the critical symptoms, such as coma, vomiting and fever, and stabilization of the pathological conditions, passive functional exercises should start. Extensive clinical observations show that passive functional exercises can start seven days after the onset of hemorrhagic wind stroke and three days after the onset of ischemic wind stroke.

Studies indicate that the muscles and loose connective tissues around the joints will become dense connective tissues, which will lead to contracture and deformity of the joints if the joints, especially the large ones, stop moving for three weeks. The passive movement of the limb on the affected side at the early stage can promote the circulation of blood, maintain the moving range of the ligaments, alleviate convulsions and stop myatrophy, prevent contracture of the muscles and ligaments as well as limited movement of the joints due to stiffness. Besides, early passive exercises can enable patients to get to know what the correct moving style is, so as to prepare for the active functional exercise stage and restoring the ability to manage their own life.

It is clinically confirmed that earlier functional exercises can reduce foot deformity, contracture and spasm of the elbow joint in movement and limited movement of the shoulder joint. Besides, earlier functional exercises can also enable most patients to walk with the aid of sticks and live without the insertion of a urinary catheter later on.

Passive functional exercises on the affected limb can be done in the 1/2 range of the movement of the joint at first, with range gradually enlarged. The following points should be borne in mind when doing passive functional exercises:

1) The manipulations of the doctor or nurse should be slow, gentle, stable and rhythmic, enabling the patients to experience the correct way of movement and the contraction of muscles.

2) The exercises should be carried out within the normal movement range of the joints. If there is pain, the exercises should stop.

3) The joint nearby should be fixated to avoid alternative movement.

4) The exercises should concentrate on the joints that tend to develop deformity (such as finger, elbow, knee and ankle joints) and the joints that have already developed deformity.

5) Each action in the exercises should be done 5-20 times. The exercises should be done at least half an hour before other treatments. It can be done one hour after the mid-day nap. It is preferable to stop the exercises at night to avoid insomnia caused by excitation.

6) Every morning, before the exercises, the blood pressure should be checked. If it fluctuates at 4kPa continuously for three days, the exercises should be reduced or stopped.

1. UPPER LIMBS

(1) Anterior bending and lifting of the shoulder joint (Fig. 4-1)

[Method] The patient lies in a supine position with a functional posture. The upper limbs are put beside the body and the palms turned upward. The doctor or nurse holds the palmar side of the wrist and the lateral side of the shoulder on the affected side with both hands to slowly extend the affected upper limb, anterior bending and lifting through 120°. After an interval of 3-5 seconds, the limb is returned to the original position. Such a manipulation is done 5-10 times.

[Effect] To train the muscles on the shoulder responsible for bending and extending of the shoulder joint, so as to prevent adhesion of the shoulder joint and spasm of the elbow joint.

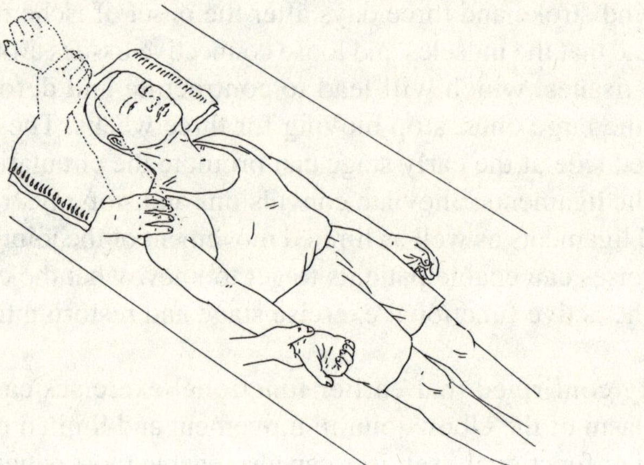

Fig. 4-1 Anterior bending and lifting of the shoulder joint

(2) Abducting and adducting the shoulder joint (Fig. 4-2)

[Method] The patient lies in a supine position with a functional posture. The upper limbs are put beside the body and the palms turned upward. The doctor or nurse holds the palmar side of the wrist and lateral side of the shoulder on the affected side with both hands to slowly extend the affected limb, abducting through 120°. After an interval of 3-5 seconds, the limb is adducted to the original position. Such a manipulation is done 5-10 times.

[Effect] To train the muscles on the shoulder responsible for abduction and adduction of the shoulder joint; and to prevent semi-dislocation of the shoulder joint and spasm of the elbow joint.

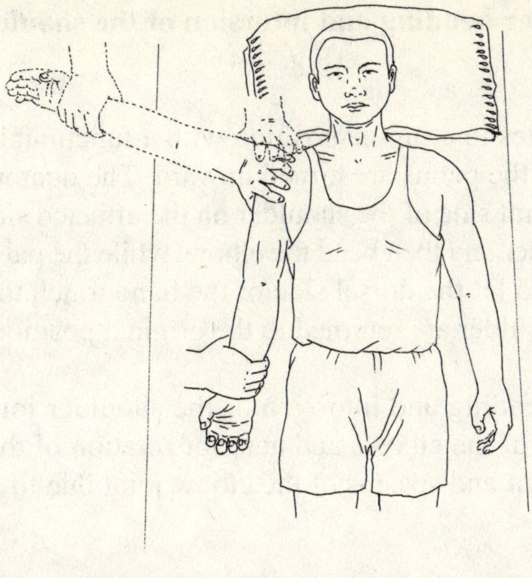

Fig. 4-2 Abducting and adducting the shoulder joint

(3) Intorsion and eversion of the shoulder joint
(Fig. 4-3)

[Method] The patient lies in a supine position with a functional posture. The upper limbs are put beside the body and the palms are turned upward. The doctor or nurse holds the dorsal side of the wrist and the lateral side of the shoulder on the affected side together to slowly abduct the shoulder and bend the elbow through about 90°. The palm is turned to the direction of the foot. The shoulder is slowly intorted and the palm is turned to the anterior and inferior direction. The shoulder is then slowly abducted and the palm is turned upward. Such a manipulation is repeated about 5-15 times and the wrist and shoulder are returned to the original positions.

[Effect] To train the abduction and adduction of the shoulder as well as the muscles responsible for bending the elbows; and to prevent the adhesion and semi-dislocation of the shoulder joint, as well as stiffness of the elbow joint.

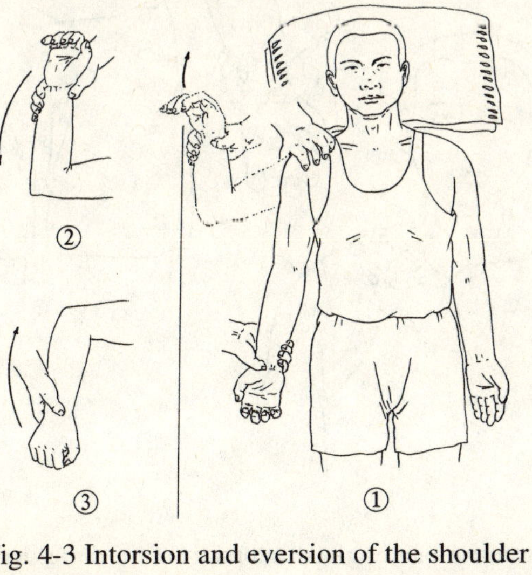

Fig. 4-3 Intorsion and eversion of the shoulder joint

(4) Anterior bending and intorsion of the shoulder joint (Fig. 4-4)

[Method] The patient lies in a supine position with a functional posture. The upper limbs are put beside the body and the palms are turned upward. The doctor or nurse holds the dorsal side of the wrist and the lateral side of the shoulder on the affected side together to slowly bend forward and intort the shoulder and then bend the elbow, while the palm is turned in the direction of the foot. It is preferable to let the dorsal side of the hand touch the shoulder on the healthy side. Then, the wrist and shoulder are returned to the original positions. Such a manipulation is repeated about 5-10 times.

[Effect] To train the bending and intorsion of the shoulder joint as well as the muscles responsible for the bending of the elbows and anterior rotation of the forearm; and to prevent adhesion of the shoulder joint and spasms of the elbow joint due to stiffness.

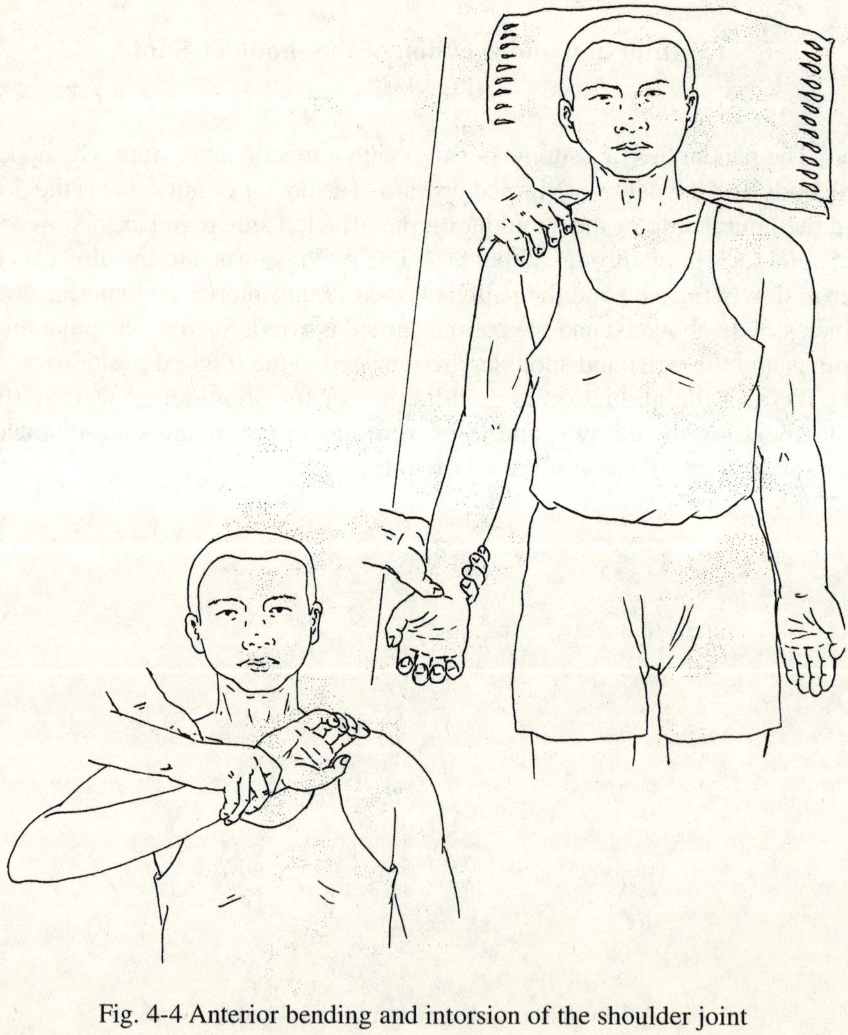

Fig. 4-4 Anterior bending and intorsion of the shoulder joint

(5) Rotation of the forearm with the bending and extending of the elbow joint (Fig. 4-5)

[Method] The patient lies in a supine position with a functional posture. The upper limbs are put beside the body and the palms are turned upward. The doctor or nurse holds the dorsal side of the wrist and the anterior and inferior side of the forearm on the affected side together to slowly bend the elbow, while the palm is turned in the direction of the foot. Then the elbow is slowly extended and the palm is turned upward. Such a manipulation is repeated about 5-15 times. Then, the wrist and forearm are returned to the original positions.

[Effect] To train the bending and extending of the elbow joint and the anterior and posterior muscles responsible for the rotation of the forearm; and to prevent spasms of the elbow joint due to stiffness.

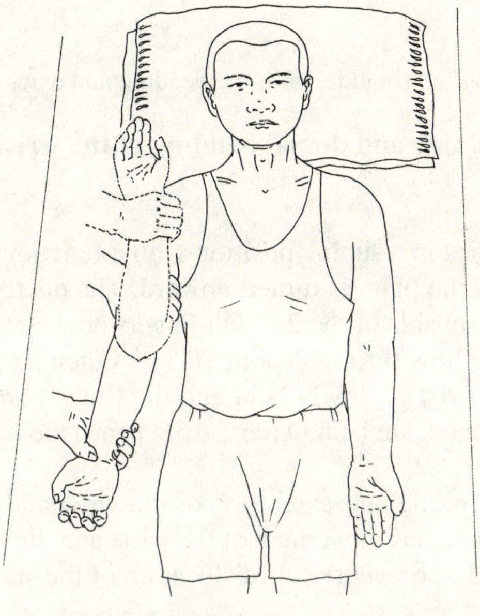

Fig. 4-5 Rotation of the forearm with the bending and extending of the elbow joint

(6) Abducting the shoulder with the bending and extending of the elbow (Fig. 4-6)

[Method] The patient lies in a supine position with a functional posture. The upper limbs are put beside the body and the palms are turned upward. The doctor or nurse holds the dorsal side of the wrist and the shoulder on the affected side together to slowly abduct the shoulder through 90°. The elbow is slowly bent and the palm is turned in the direction of the foot. The elbow is then extended and the palm is turned upward. Such a manipulation is repeated about 5-15 times. Then, the wrist and shoulder are returned to the original positions.

[Effect] To train the abduction of the shoulder joint, the bending and extending of the elbow joint and the anterior and posterior muscles responsible for the rotation of the forearm; and to prevent semi-dislocation of the shoulder joint and alleviate the spasms and stiffness of the elbow joint.

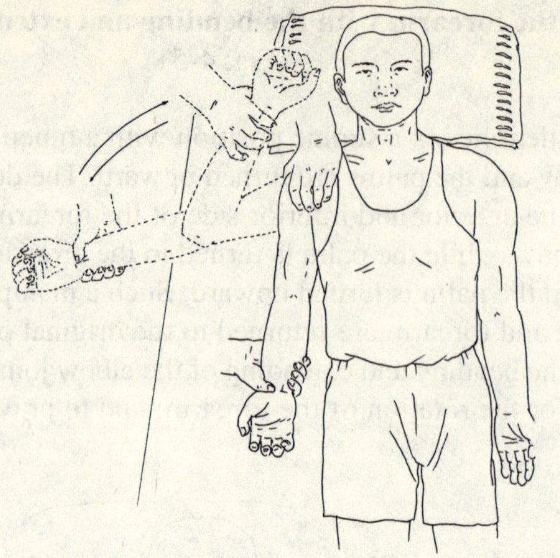

Fig. 4-6 Abducting the shoulder with the bending and extending of the elbow

(7) Palmar and dorsal bending of the wrist joint
(Fig. 4-7)

[Method] The patient lies in a supine position with a functional posture. The upper limbs are put beside the body and the palm is turned upward. The doctor or nurse holds the palmar side of the wrist and the dorsal side of the 2nd-5th fingers on the affected side to slowly abduct the shoulder and bend the elbow through about 90°, and then fixates it with the palm turned toward the foot. Then, the wrist is slowly bent and the fingers are extended, after which the wrist is extended and the fingers are bent. After 5-15 repeats, the wrist and fingers are returned to the original position.

[Effect] To train the bending and extending of the wrist and muscles around the digital joints; to separate the simultaneous movement of the wrist and digital joints to alleviate spasms of the wrist and fingers; and to prevent semi-dislocation of the shoulder joint.

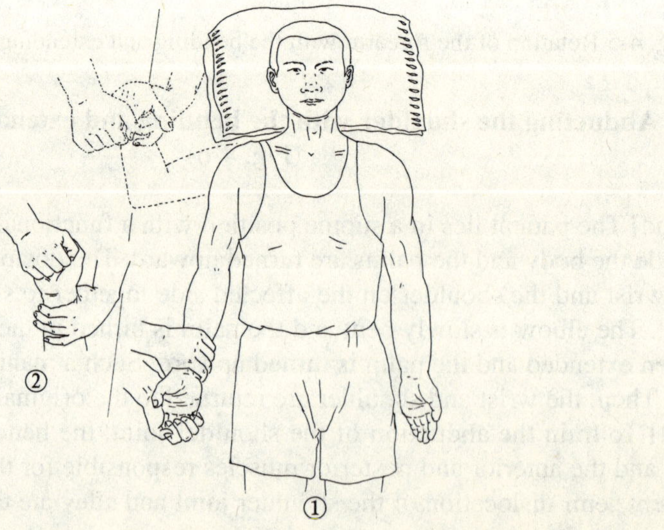

Fig. 4-7 Palmar and dorsal bending of the wrist joint

(8) Ulnar and radial bending of the radiocarpal joint (Fig. 4-8)

[Method] The patient lies in a supine position with a functional posture. The upper limbs are put beside the body and the palms are turned upward. The doctor or nurse holds the palmar side of the wrist and dorsal side of the metacarpal part on the affected side with the thumb kept laterally. The shoulder is slowly abducted and the elbow is bent through about 90° and fixated with the palm turned toward the foot. Then, the hand is slowly adducted and abducted. After such a manipulation is repeated 5-15 times, the limbs are returned to their original position.

[Effect] To train the abduction and adduction of the muscles on the rediocarpal joint; and to prevent semi-dislocation of the shoulder joint, droop of the wrist and spasm of the fingers.

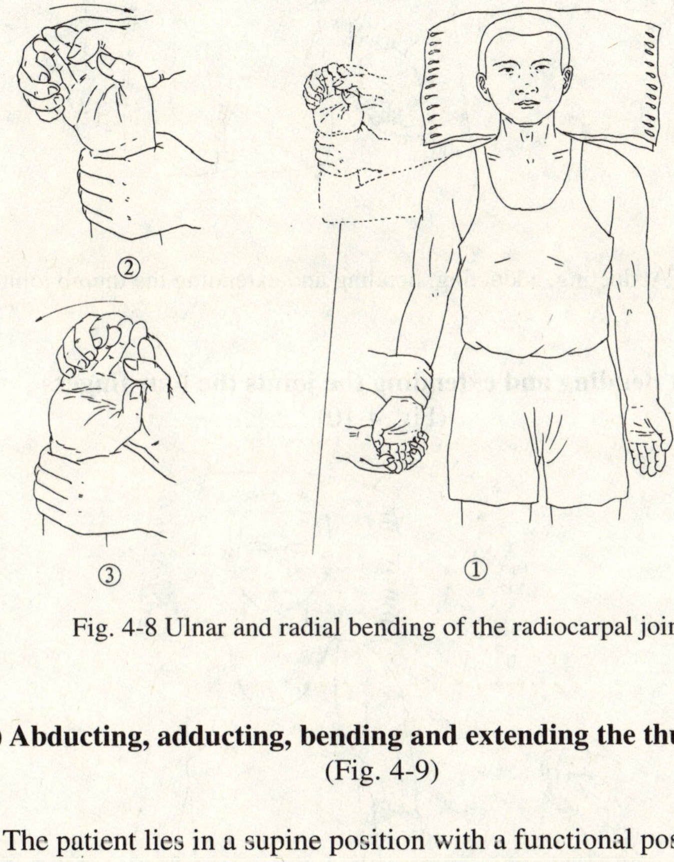

Fig. 4-8 Ulnar and radial bending of the radiocarpal joint

(9) Abducting, adducting, bending and extending the thumb joint (Fig. 4-9)

[Method] The patient lies in a supine position with a functional posture. The upper limbs are put beside the body and the palms are turned upward. The doctor or nurse holds the palmar side of the wrist and the dorsal side of the 2nd-5th fingers on the affected side to slowly abduct the shoulder and bend the elbow through about 90° and fixates it with the palm turned toward the foot. Then, the thumb and index finger of one hand hold the thumb of the affected side of the patient to slowly abduct, adduct, bend and extend the thumb. After such a manipulation is repeated about 5-20 times, the limbs are returned to their original positions.

[Effect] To train the abduction, adduction, bending and extending of the muscles on the thumb joint, regulate the reflex of the cerebral functions, and promote the restoration of the functions of the fingers; and to prevent semi-dislocation of the shoulder joint and droop of the wrist.

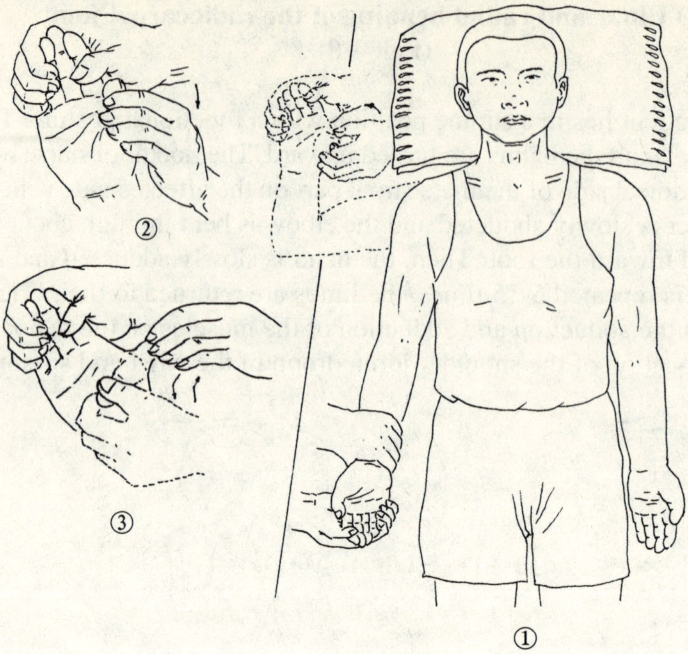

Fig. 4-9 Abducting, adducting, bending and extending the thumb joint

(10) Bending and extending the joints the four fingers
(Fig. 4-10)

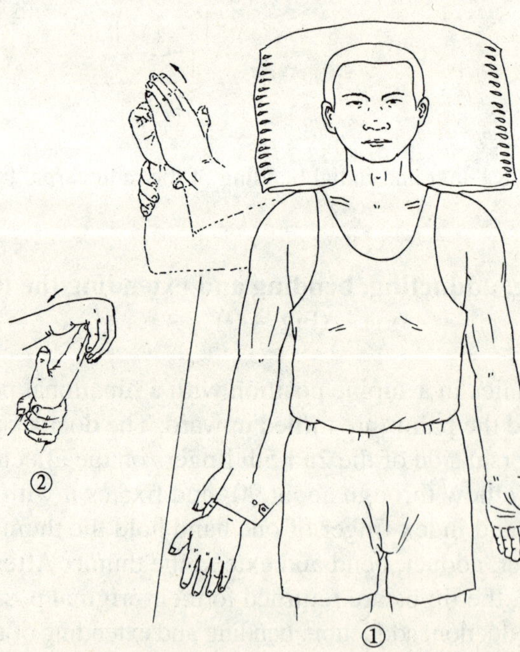

Fig. 4-10 Bending and extending the joints of the four fingers

[Method] The patient lies in a supine position with a functional posture. The upper limbs are put beside the body and the palms are turned upward. The doctor and nurse holds the dorsal side of the wrist with one hand and the tips of the 2nd-5th fingers with the other on the affected side to slowly abduct the shoulder and bend the elbow through about 90°. Such a position is fixated with the palm turned toward the foot. The doctor or nurse should slowly and gently rub with the palms, while the finger joints of the patient are bent and extended accordingly. Such a manipulation is repeated 5-20 times. Then, the limbs are returned to their original positions.

[Effect] To train the muscles responsible for bending and extending the fingers, regulate the reflex of the cerebral functions, and promote the restoration of the normal functions of the fingers; and to prevent semi-dislocation of the shoulder joint and droop of the wrist.

(11) Adducting and abducting the joints of the four fingers (Fig. 4-11)

[Method] The patient lies in a supine position with a functional posture. The upper limbs are put beside the body and the palms are turned upward. The doctor or nurse holds the dorsal side of the wrist on the affected limb with one hand and uses the finger pad to press the finger pad of the patient. Then, the shoulder is slowly abducted and the elbow is bent through about 90°, and is fixated with the palm turned toward the foot. The doctor or nurse adducts and abducts the fingers, and the fingers of the patient are adducted and abducted accordingly. Such a manipulation is repeated 5-20 times. Then, the limbs are slowly returned to the original positions.

[Effect] To train the muscles responsible for adducting and abducting the fingers, regulate the reflex of the cerebral functions, and promote the restoration of the normal functions of the fingers; and to prevent semi-dislocation of the shoulder joint and droop of the wrist.

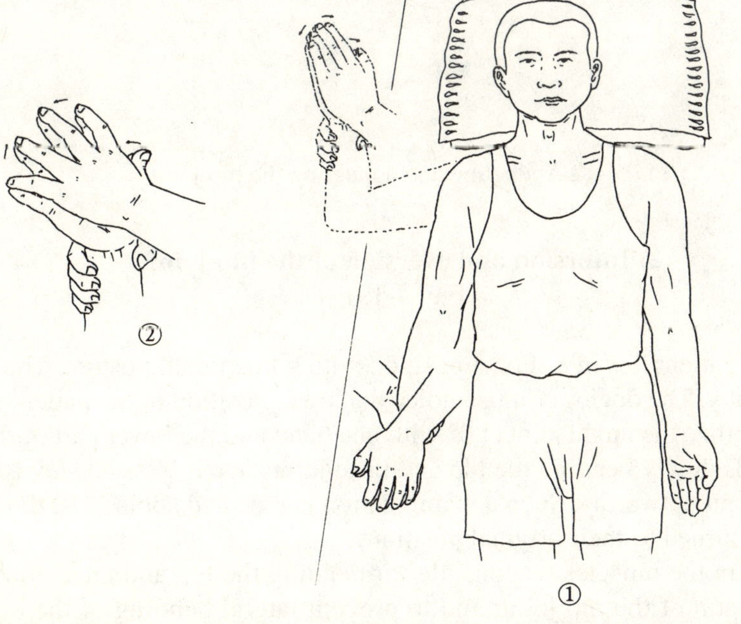

Fig. 4-11 Adducting and abducting the joints of the four fingers

2. LOWER LIMBS

(1) Abducting and adducting the hip joint
(Fig. 4-12)

[Method] The patient lies in a supine position with a functional posture. The lower limbs are extended naturally. The doctor or nurse holds the posterior part of the ankle on the affected limb and stabilizes the ankle joint in a position of 0° with one hand, holds the lower part of the knee to extend the knee joint, slightly lifts the affected limb, abducts the hip (be careful not to move the healthy lower limb) and adducts the hip with the other hand. Such a manipulation is repeated 5-6 times. Then, the limbs are slowly returned to their original positions.

[Effect] To train the muscles responsible for abducting and adducting the hip joint; and to prevent contracture of the hip and knee joints, foot droop and strephenopodia.

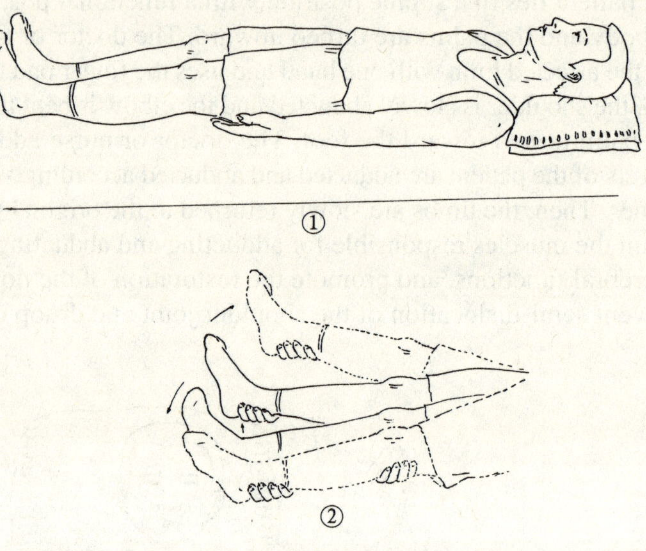

Fig. 4-12 Abducting and adducting the hip joint

(2) Intorsion and eversion of the hip joint
(Fig. 4-13)

[Method] The patient lies in a supine position with a functional posture. The lower limbs are extended naturally. The doctor or nurse holds the lower position of the patient's foot on the affected side to stabilize the ankle joint at 0° with one hand and the lower part of the knee joint with the other hand, slowly bending the hip and knee joints about 90° and slowly rotating the hip joint inwardly and outwardly. Such a manipulation is repeated about 5-10 times. Then, the limbs are slowly returned to their original positions.

[Effect] To train the muscles responsible for bending the hip and knee joints as well as intorsion and eversion of the hip joint; and to prevent lateral bending of the hip joint, foot droop and strephenopodia.

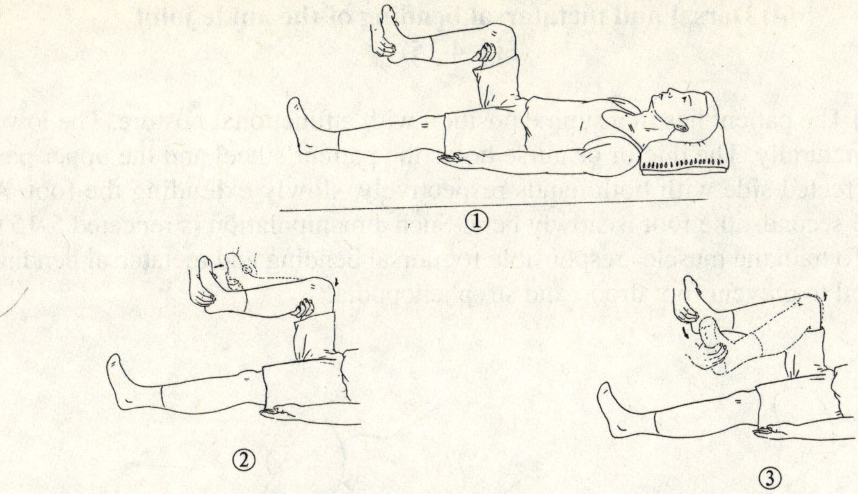

Fig. 4-13 Intorsion and eversion of the hip joint

(3) Bending and extending the hip and knee joints
(Fig. 4-14)

[Method] The patient lies in a supine position with a functional posture. The lower limbs are extended naturally. The doctor or nurse holds the middle part of the patient's sole on the affected side to stabilize the ankle joint at 0° with one hand, and the lower part of the knee joint with the other, slowly bending the hip and knee joints about 120°. After an interval of 3-5 seconds, the knee is slowly extended and then the hip joint is slowly stretched. Such a manipulation is repeated 5-10 times. Then, the limbs are returned to their original positions.

[Effect] To train the muscles responsible for bending and extending the hip and knee joints; and to prevent spasms and stiffness of the hip and knee joints, as well as foot droop and strephenopodia.

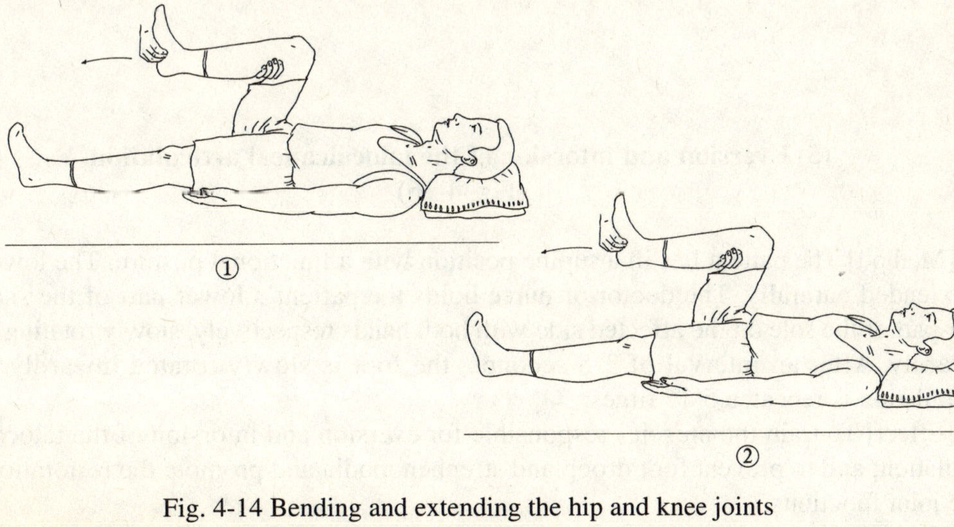

Fig. 4-14 Bending and extending the hip and knee joints

(4) Dorsal and metatarsal bending of the ankle joint (Fig. 4-15)

[Method] The patient lies in a supine position with a functional posture. The lower limbs are extended naturally. The doctor or nurse holds the patient's heel and the upper part of the sole on the affected side with both hands respectively, slowly extending the foot. After an interval of 3-5 seconds, the foot is slowly bent. Such a manipulation is repeated 5-15 times.

[Effect] To train the muscles responsible for dorsal bending and metatarsal bending of the ankle joint; and to prevent foot droop and strephenopodia.

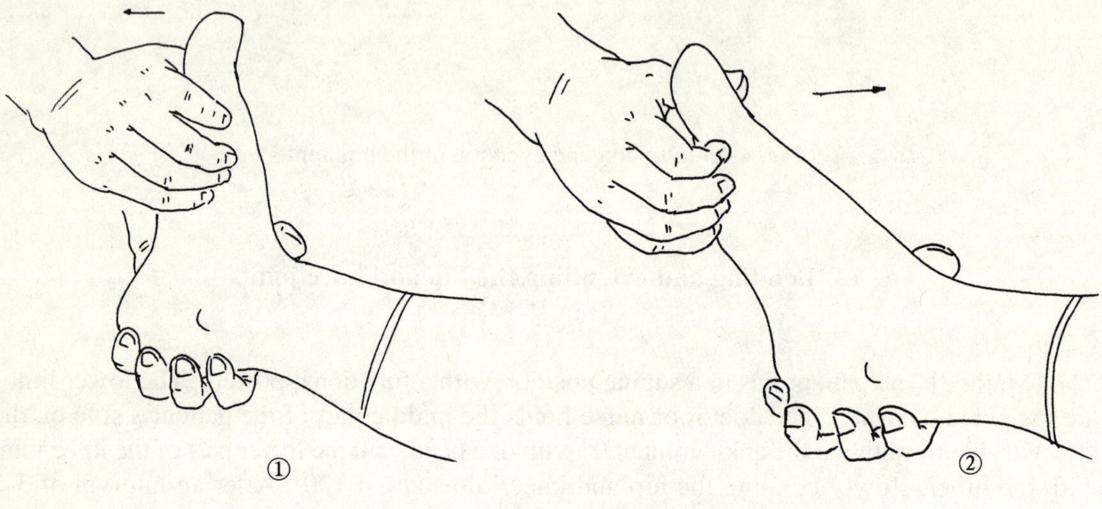

Fig. 4-15 Dorsal and metatarsal bending

(5) Eversion and intorsion of the talocalcaneal articulation (Fig. 4-16)

[Method] The patient lies in a supine position with a functional posture. The lower limbs are extended naturally. The doctor or nurse holds the patient's lower part of the shank and upper part of the sole on the affected side with both hands respectively, slowly rotating the foot outwardly. After an interval of 3-5 seconds, the foot is slowly rotated inwardly. Such a manipulation is repeated 5-15 times.

[Effect] To train the muscles responsible for eversion and intorsion of the talocalcaneal articulation; and to prevent foot droop and strephenopodia and promote the restoration of the ankle joint functions.

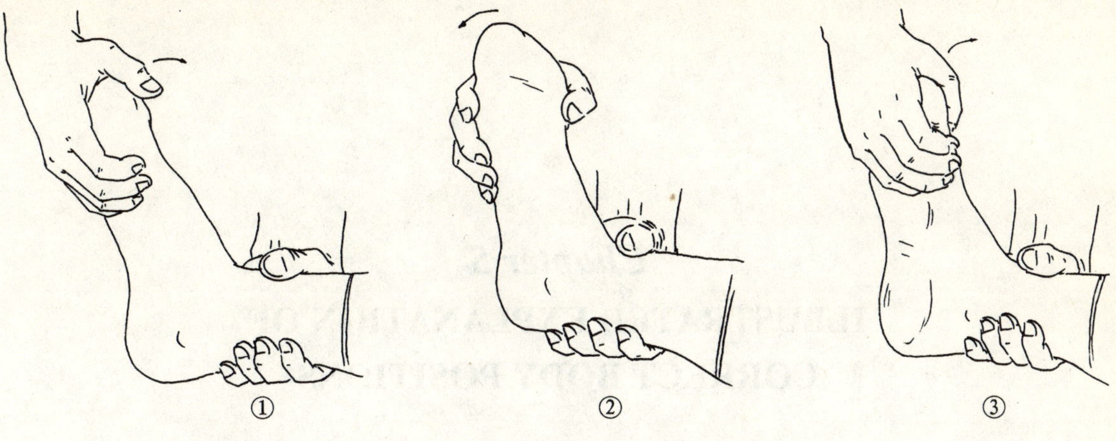

Fig. 4-16 Eversion and intorsion

(6) Extending and bending the metatarsophalangeal joint
(Fig.4-17)

[Method] The patient lies in a supine position with a functional posture. The lower limbs are extended naturally. The doctor or nurse holds the patient's foot dorsum with one hand to stabilize the ankle joint at 0° and the last knuckle of the toes on the affected side with the other hand, slowly extending and bending the phalangeal joints. Such a manipulation is repeated 5-20 times.

[Effect] To train the muscles responsible for bending and extending the metatarsophalangeal joint, regulate the reflex of the cerebral functions, and promote the restoration of functions of the toes; and to prevent foot droop and strephenopodia.

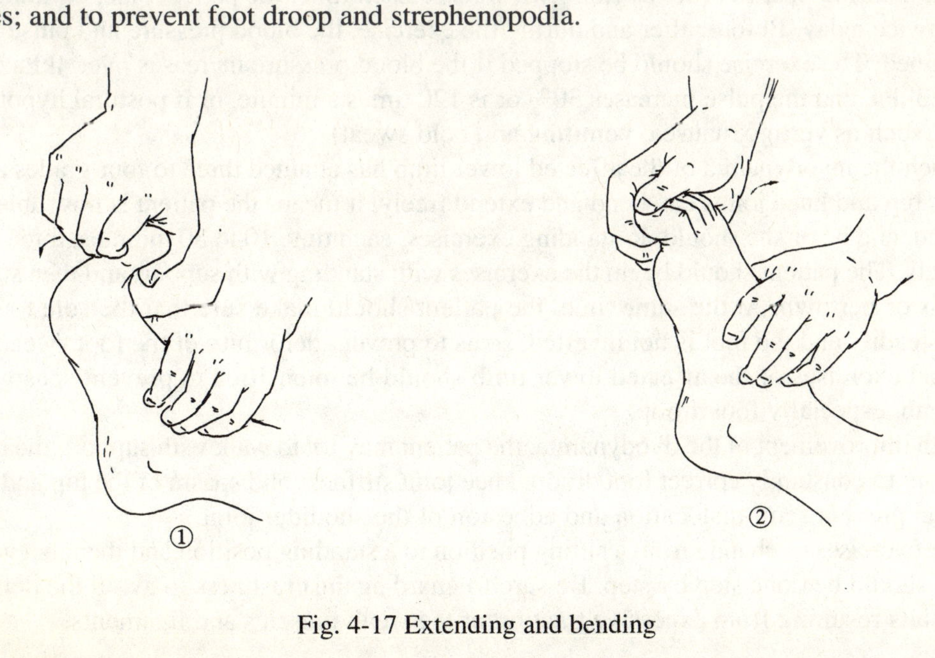

Fig. 4-17 Extending and bending

Chapter 5

ILLUSTRATED EXPLANATION OF CORRECT BODY POSITIONS

The patient needs to change the body position after a period of treatment to prevent secondary dysfunction due to long-term lying on the bed. The body can be changed gradually from a lying position to a sitting position, and from a sitting position to a standing position and from a standing position to a walking position. In this way, the patient is eventually able to walk and go up and down stairs with ease.

The change of body position is not simply a matter of sitting or standing up. Such a change should be scientific. Changing the body position too early or too late will increase the possibility and degree of disablement. Besides, a premature change of the body position may lead to wind stroke and death.

Generally speaking, the change from a lying to a sitting position can be done after the acute stage (two weeks after ischemic wind stroke, 3-4 weeks after hemorrhagic wind stroke). If the patient is conscious and the myodynamia of the affected lower limbs is two to three grades, he or she may do sitting exercises from angles of 30°, 45°, 60° and 80°, and reaching the highest sitting position (80°) within two weeks. Each time, the patient sits 30 minutes and once or twice a day. Before, after and during the exercise, the blood pressure and pulse should be examined. The exercise should be stopped if the blood pressure increases over 4kPa or falls below 1.3kPa, and the pulse increases 30% or is 120 times a minute, or if postural hypotension appears (such as vertigo, nausea, vomiting and cold sweat).

When the myodynamia of the affected lower limb has attained three to four grades and the patient's hip and knee joints can bend and extend freely, it means the patient is now able to get out of bed, and he or she should do standing exercises, each time 10 to 30 minutes, three to four times daily. The patient should begin the exercises with standing with support and then standing all on his or her own. At the same time, the patient should make sure that the sole touch the ground steadily and the foot is not inverted, so as to prevent deformity of the foot. Meanwhile, functional exercises of the affected lower limb should be intensified to prevent spasm of the lower limb, especially foot droop.

With improvement of the dyodynamia, the patient may try to walk with support, meanwhile taking care to constantly correct foot droop, knee joint stiffness and spasm of the hip and elbow joints and prevent semi-dislocation and adhesion of the shoulder joint.

The exercises of change from a sitting position to a standing position and then to a walking position should be done step by step. Be sure to guard against rashness to avoid the deformity of the joints resulting from excessive traction of the weak muscles and ligaments.

1. FUNCTIONAL SITTING POSITION
(Fig. 5-1)

[Method] The patient sits straight on the chair (without leaning against the back). The upper part of the body stretches as much as possible. The head is not deviated to the healthy side. The hips and knees are bent at an angle of 90°. The feet are placed in a stable position on the ground with the same width of the shoulders. In doing functional exercise, the hands are placed on the thighs to keep a balanced sitting position. The affected upper limb is usually suspended with a triangular bandage in front of the chest.

[Effect] To exercise muscles responsible for extension of the spine; to prevent anterior bending of the body, stiffness of the hip and knee joints and droop and inversion of the foot; and to improve cardiocerebrovascular functions.

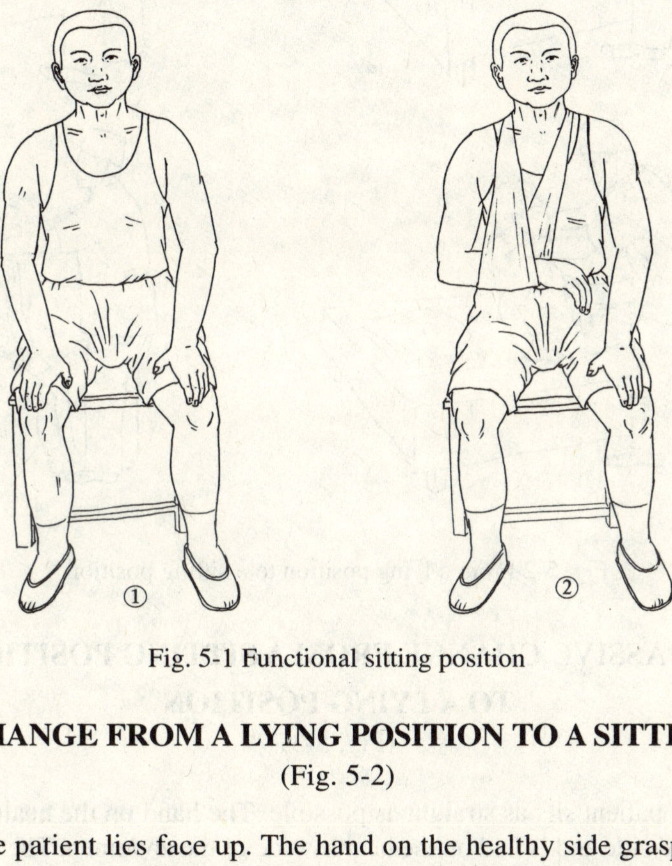

Fig. 5-1 Functional sitting position

2. PASSIVE CHANGE FROM A LYING POSITION TO A SITTING POSITION
(Fig. 5-2)

[Method] The patient lies face up. The hand on the healthy side grasps the hand on the affected side and is laid on the abdomen. The foot on the healthy side is placed beneath the foot on the affected side in a crossover position. The doctor or nurse stands on the healthy side of the patient with both hands on the patient's shoulders, turning the body slowly to the healthy side and pulling the shoulders upward. At the same time, the patient bends the elbow on the healthy side to support the body and then, with the palms resting on the bed, extends the elbow on the healthy side as the upper part of the body is being pulled up. The foot on the healthy side moves the affected lower limb to a lower place of the bed and both feet are placed evenly on the ground. Then, the patient stays in a functional posture.

[Effect] To exercise the muscles responsible for extending the shoulder and elbow joint and stretching the hip joint on the healthy side, as well as the neck, back, waist and abdominal muscles; and to prevent atrophy due to disuse. The other effects are the same as those of the functional sitting.

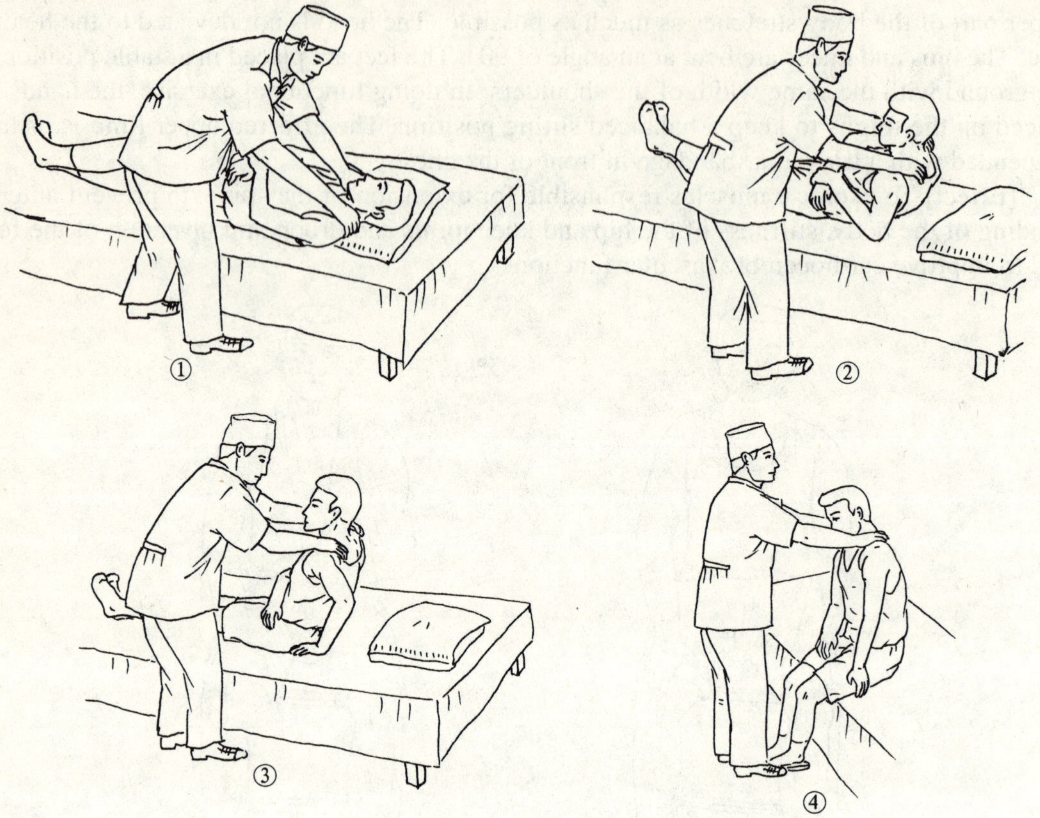

Fig. 5-2 From a lying position to a sitting position

3. PASSIVE CHANGE FROM A SITTING POSITION TO A LYING POSITION

(Fig. 5-3)

[Method] The patient sits as straight as possible. The hand on the healthy side grasps the hand on the affected side and is laid on the healthy side of the abdomen. The foot on the healthy side is placed in a position posterior to the foot on the affected side. The doctor or nurse stands before the patient and holds the patient's shoulders with both hands, slowly turning the body to the healthy side and bending the elbow on the healthy side to support it. At the same time, the foot on the healthy side leads the foot on the affected side to lift up. The doctor or nurse helps the patient to move the lower limbs to the bed with one hand, and prevents the patient's upper part of the body from leaning continuously backward with the other hand. This enables the patient to lie on the bed gradually and sequentially with his waist, back, shoulders and head. The patient then stays in a functional lying position.

[Effect] To exercise the muscles responsible for bending the shoulder and elbow joints and adducting and bending the hip joint on the healthy side, as well as the neck, back, waist and abdominal muscles; and to prevent atrophy due to disuse.

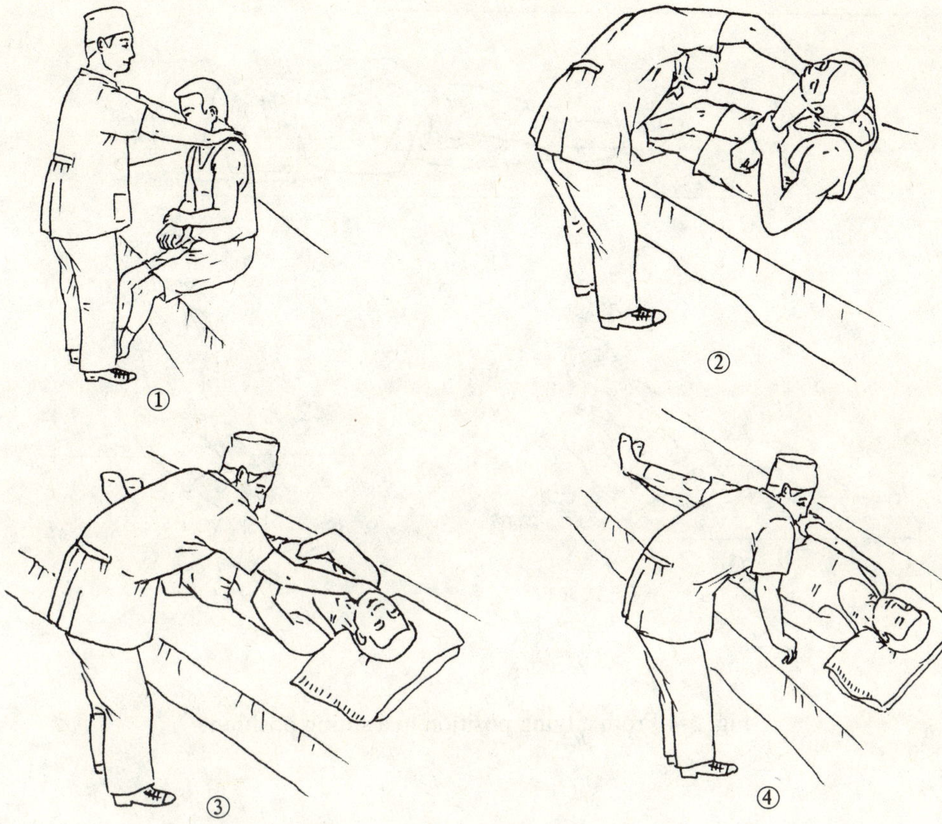

Fig. 5-3 From a sitting position to a lying position

4. ACTIVE CHANGE FROM A LYING POSITION TO A SITTING POSITION

(Fig. 5-4)

[Method] The patient lies face up. The hand on the healthy side grasps the hand on the affected side and is laid on the abdomen. The foot on the healthy side is put under the foot on the affected side in a crossover position. The former leads the lower limb on the affected side to the edge of the bed and turns toward the healthy side with the elbow on the healthy side supporting the upper part of the body. At the same time, the lower limbs continue to move out of the bed. When the lower limbs touch the ground, the patient stands up with both feet evenly on the ground. The doctor or nurse helps the patient keep a functional sitting position.

[Effect] To fully exercise the muscles responsible for extending the shoulder and elbow joints and stretching and abducting the hip joint on the healthy side as well as the neck, back, waist and abdominal muscles; to prevent atrophy from disuse; and to adjust and improve functions of the internal organs. The other effects are the same as those of the functional sitting.

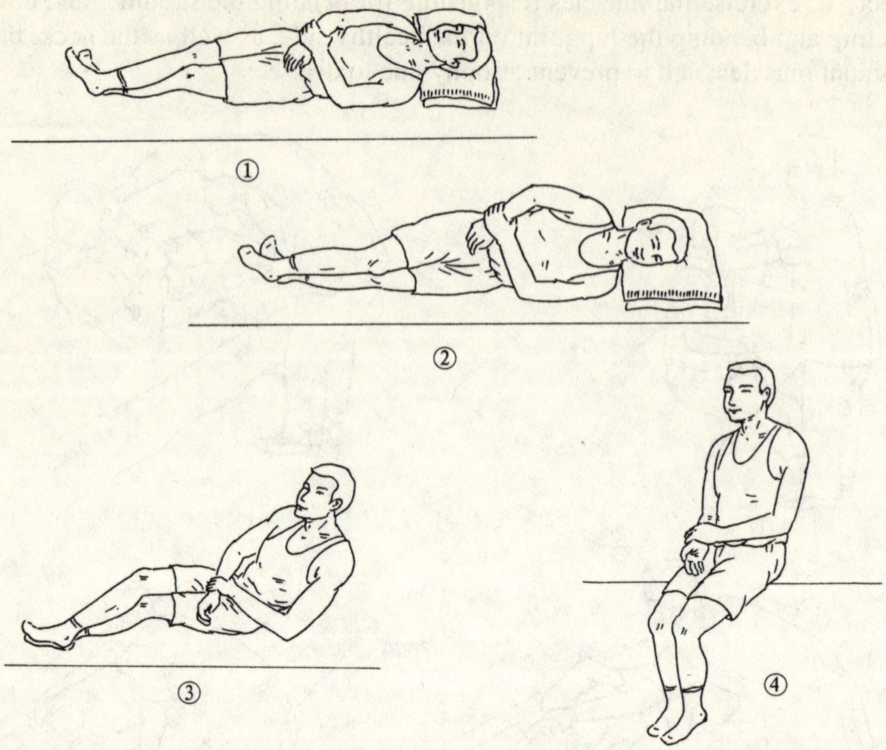

Fig. 5-4 From a lying position to a sitting position

5. ACTIVE CHANGE FROM A SITTING POSITION TO A LYING POSITION

(Fig. 5-5)

[Method] The patient sits straight with the affected hand laid on the abdomen, the healthy hand on the bed and the healthy foot put behind the affected foot in a crossover position. Then, the patient slowly bends the healthy elbow to support the upper part of the body and enable it to lean slowly toward the healthy side. At the same time, the healthy foot leads the affected lower limb to the bed. Then, the patient continues to lean backward to enable the waist, back, shoulder and head to touch the bed sequentially. The doctor or nurse helps the patient keep a functional supine position.

[Effect] To exercise the muscles responsible for bending the shoulder and elbow joint and adducting and bending the hip joint on the healthy side as well as the neck, back, waist and abdominal muscles; to prevent atrophy from disuse; and to adjust and improve functions of the heart and brain vessels.

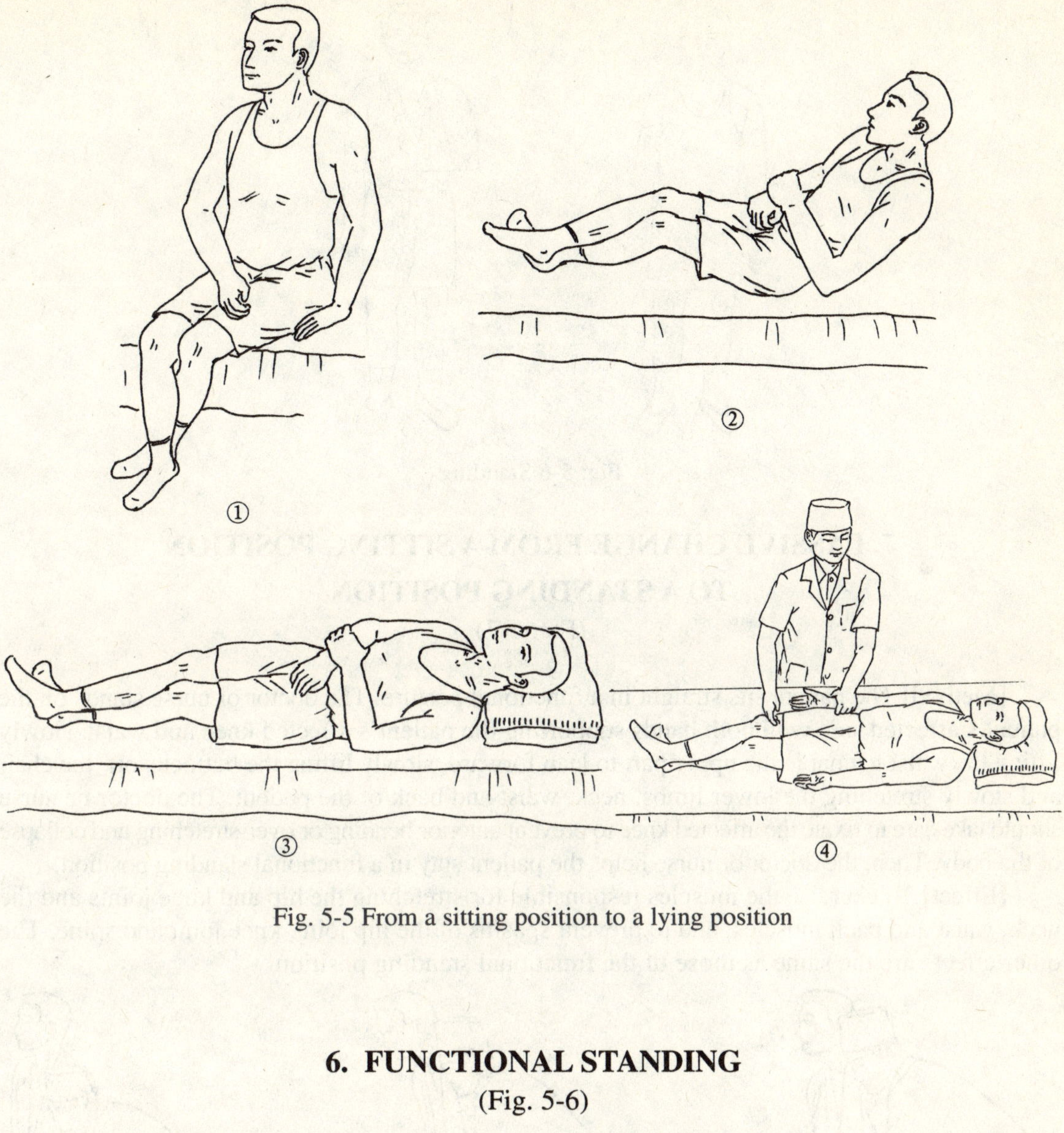

Fig. 5-5 From a sitting position to a lying position

6. FUNCTIONAL STANDING

(Fig. 5-6)

[Method] The patient keeps both feet the same width as the shoulders; the feet are placed in a stable position on the ground. This is followed by stretching of the lower limbs, waist and back. The patient slightly raises the head and stares ahead without deviating the head and neck toward the healthy side; the lower limbs support the body in a balanced way. In doing functional exercise, the upper limbs hang down in a natural manner. At ordinary times, the affected limb is suspended before the chest with a triangular towel. In the early period, the patient can stand up with the healthy hand grasping a supporter.

[Effect] To train the balancing function of the brain; to strengthen the myodynamia of the lower limbs, back and waist; to prevent atrophy from disuse, deformity of the lower limbs and foot droop and inversion; and to adjust and improve the functions of the internal organs, especially the heart and brain vessels.

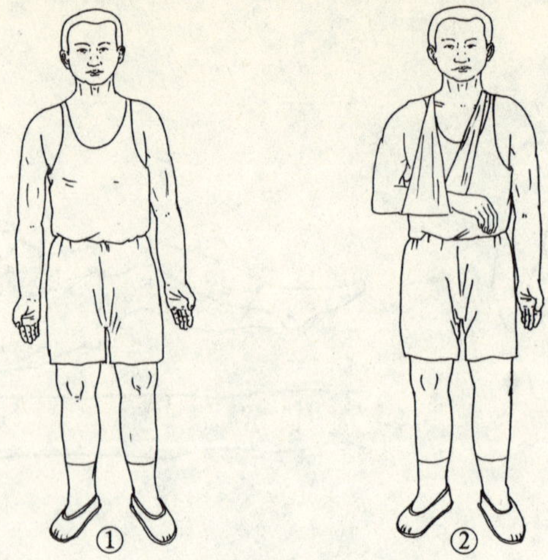

Fig. 5-6 Standing

7. PASSIVE CHANGE FROM A SITTING POSITION TO A STANDING POSITION

(Fig. 5-7)

[Method] The patient sits straight in a functional posture. The doctor or nurse stands on the patient's affected side with both hands supporting the patient's affected knee and waist, slowly lifting the waist to enable the upper part to lean forward, slowly lifting the buttocks off the chair and slowly stretching the lower limbs, neck, waist and back of the patient. The doctor or nurse should take care to fixate the affected knee to prevent anterior bending or over-stretching and collapse of the body. Then, the doctor or nurse helps the patient stay in a functional standing position.

[Effect] To exercise the muscles responsible for stretching the hip and knee joints and the neck, waist and back muscles; and to prevent spasms of the hip joint, knee joint and spine. The other effects are the same as those of the functional standing position.

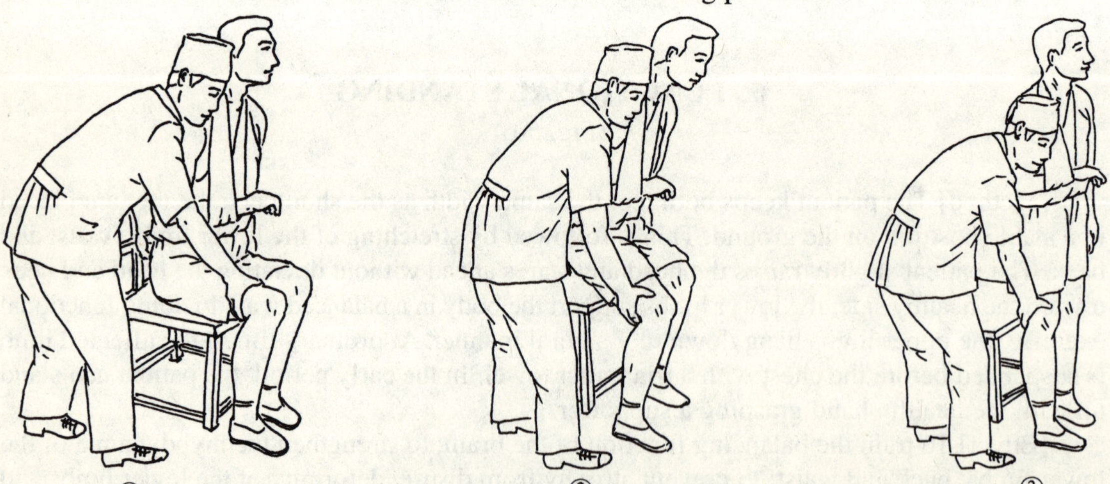

Fig. 5-7 From a sitting position to a standing position

8. PASSIVE CHANGE FROM A STANDING POSITION TO A SITTING POSITION

(Fig. 5-8)

[Method] The patient stands in a stable position in a functional posture. The doctor or nurse stands on the affected side of the patient and holds the affected knee and waist with both hands. The patient slowly bends the head and the waist, leaning the upper part of the body forward, slowly bending the hip and knee, shifting the body in a posterior direction and slowly sitting down. The doctor or nurse helps the patient to remain in a functional sitting position.

[Effect] To exercise the muscles responsible for bending the hip and knee joints and the waist muscles and to improve the functions of the joints on the lower limbs. The other effects are the same as those of the functional sitting position.

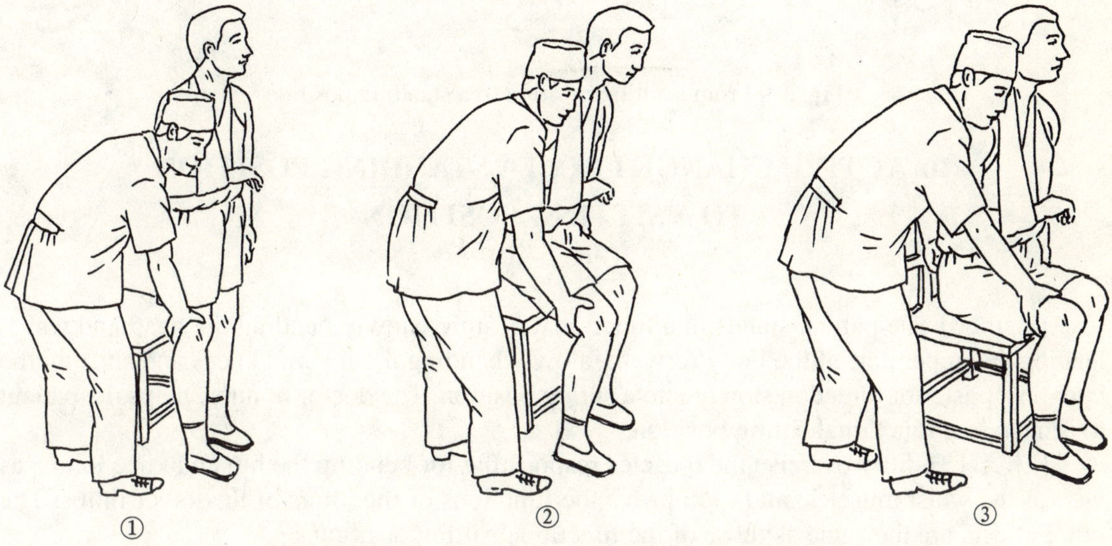

Fig. 5-8 From a standing position to a sitting position

9. ACTIVE CHANGE FROM A SITTING POSITION TO A STANDING POSITION

(Fig. 5-9)

[Method] The patient sits straight in a functional posture. The affected upper limb is suspended before the chest, keeping it from deviating medially and laterally. The patient bends the head and waist, leaning the upper part of the body forward and lifting the buttocks off the chair, stretching as hard as possible the hip and knee, raising the head, and slowly straightening the waist into a standing position. The doctor or nurse helps the patient to remain in a functional standing position.

[Effect] To fully exercise the muscles responsible for extending the hip and knee joints as well as the neck, waist, back and abdominal muscles; and to prevent stiffness and spasms of the joints of the lower limbs.

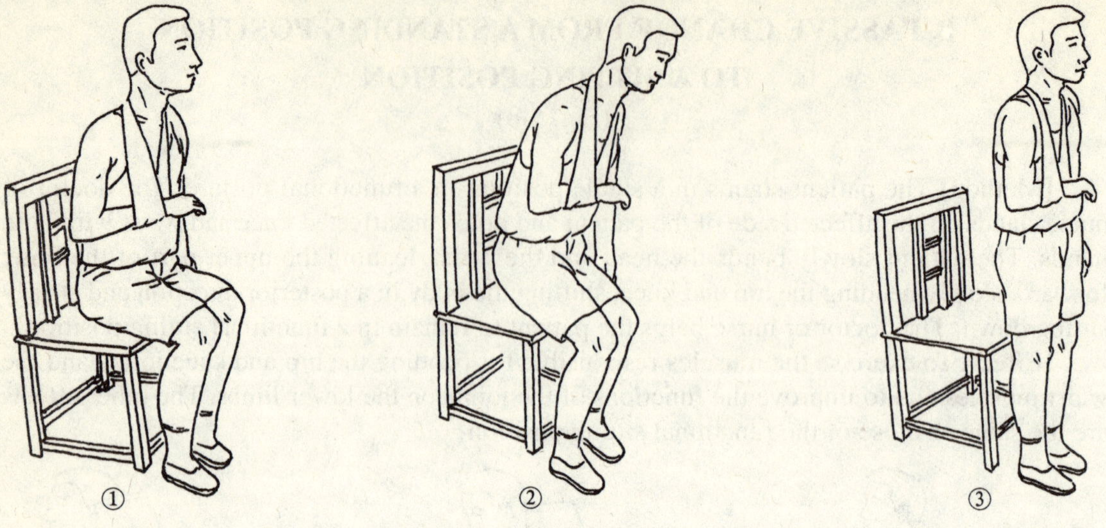

Fig. 5-9 From a sitting position to a standing position

10. ACTIVE CHANGE FROM A STANDING POSITION TO A SITTING POSITION

(Fig. 5-10)

[Method] The patient stands in a functional posture, slowly bending the head and waist, leaning the upper part of the body forward, slowly bending the hip and knees and shifting the body in a posterior direction slowly into a sitting position. The doctor or nurse helps the patient to remain in a functional sitting position.

[Effect] To fully exercise the muscles responsible for bending the hip and knee joints, as well as the waist muscles; and to improve the functions of the joints of the lower limbs. The other effects are the same as those of the functional sitting position.

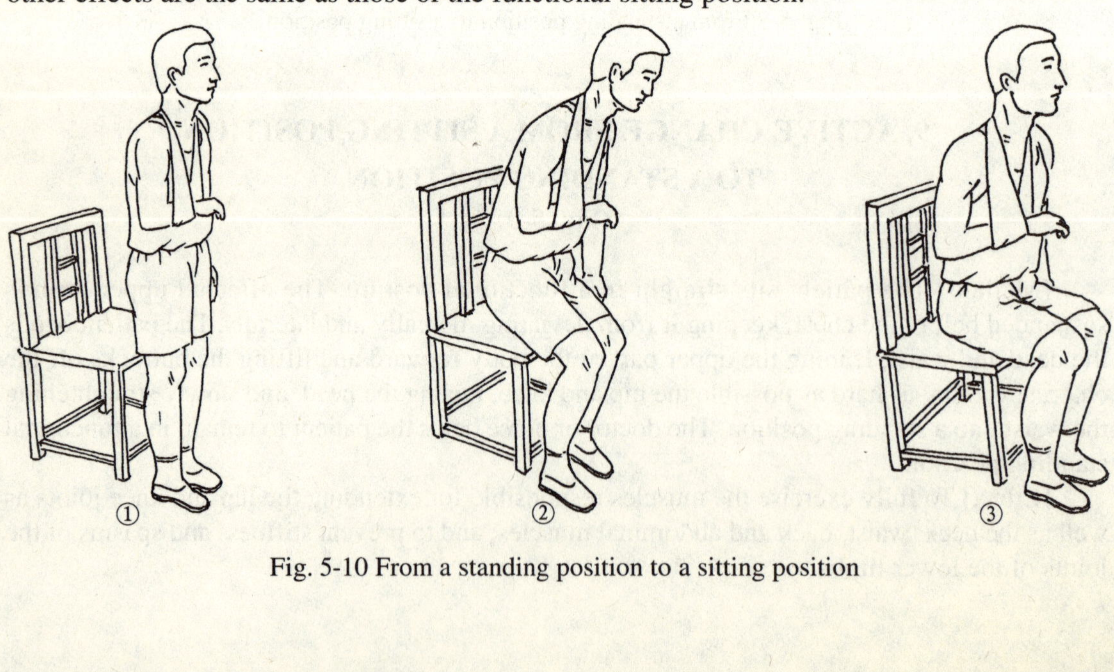

Fig. 5-10 From a standing position to a sitting position

11. FUNCTIONAL WALKING

(Fig. 5-11)

[Method] The patient suspends the affected upper limb with a triangular towel before the chest; the center of the body is shifted to the healthy side, raising the head, stretching the waist, bending the affected hip and knee, lifting the foot, dorsally bending the ankle joint as much as possible, taking a small step forward, stretching the hip and knee with the sole in a stable position put on the ground, swinging the healthy arm forward and shifting the center of the body to the affected side. With the same method, the healthy lower limb takes a big step forward. The center of the body is shifted to the healthy side and the affected lower limb is swung forward parallel to the healthy lower limb. The affected lower limb takes another small step forward with the repetition of the methods above to walk straight forward while maintaining balance.

[Effect] To fully exercise the muscles responsible for bending the hip, knee and ankle joints, and improve the physiological functions of the brain, especially the balance and directional functions.

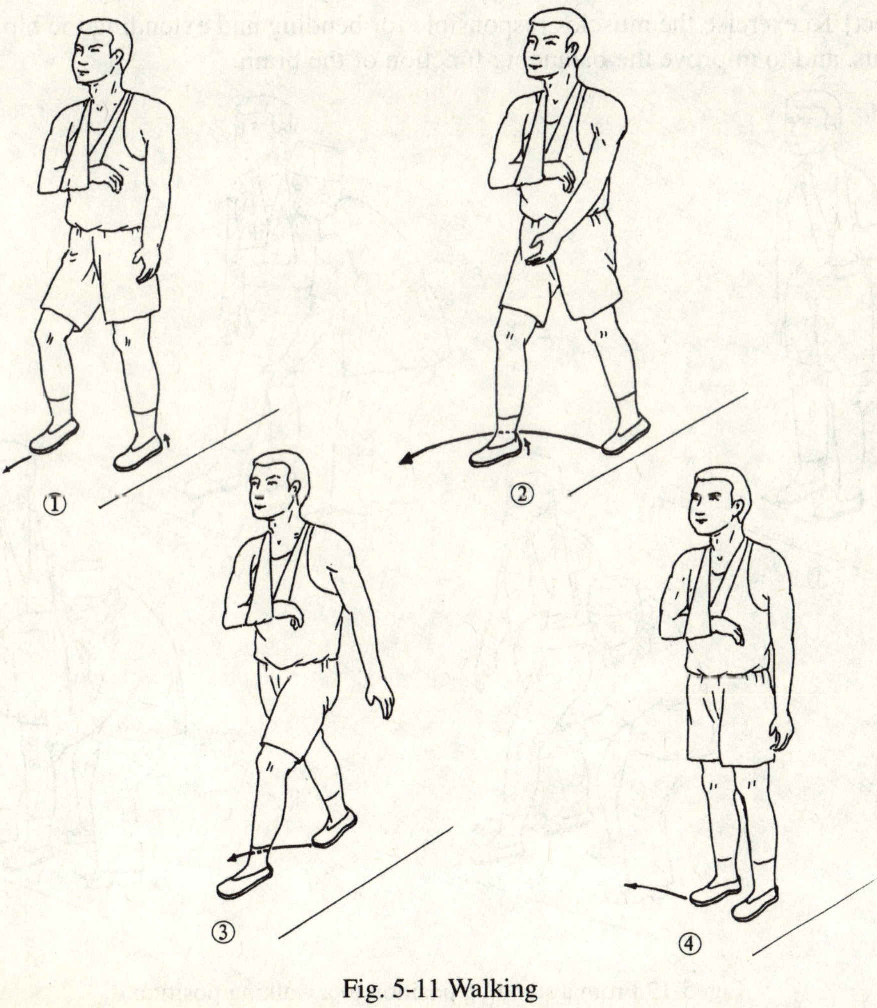

Fig. 5-11 Walking

12. PASSIVE CHANGE FROM A STANDING POSITION TO A WALKING POSITION

(Fig. 5-12)

[Method] The patient stands in a functional posture with the affected upper limb suspended before the chest and the center of the body shifted to the healthy side. The doctor or nurse stands by the patient's affected side with both hands holding the knee and waist on the affected side to help the patient slowly bend the affected hip and knee, lift the foot and dorsally bend the ankle joint as much as possible. The patient then slowly takes a step forward, extends the hip and knee with the sole in a stable position on the ground. At the same time, the healthy arm is swung forward and the center of the body is shifted toward the affected side. Then, the healthy lower limb takes two small steps forward to keep parallel to the affected lower limb. The doctor or nurse should take measures to fixate the affected knee to prevent it from anterior bending or over-stretching and leaning to the affected side. The patient then walks in a stable manner forward, with the repetition of "affected side, healthy side, healthy side; affected side, healthy side, healthy side…"

[Effect] To exercise the muscles responsible for bending and extending the hip, knee and ankle joints, and to improve the balancing function of the brain.

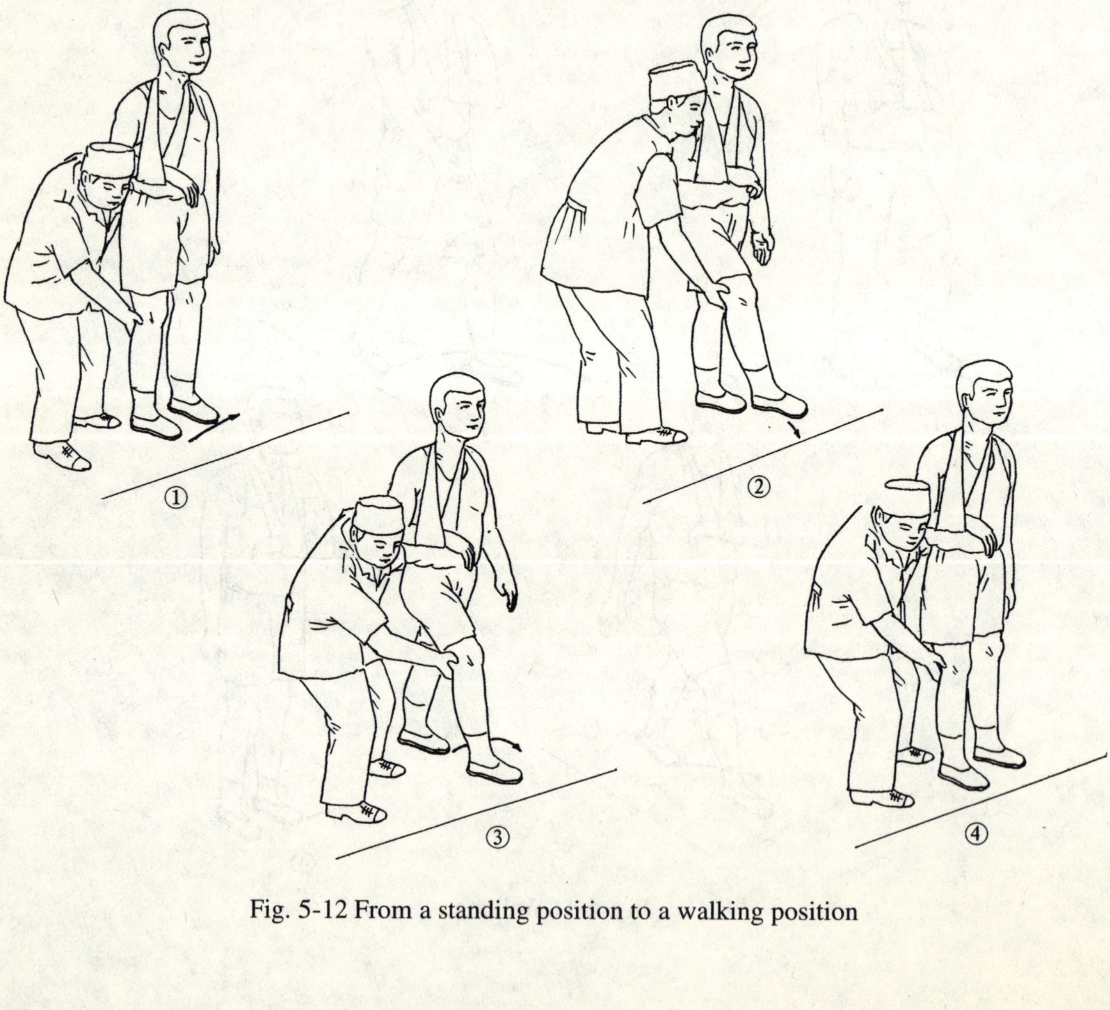

Fig. 5-12 From a standing position to a walking position

13. ACTIVE CHANGE FROM A STANDING POSITION TO A WALKING POSITION

(Fig. 5-13)

[Method] The patient stands in a functional posture with the affected upper limb suspended before the chest. At the beginning, the patient holds a fixated transverse pole with the healthy hand and walks forward with the affected limb in the fashion mentioned above (see the section on functional walking). Gradually the patient walks alone without support of the pole. The doctor or nurse should walk by the affected side to take care of the patient.

[Effect] To fully exercise the muscles responsible for bending and extending the hip, knee and ankle joints; and to adjust and improve physiological functions, especially the balance and directional functions of the brain.

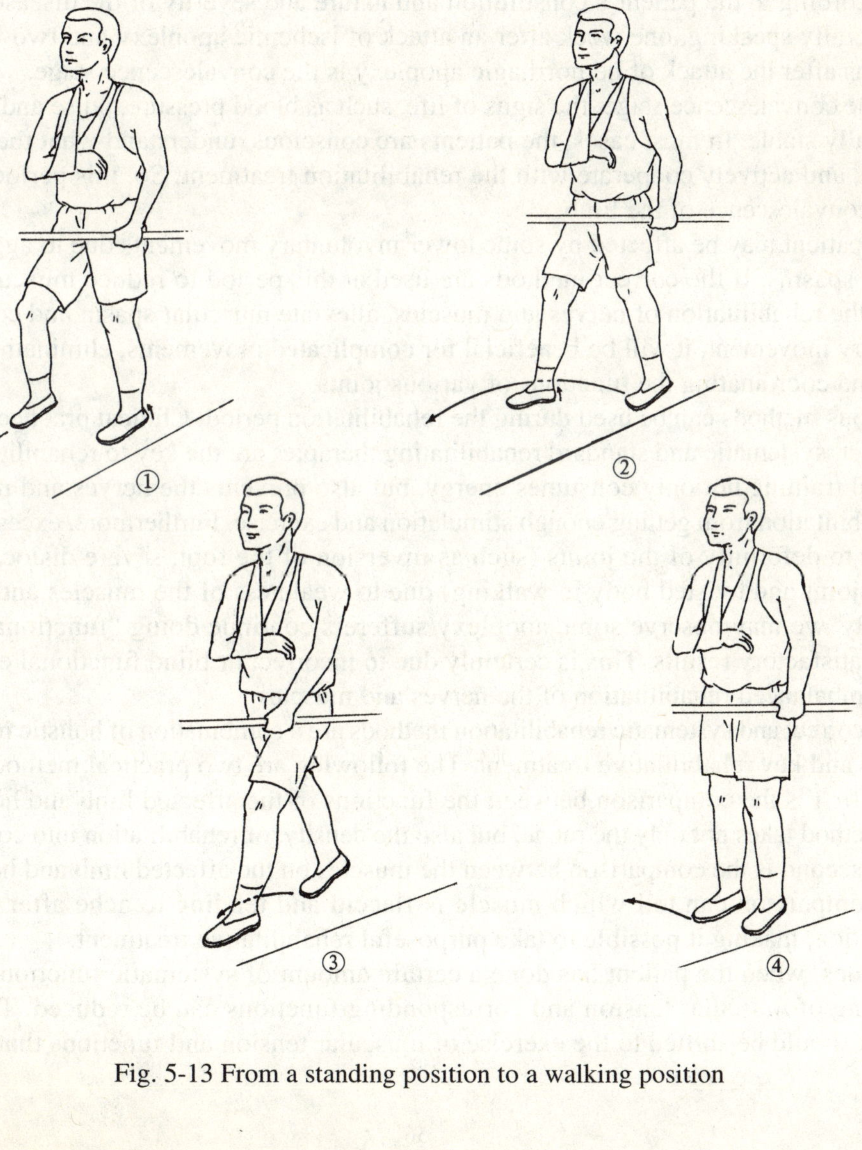

Fig. 5-13 From a standing position to a walking position

Chapter 6
ILLUSTRATED REHABILITATIVE TECHNIQUES AT THE CONVALESCENCE STAGE

The time needed to progress from apoplexy in the acute stage to the convalescence stage varies according to the patient's constitution and nature and severity of the disease.

Generally speaking, one week after an attack of ischemic apoplexy and two weeks up to six months after the attack of hemorrhagic apoplexy is the convalescence stage.

At the convalescence stage, the signs of life, such as blood pressure, pulse and respiration, are basically stable. In most cases, the patients are conscious, understand what the doctor and nurse say, and actively cooperate with the rehabilitation treatment. So, this period is the best time for convalescence of the limbs.

The patient may be affected by some lower involuntary movements due to aggravation of muscular spasms. If the correct methods are used at this period to reduce muscular tension, promote the rehabilitation of nerves and muscles, alleviate muscular spasm and control lower involuntary movement, it will be beneficial for complicated movements, eliminating muscular spasms and coordinating the functions of various joints.

Various methods can be used during the rehabilitation period. Clinical practice has proved that correct, systematic and standard rehabilitating therapies are the key to rehabilitation. Blind functional training not only consumes energy, but also prevents the nerves and muscles that need rehabilitation from getting enough stimulation and exercise. Furthermore, excessive pulling may lead to deformity of the joints (such as inversion of the foot, severe dislocation of the shoulder joint and twisted body in walking) due to weakness of the muscles and ligaments. Frequently, we may observe some apoplexy sufferers continue doing "functional exercise" without satisfactory results. This is certainly due to incorrect or blind functional exercise that leads to imbalanced rehabilitation of the nerves and muscles.

The correct and systematic rehabilitation methods are a combination of holistic rehabilitative treatment and key rehabilitative treatment. The following are two practical methods.

The first is the comparison between the functions of the affected limb and healthy limb. Such a method takes not only the range, but also the density, of rehabilitation into consideration.

The second is the comparison between the muscles on the affected limb and healthy limb. Such a comparison can tell which muscle is flaccid and tending to ache after a period of rehabilitation, making it possible to take purposeful rehabilitative treatment.

Besides, when the patient has done a certain amount of systematic functional exercise, the training of muscular tension and corresponding functions can be reduced. The focus of treatment should be shifted to the exercise of muscular tension and functions that are not yet restored.

1. PASSIVE FUNCTIONAL EXERCISE DONE BY THE PATIENTS THEMSELVES

Passive functional exercise means that the patient helps the affected limb move with the healthy limb. Such an exercise is applicable to patients with 1-2 grades of muscular tension of the affected limb. This kind of exercise will not only fully exercise the muscles on the affected side, but also prevent atrophy from disuse, promote blood circulation throughout the body, and adjust and improve visceral functions on the healthy side.

The following points should be noted in doing passive exercise:

a. The doctor or nurse should help the patient to do exercise that is difficult for him or her to do alone.

b. The patient should be gentle and rhythmic in doing exercise, avoiding making rough actions and overstraining. The movement in exercise should be limited to half of the normal range at the beginning. It can be gradually enlarged without producing any pain.

c. The patient may repeat the exercise 5-20 times twice a day according to his or her constitution. There should be an interval of rest between the two actions.

d. The density of movement can be monitored to the degree that there is no fatigue the next day. The frequency of each action can be modified at random but it should not be stopped.

e. Each time, the affected limb should do muscular contraction as much as possible. This is beneficial to activation of the nerve metabolism, promotion of formation of the nerve passage and increase of muscular tension.

(1) Upper limbs (lying position)

1) Anterior bending and upward lifting of the shoulder joint (Fig. 6-1)

[Method] The patient lies in a supine position in a functional posture with the healthy hand grasping the wrist of the affected hand to turn the palm upwards and extend the elbow. The patient inhales and slowly bends in an anterior direction and lifts the affected shoulder toward the head. After a 3-5 seconds interval, the patient exhales and slowly lowers the hand. Such a movement is repeated 5-10 times and then the patient returns to the normal position again.

[Effect] To exercise the muscles responsible for bending and extending the shoulder, and to prevent adhesion of the shoulder joint and spasm of the elbow point.

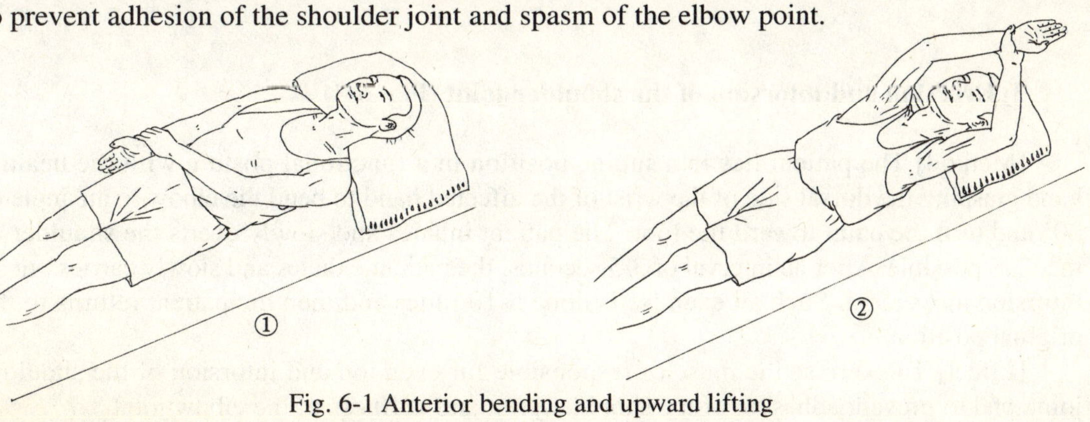

Fig. 6-1 Anterior bending and upward lifting

2) Abducting and adducting the shoulder joint (Fig. 6-2)

[Method] The patient lies in a supine position in a functional posture with the healthy hand grasping the wrist of the affected hand to turn the palm upward and extend the elbow. The patient inhales and slowly abducts the affected shoulder as much as possible. After an interval of 3-5 seconds, the patient exhales and slowly adducts. Such a movement is repeated 5-10 times and then the patient returns to the original position.

[Effect] To exercise the muscles responsible for abduction and adduction of the shoulder joint, and to prevent semiluxation of the shoulder joint and spasm of the elbow joint.

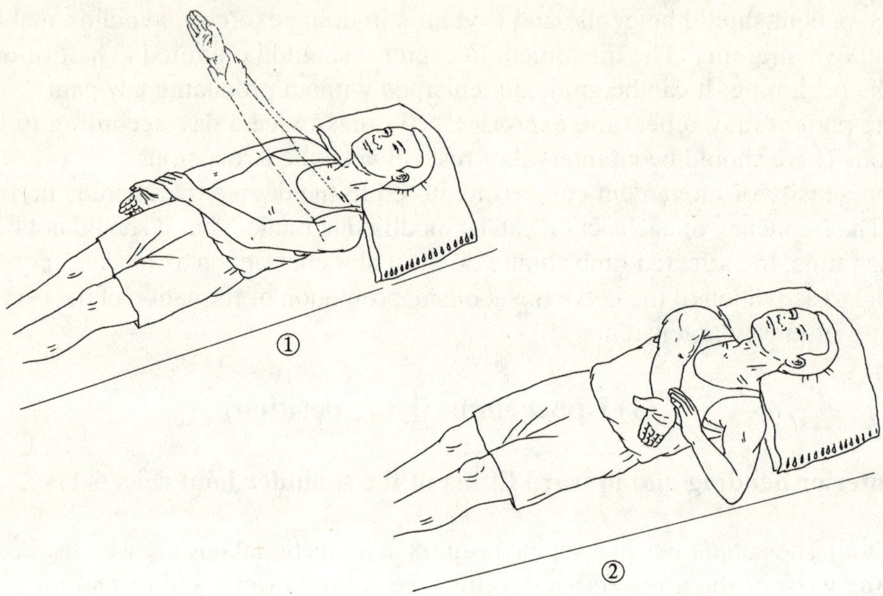

Fig. 6-2 Abduction and adduction

3) Eversion and intorsion of the shoulder joint (Fig. 6-3)

[Method] The patient lies in a supine position in a functional posture with the healthy hand grasping the dorsal side of the wrist of the affected hand to bend the elbow to an angle of 90° and turn the palm toward the foot. The patient inhales and slowly everts the shoulder as much as possible. After an interval of 3-5 seconds, the patient exhales and slowly carries out an intorsion movement. Such an exercise is done 5-10 times and then the patient returns to the original position.

[Effect] To exercise the muscles responsible for eversion and intorsion of the shoulder joint, and to prevent adhesion of the shoulder joint and stiffness of the elbow joint.

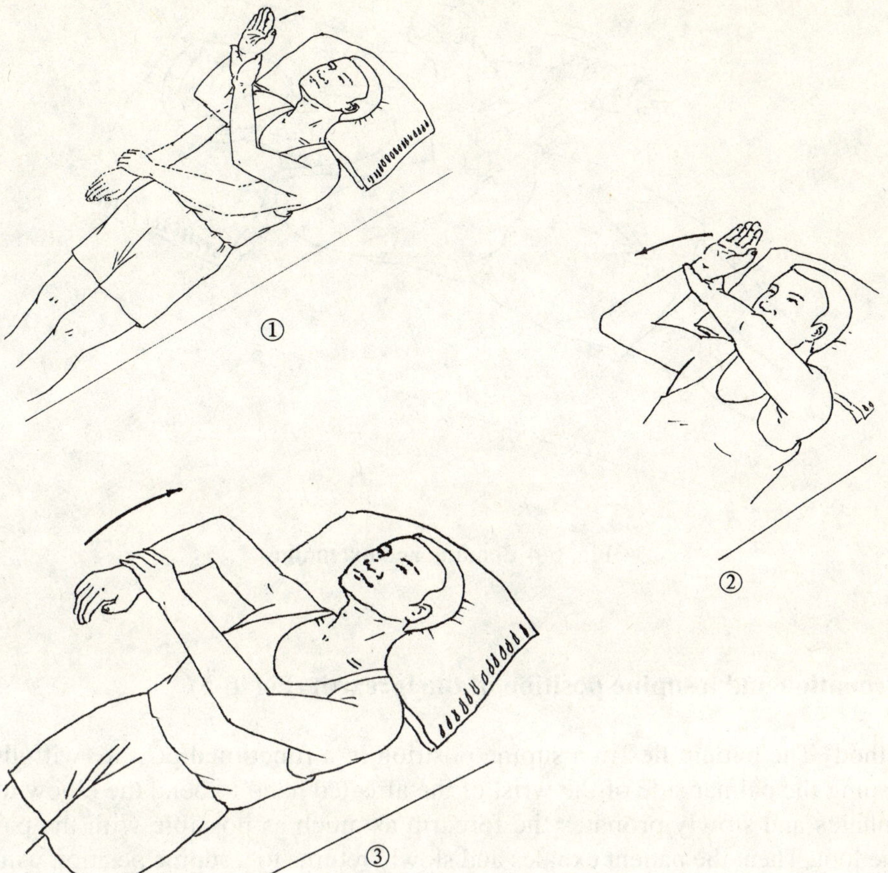

Fig. 6-3 Eversion and intorsion

4) Bending and extending the elbow joint (Fig. 6-4)

[Method] The patient lies in a supine position in a functional posture with the healthy hand grasping the palmar side of the wrist of the affected hand. The patient inhales and slowly extends the elbow as much as possible to turn the palm upward and bend the shoulder. The patient then exhales and slowly does bending movement with the palm turned toward the foot and the shoulder extended. Such an exercise is done 5-15 times and then the patient returns to the original position.

[Effect] To exercise the muscles responsible for bending and extending the elbow and shoulder joints as well as the muscles responsible for pronation and a supine position of the forearm; to separate the bending and extending movement of the elbow and forearm to reduce spasm of the elbow; and to prevent adhesion of the shoulder joint.

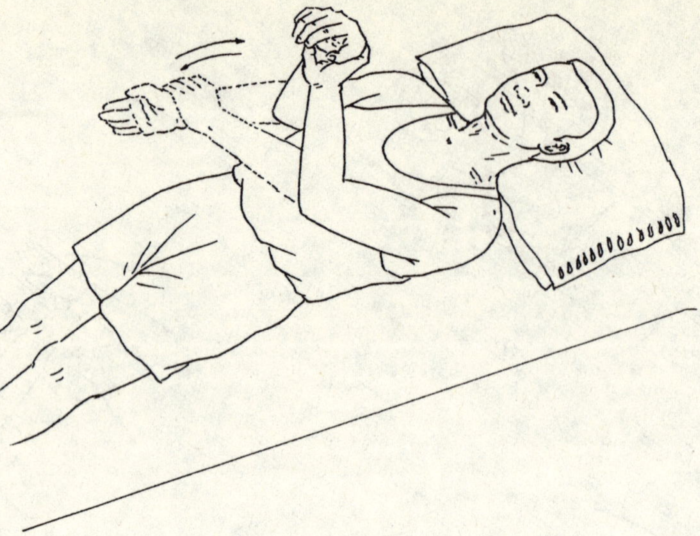

Fig. 6-4 Bending and extending

5) Pronation and a supine position of the forearm (Fig. 6-5)

[Method] The patient lies in a supine position in a functional posture with the healthy hand grasping the palmar side of the wrist of the affected hand to bend the elbow to 90°. The patient inhales and slowly pronates the forearm as much as possible with the palm turned toward the foot. Then, the patient exhales and slowly returns to a supine position with the palm turned to the head. Such an exercise is done 5-20 times and then the patient returns to the original position. In the whole course of exercise, the wrist is slightly bent dorsally.

[Effect] To exercise the muscles responsible for pronation and a supine position of the forearm, and to prevent spasm of the forearm and droop of the wrist.

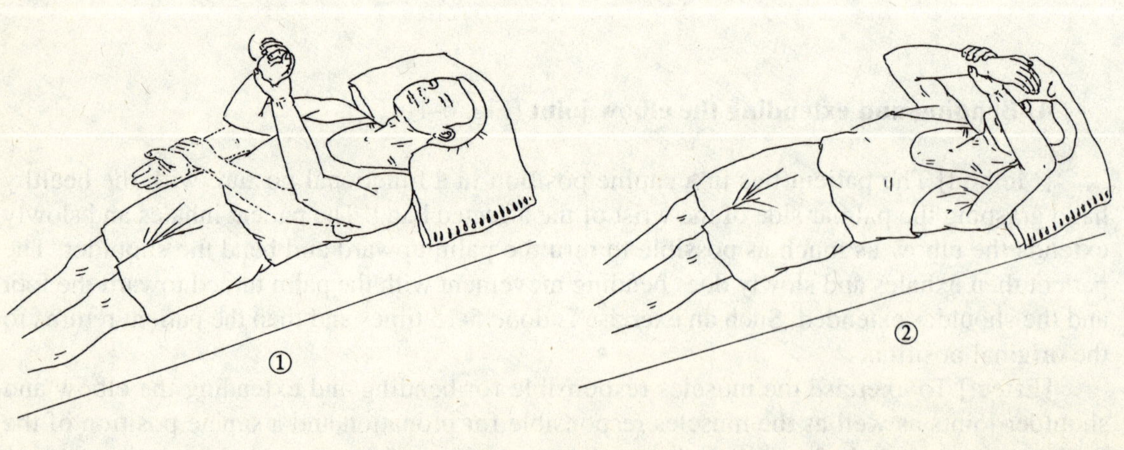

Fig. 6-5 Pronation and a supine position

6) Dorsal and palmar bending of the wrist joint (Fig. 6-6)

[Method] The patient lies in a supine position in a functional posture with the healthy hand grasping the dorsum of the affected hand and the elbow bent to 90o. The patient inhales and slowly extends the wrist with the palm turned upward, the fingers bent and the dorsum of the fingers turned toward the foot. Then, the patient exhales and slowly bends the palm downward and the fingers toward the foot. Such an exercise is done 5-15 times and then the patient returns to the original position.

[Effect] To exercise the muscles responsible for extending and bending the wrist and finger joints as well as pronation and a supine position of the forearm; to separate the bending and extending movements of the forearm and the wrist as well as the wrist and the fingers in order to reduce spasms.

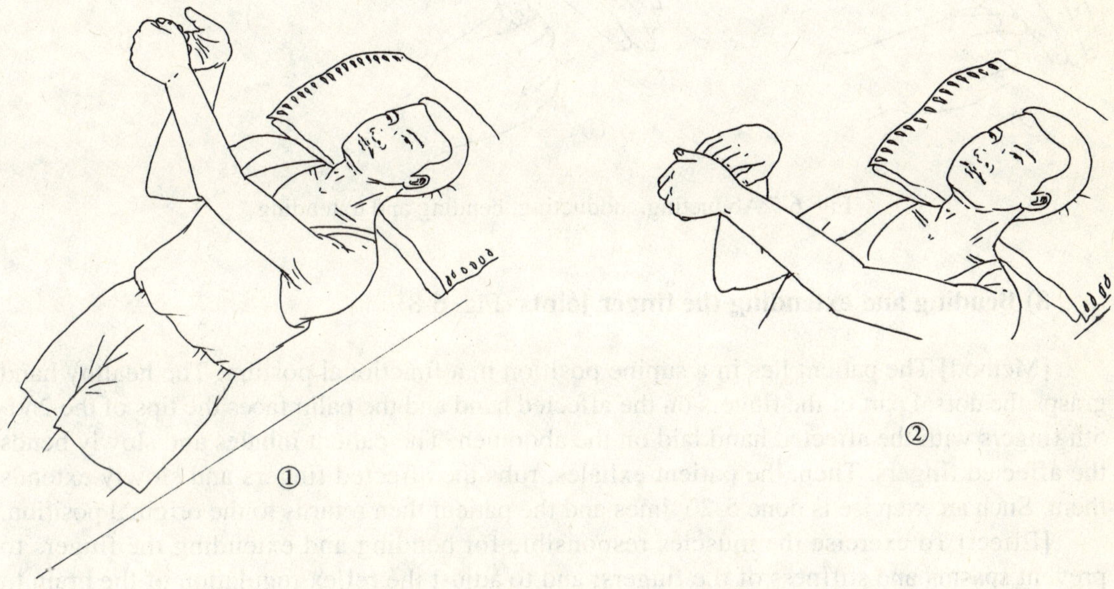

Fig. 6-6 Dorsal and palmar bending

7) Abducting, adducting, bending and extending the thumb joint (Fig. 6-7)

[Method] The patient lies in a supine position in a functional posture with the thumb and index finger of the healthy hand holding the end of the thumb on the affected hand. The hand is put on the abdomen. The patient inhales and slowly abducts and adducts the thumb on the affected hand. Then, the patient exhales and slowly bends and extends the thumb. Such a movement is done 5-20 times and then the patient returns to the original position.

[Effect] To exercise the muscles responsible for abduction, adduction, bending and extending of the thumb to prevent spasm and flaccidity of the thumb; and to adjust reflex regulation of the brain to promote restoration of the functions of the fingers.

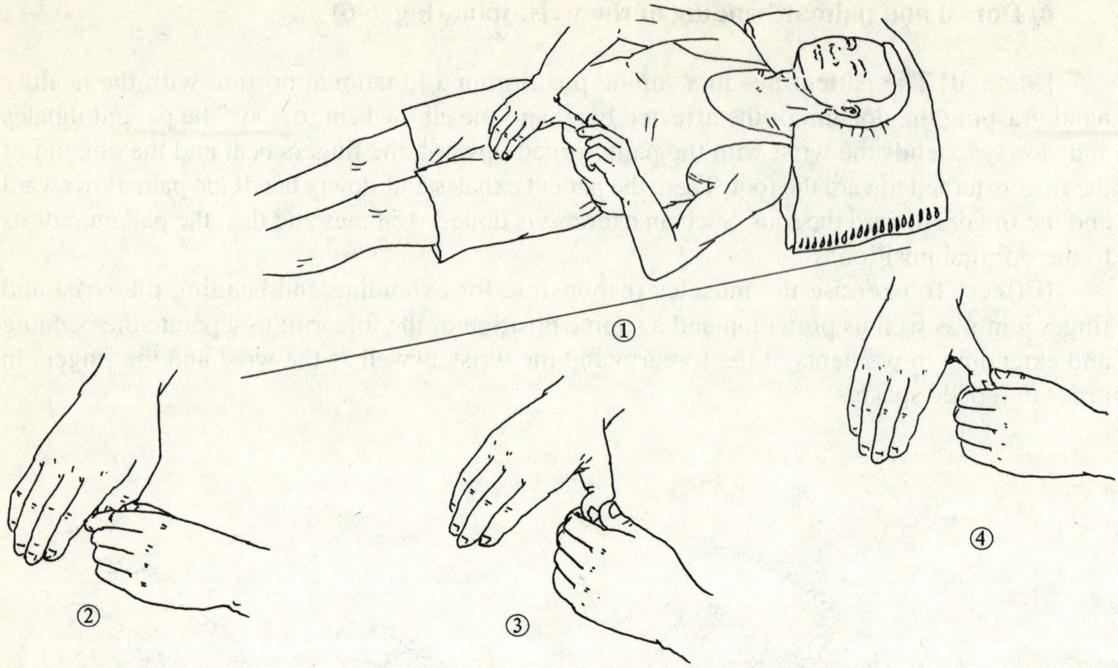

Fig. 6-7 Abducting, adducting, bending and extending

8) Bending and extending the finger joints (Fig. 6-8)

[Method] The patient lies in a supine position in a functional posture. The healthy hand grasps the dorsal part of the fingers on the affected hand and the palm faces the tips of the 2nd-5th fingers with the affected hand laid on the abdomen. The patient inhales and slowly bends the affected fingers. Then, the patient exhales, rubs the affected fingers and slowly extends them. Such an exercise is done 5-20 times and the patient then returns to the original position.

[Effect] To exercise the muscles responsible for bending and extending the fingers to prevent spasms and stiffness of the fingers; and to adjust the reflex regulation of the brain to promote restoration of finger functions.

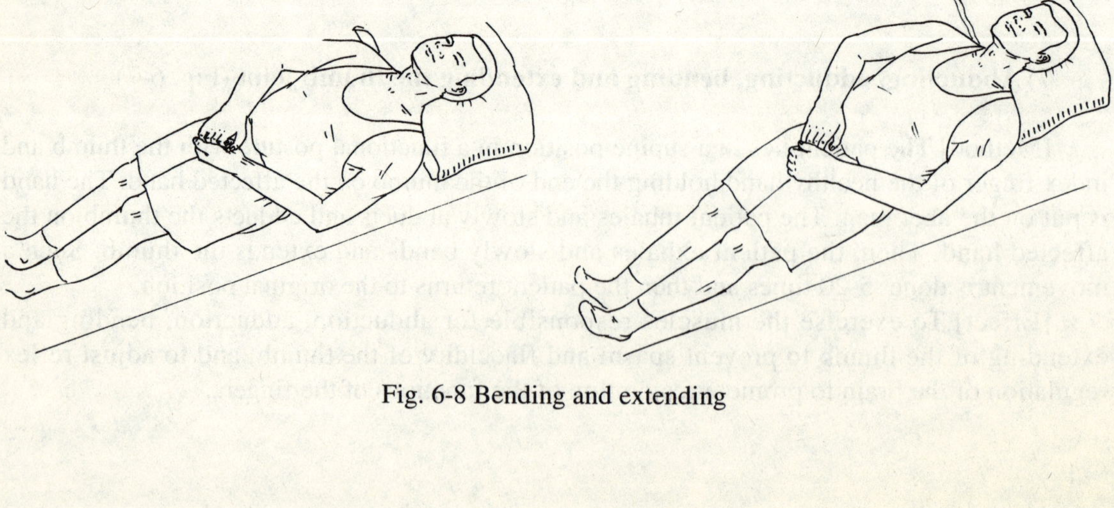

Fig. 6-8 Bending and extending

(2) Lower limbs (lying position)

1) Bending and extending the hip joint (Fig. 6-9)

[Method] The patient lies in a supine position in a functional posture. The dorsum of the healthy foot is put behind the heel of the affected foot and the knee on the affected side is extended. The patient inhales and slowly bends the hip joint. Then, the patient exhales and slowly lowers the hip. Such an exercise is done 5-10 times and then the patient returns to the original position.

[Effect] To exercise the muscles responsible for bending and extending the hip joint and waist and abdominal muscles, and to prevent stiffness of the hip joint.

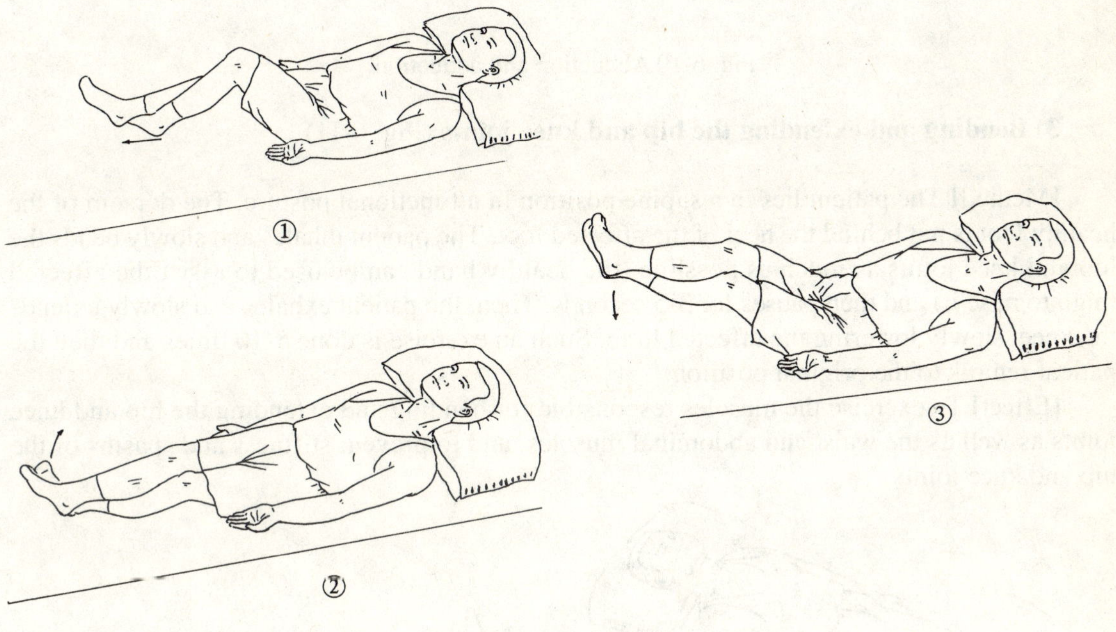

Fig. 6-9 Bending and extending

2) Abducting and adducting the hip joint (Fig. 6-10)

[Method] The patient lies in a supine position in a functional posture. The dorsum of the healthy foot is put behind the heel of the affected foot with the lower limbs slightly raised. The patient inhales and slowly abducts the hip joint. Then, the patient exhales and slowly adducts the hip joint. Such an exercise is done 5-10 times and then the patient returns to the original position.

[Effect] To exercise the muscles responsible for bending and extending the hip joint and prevent looseness of the hip joint.

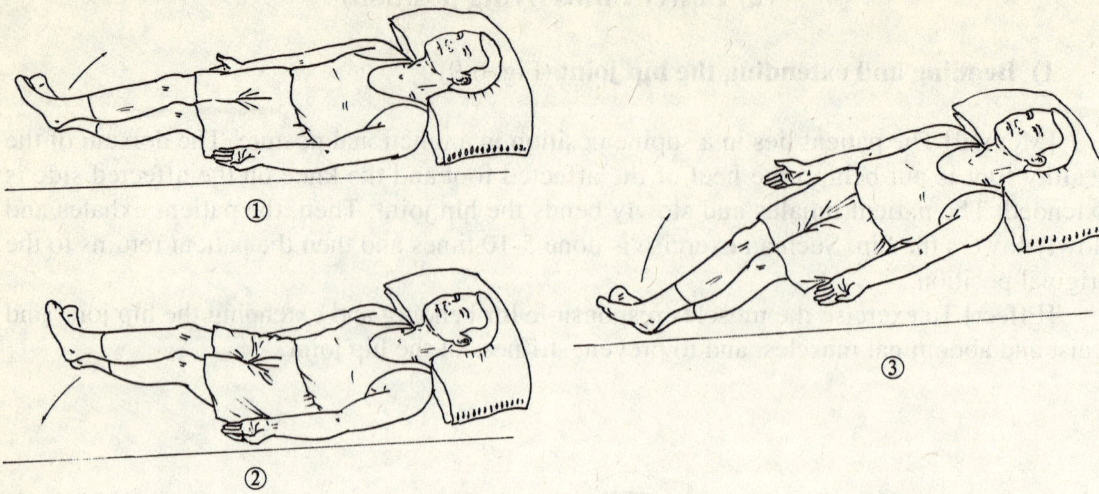

Fig. 6-10 Abduction and adduction

3) Bending and extending the hip and knee joints (Fig. 6-11)

[Method] The patient lies in a supine position in a functional posture. The dorsum of the healthy foot is put behind the heel of the affected foot. The patient inhales and slowly bends the hip and knee joints as much as possible (the healthy hand can be used to assist the affected thigh to raise it) and then pauses for 3-5 seconds. Then, the patient exhales and slowly extends the knee, slowly lowering the affected limb. Such an exercise is done 5-10 times and then the patient returns to the original position.

[Effect] To exercise the muscles responsible for bending and extending the hip and knee joints as well as the waist and abdominal muscles, and to prevent stiffness and spasms of the hip and knee joints.

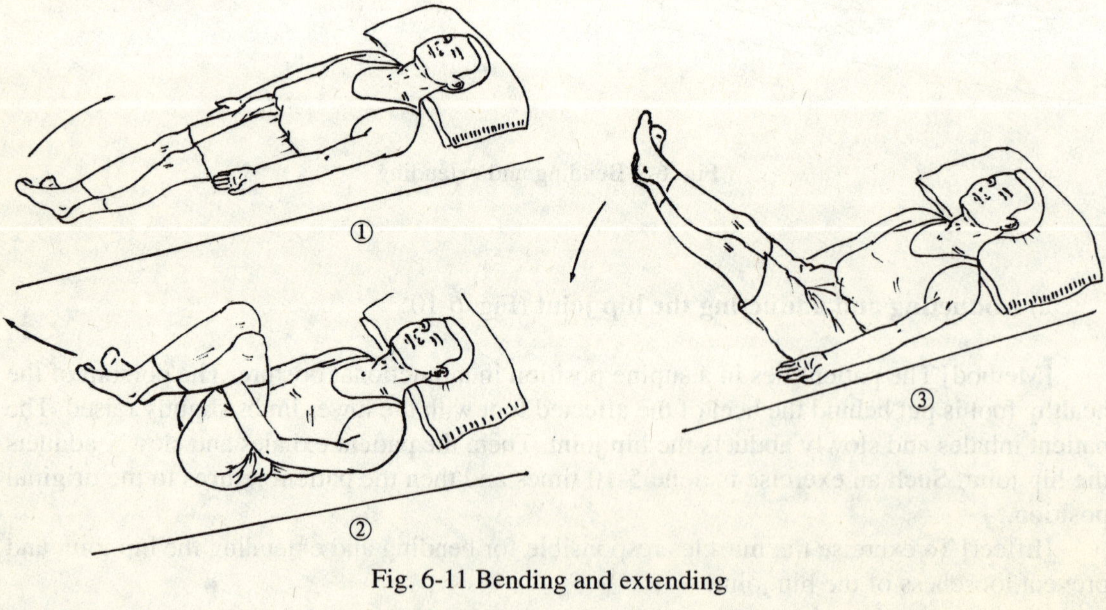

Fig. 6-11 Bending and extending

4) Dorsal bending and extroversion of the ankle (Fig. 6-12)

[Method] The patient lies in a supine position in a functional posture. The dorsum of the healthy foot is put lateral to the heel of the affected foot. The anterior part of the dorsum of the healthy foot is put at the anterior part of the sole of the affected foot in a crossover state. The patient inhales, slowly bends dorsally and turns the ankle joint on the affected limb in an external direction as hard as possible, followed by a break of 3-5 seconds. After that, the patient exhales and returns to 0°. Such an exercise is done 5-20 times and then the patient returns to the original position.

[Effect] To exercise the muscles responsible for dorsal bending and external rotation of the ankle joint and to prevent strephenopodia.

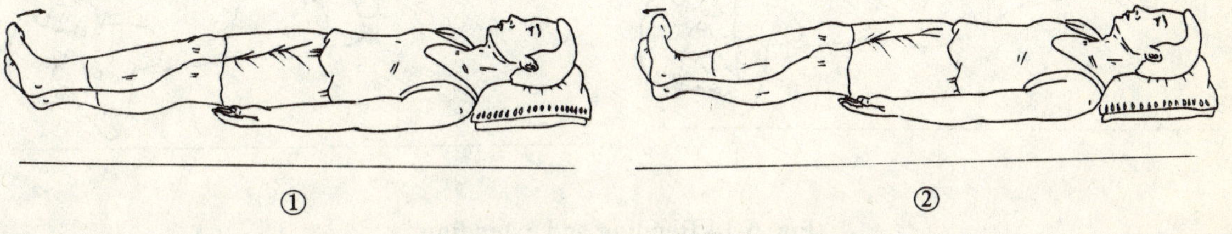

Fig. 6-12 Dorsal bending and extroversion

5) Sit-ups (Fig. 6-13)

[Method] The patient lies in a supine position in a functional posture with both lower limbs naturally extended and the healthy hand grasping one end of the rope tied around the other side of the bed. The patient inhales and slowly pulls the rope as hard as possible to enable the upper part of the body to lift up from the bed as much as possible. Then the patient exhales and slowly lies down. Such an exercise is done 5-10 times.

[Effect] To exercise the muscles responsible for bending and extending the hip joints and spine; to prevent deformity of the spine; and to improve the functions of the heart and lungs.

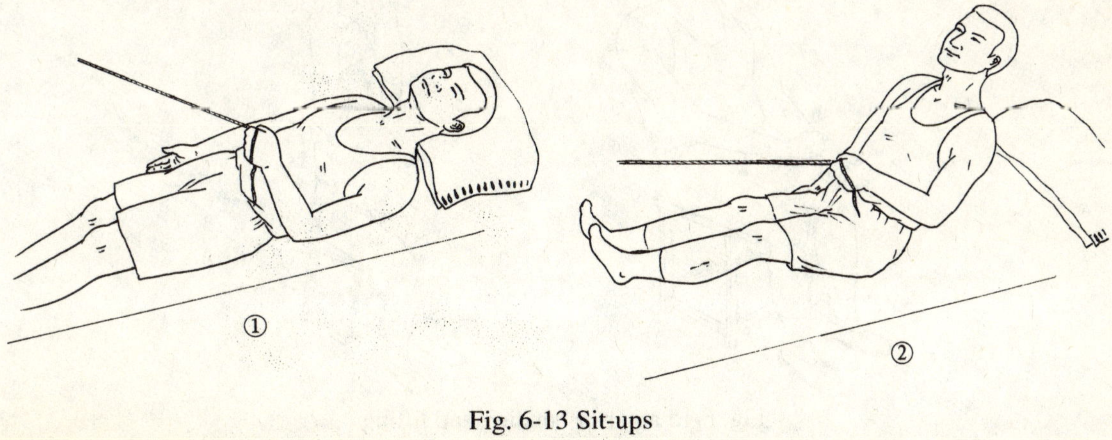

Fig. 6-13 Sit-ups

6) Bending and extending the knee joint (Fig. 6-14)

[Method] The patient lies prostrate in a functional posture. The heel of the healthy foot is put behind the dorsam of the affected foot. The patient inhales and slowly bends the knee joint as hard as possible (the buttocks should not be raised up). After a break of 3-5 seconds, the patient exhales and slowly extends the knee joint. Such an exercise is done 5-20 times.

[Effect] To exercise the muscles responsible for bending and extending the knee joint; to separate the common bending and extending activity of the hip and knee joints; and to reduce spasm of the hip and knee joints.

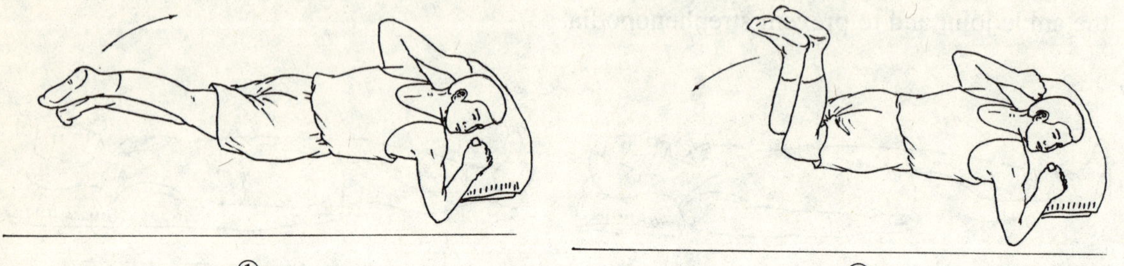

①　　②

Fig. 6-14 Bending and extending

(3) Upper limbs (sitting position)

1) Anterior bending and lifting of the shoulder joint (Fig. 6-15)

[Method] The patient sits as straight as possible in a functional posture. The healthy hand grasps the wrist of the affected hand to turn the palm upward and extend the elbow. The patient inhales, slowly bends in an anterior way and raises the shoulder above the head as hard as

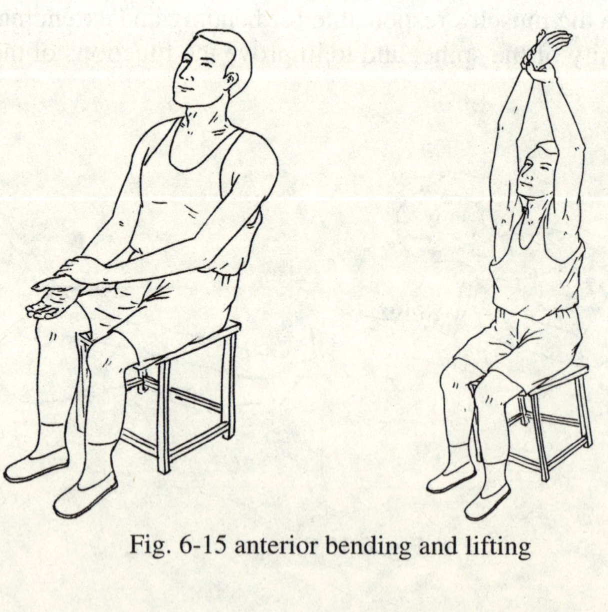

Fig. 6-15 anterior bending and lifting

possible. After a 3-5 seconds' interval, the patient exhales and slowly lowers the hand. Such an exercise is done 5-10 times and then the patient returns to the original position.

[Effect] To exercise the muscles responsible for bending and extending the shoulder and intercostal muscles; to prevent adhesion of the shoulder joint and spasm of the elbow joint; and to improve the functions of the heart and lungs.

2) Anterior bending, abducting and adducting of the shoulder joint (Fig. 6-16)

[Method] The patient sits as straight as possible in a functional posture. The healthy hand grasps the wrist of the affected hand to turn the palm upward and extend the elbow. The patient inhales, slowly bends the shoulder about 90° and then slowly abducts it as hard as possible. Then, the patient exhales and slowly performs adduction. Such an exercise is done 5-10 times and then the patient returns to the original position.

[Effect] To exercise the muscles responsible for bending, extending, abducting and adducting the shoulder joint; to prevent adhesion and semiluxation of the shoulder joint, spasm of the elbow joint and deformity of the spine.

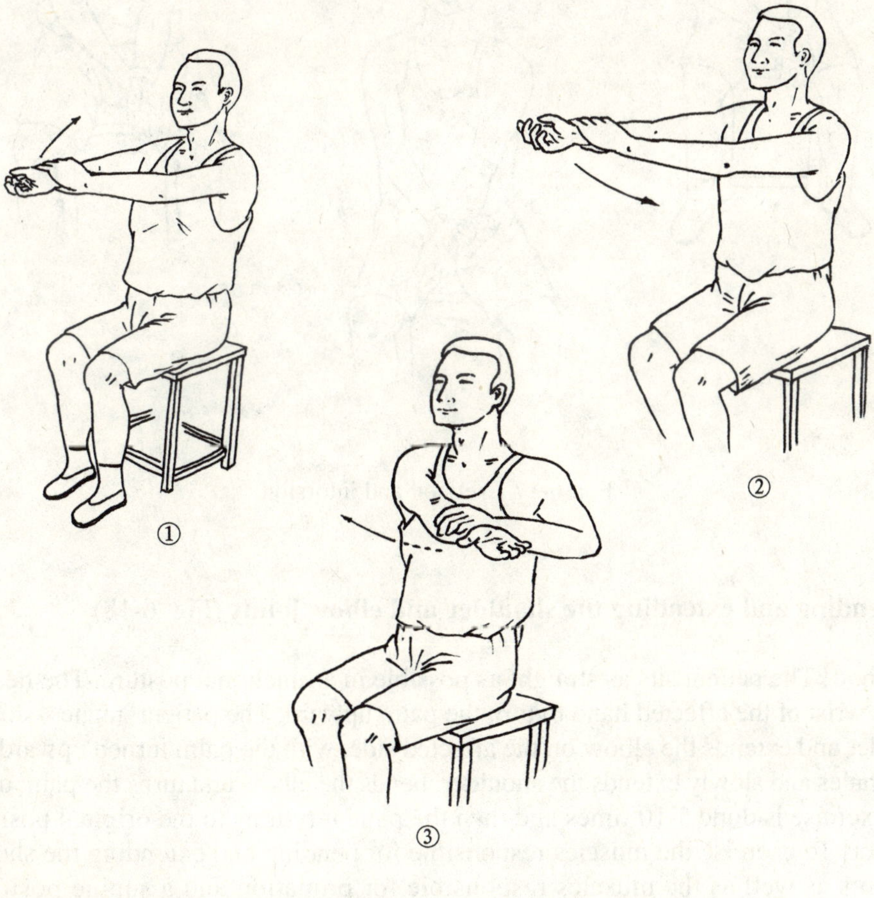

Fig. 6-16 Anterior bending, abducting and adducting

3) Eversion and intorsion of the shoulder joint (Fig. 6-17)

[Method] The patient sits as straight as possible in a functional posture. The healthy hand grasps the wrist of the affected hand to turn the palm upward and extend the elbow. The patient inhales and slowly rotates the shoulder outwardly as much as possible. After a 3-5 seconds' interval, the patient exhales and slowly performs intorsion of the shoulder joint. Such an exercise is done 10-20 times.

[Effect] To exercise the muscles responsible for eversion and intorsion of the shoulder joint, and to prevent adhesion of the shoulder joint and spasm of the elbow joint.

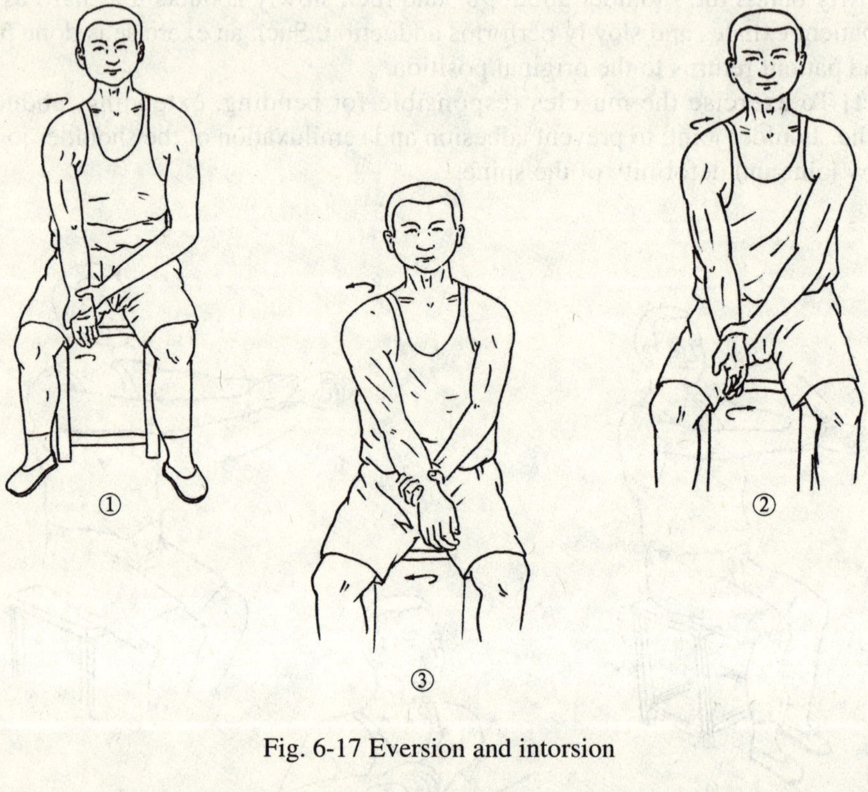

Fig. 6-17 Eversion and intorsion

4) Bending and extending the shoulder and elbow joints (Fig. 6-18)

[Method] The patient sits as straight as possible in a functional posture. The healthy hand grasps the wrist of the affected hand to turn the palm upward. The patient inhales, slowly bends the shoulder and extends the elbow on the affected side, with the palm turned upward. Then the patient exhales and slowly extends the shoulder, bends the elbow and turns the palm downward. Such an exercise is done 5-10 times and then the patient returns to the original position.

[Effect] To exercise the muscles responsible for bending and extending the shoulder and elbow joints as well as the muscles responsible for pronation and a supine position of the forearm; to separate the common bending and extending of the shoulder and elbow joints to reduce their spasm; and to prevent adhesion of the shoulder joint.

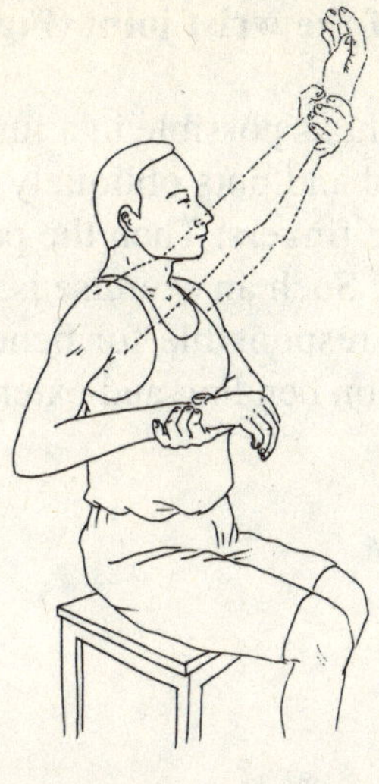

Fig. 6-18 Bending and extending

5) Bending and extending the elbow joint (Fig. 6-19)

[Method] The patient sits as straight as possible in a functional posture. The healthy hand grasps the wrist of the affected hand. The patient inhales and slowly bends the elbow joint with the palm turned in an anterior way. Then the patient exhales and slowly extends the elbow with the palm turned upward. Such an exercise is done 10-20 times.

[Effect] To exercise the muscles responsible for bending and extending the elbow joint as well as the muscles responsible for pronation and a supine position of the forearm; to separate the common bending and extending of the elbow joint and the forearm to reduce spasm of the elbow joint; and to prevent stiffness of the elbow joint.

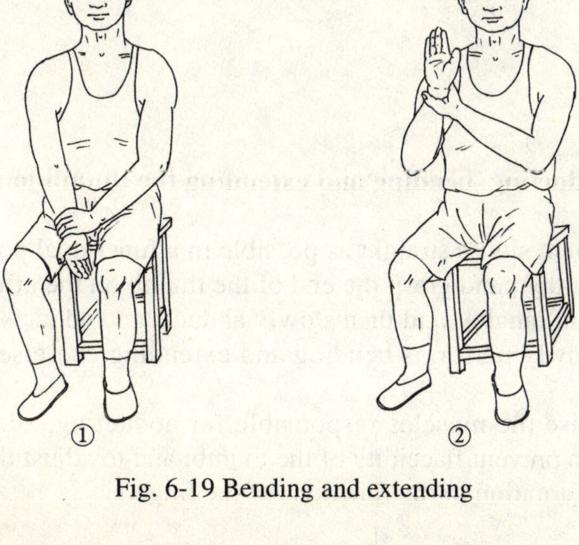

Fig. 6-19 Bending and extending

6) Palmar and dorsal bending of the wrist joint (Fig. 6-20)

[Method] The patient sits as straight as possible in a functional posture. The healthy hand grasps the dorsum of the affected hand and puts obliquely on the thigh. The patient inhales, slowly bends the wrist and extends the fingers. Then the patient exhales and slowly extends (dorsal bending) and bends the fingers. Such an exercise is done 10-20 times.

[Effect] To exercise the muscles responsible for bending and extending the wrist and finger joints; and to separate the common bending and extending of the wrist and finger joints to reduce spasm.

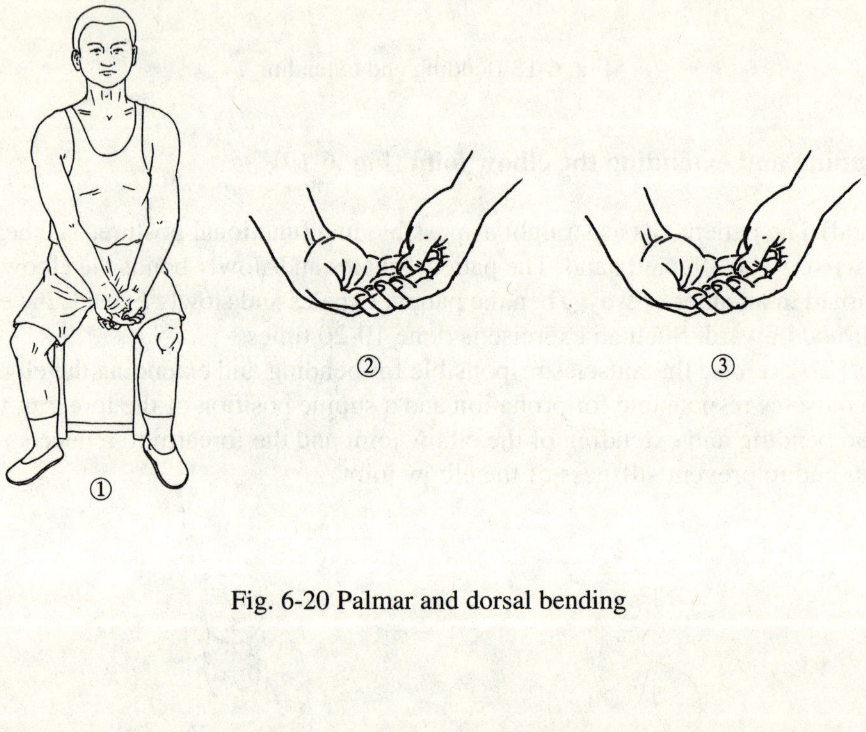

Fig. 6-20 Palmar and dorsal bending

7) Abducting, adducting, bending and extending the thumb joint (Fig. 6-21)

[Method] The patient sits as straight as possible in a functional posture. The thumb and index finger on the healthy hand grasp the end of the thumb on the affected hand and is laid on the thigh. The patient inhales, and then slowly abducts and adducts the thumb. Then, the patient exhales and slowly performs bending and extending exercise. Such an exercise is done 10-20 times.

[Effect] To exercise the muscles responsible for abducting, adducting, bending and extending the thumb; to prevent flaccidity of the thumb; and to adjust the reflex regulation of the brain to promote restoration of the functions of the fingers.

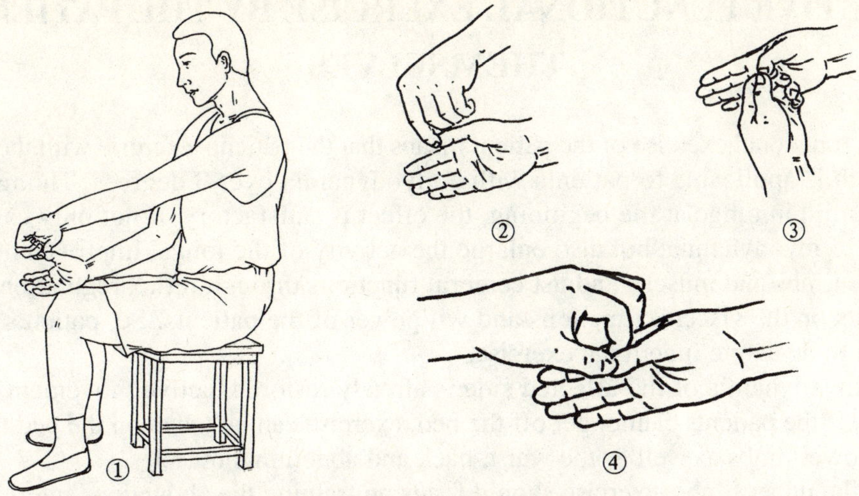

Fig. 6-21 Abducting, adducting, bending and extending

8) Bending and extending the joints of the four fingers (Fig. 6-22)

[Method] The patient sits as straight as possible in a functional posture. The healthy hand grasps the dorsal part of the fingers on the affected hand and the palm faces the tips of the 2nd-5th fingers. The affected hand is put obliquely on the thigh. The patient inhales and slowly bends the fingers. Then, the patient exhales, rubs the affected fingers and slowly extends them. Such an exercise is done 10-20 times.

[Effect] To exercise the muscles responsible for bending and extending the fingers; to prevent spasms and stiffness of the finger joints; and to adjust the reflex regulation of the brain to promote restoration of the functions of the fingers.

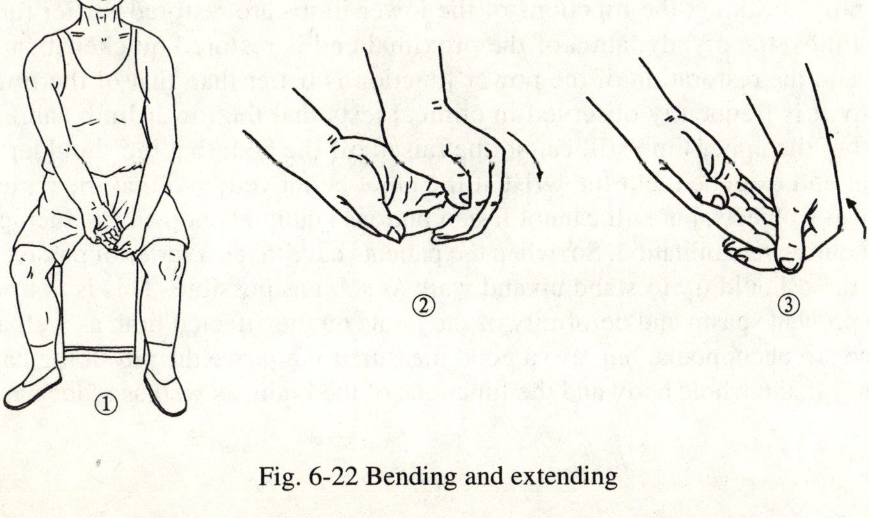

Fig. 6-22 Bending and extending

2. ACTIVE FUNCTIONAL EXERCISE BY THE PATIENTS THEMSELVES

Active functional exercise of the patient means that the patients exercise with their affected limbs, which is applicable to patients with a myodynamia over 3 degrees. Though such an exercise is mild in range at the beginning, the effect is satisfactory. It not only can promote restoration of myodynamia, but also enlarge the activity of the joints, improve coordination between the limbs and muscles, adjust cerebral functions through reflex regulation and exert better effects on the visceral functions and willpower of the patients. So, patients should be encouraged to do active functional exercise.

If the myodynamia of the affected side is already restored, active movement should be undertaken. If the patients cannot get off the bed, exercise can be taken on the bed to train the upper and lower limbs as well as the waist, back and abdominal muscles.

a. For the upper limbs, exercise should focus on training the abduction, anterior bending and lifting of the shoulder joint, bending and extending of the elbow joint, dorsal bending and extending of the wrist joint and extending of the finger joints. Functional exercise of the thumb joint is especially important.

b. For the lower limbs, the exercise should focus on adduction and medial rotation of the hip joint, bending of the hip and knee joints as well as dorsal bending and extending of the ankle joint.

c. The exercise can be repeated 10-30 times and twice a day. The amount of exercise should be monitored to ensure patients do not feel fatigue next day. After exercise, there will naturally be aching, distension and pain in the affected side, which can be alleviated by self massage and Tuina, or fumigation with Chinese medicinal herbs or moxibustion to promote metabolism of acid waste substances and rehabilitation of the limbs.

d. When the affected limb has rehabilitated to a certain degree, anti-resistance exercise (for instance, the patient stays in a lying position and the doctor presses the sole of the affected limb and asks the patient to extend the hip and knee joints as much as possible, or the doctor grasps the patient's hand and asks the patient to bend the elbow and extend the shoulder as much as possible, etc.) should be done.

Generally speaking, the functions of the lower limbs are restored earlier than those of the upper limbs, the myodynamia of the proximal end is restored quicker than that of the distal end and the restoration of the power function is better than that of the fine function. That is why it is frequently observed in clinical tests that the lower limb can be bent and extended, but the upper limb still cannot be raised off the bed; that the shoulder and elbow can be bent and extended, but the wrist still cannot be moved; and that the patient already can hold heavy objects, but still cannot fasten buttons and hold chopsticks. Such phenomena are normal during rehabilitation. So, when the patients have taken a series of passive functional exercises, they should try to stand up and walk as soon as possible. This is not only a good method to prevent spasm and deformity of the joints on the affected limb as well as droop of the foot and strephenopodia, but also a good measure to improve the physiological functions of the organs in the whole body and the functions of the brain, as well as reduce and alleviate disability.

(1) Head and neck (lying position)

1) Anterior bending and posterior extending of the neck (Fig. 6-23)

[Method] The patient lies in a supine position in a functional posture with a pillow beneath the shoulder and back. The patient inhales and slowly bends the head and neck in an anterior direction. Then, the patient exhales and slowly extends the head and neck in a posterior direction. Such an exercise is repeated 10-15 times.

[Effect] To exercise the muscles responsible for bending and extending atlantooccipital articulation; to prevent spasm and stiffness of muscles on the neck; and to improve cerebral blood circulation.

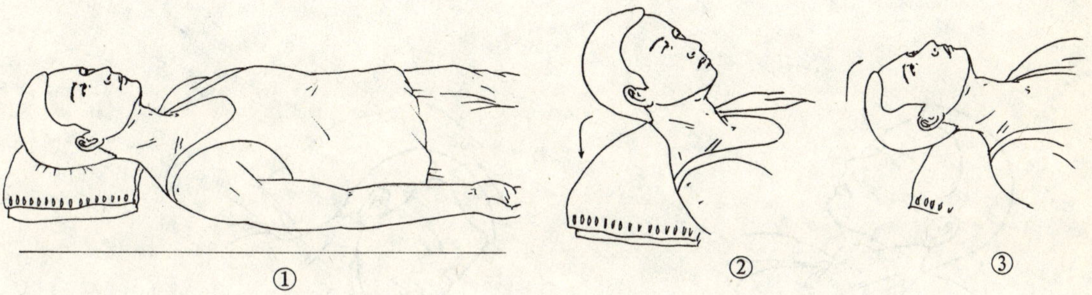

Fig. 6-23 Anterior bending and posterior extending

2) Bilateral bending of the neck (Fig. 6-24)

[Method] The patient lies in a supine position in a functional posture with a pillow beneath the shoulder and back. The patient inhales and slowly bends the neck to the affected side. After an interval of 3-5 seconds, the patient exhales and slowly bends the neck to the healthy side. Such an exercise is repeated 10-15 times.

[Effect] To exercise the muscles responsible for lateral bending of atlantooccipital articulation; to prevent spasms of the neck muscles; and to improve cerebral blood supply.

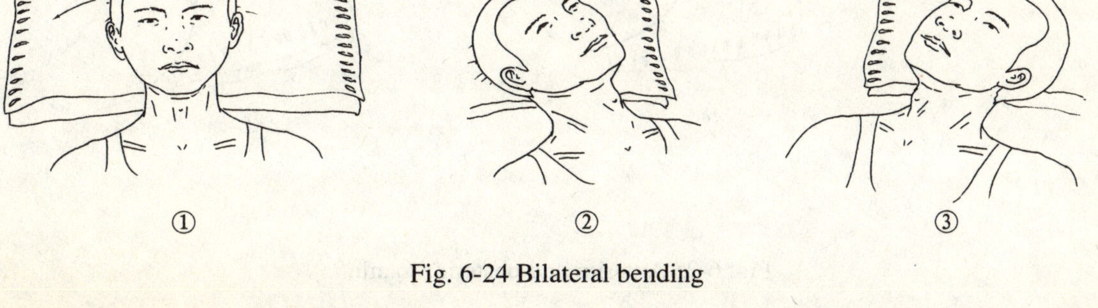

Fig. 6-24 Bilateral bending

3) Anterior and posterior rotation of the neck (Fig. 6-25)

[Method] The patient lies in a supine position in a functional posture with a pillow beneath the shoulder and back. The patient inhales and slowly rotates the head from the front of the neck to the affected side and the posterior part of the neck. After an interval of 3-5 seconds, the patient exhales and slowly rotates the head from the posterior part of the neck to the healthy side and the front of the neck. Such an exercise is repeated 10-15 times (the patient may close the eyes in rotating the head).

[Effect] To exercise the muscles responsible for rotation and lateral bending as well as bending and extending atlantooccipital articulation; to prevent spasms and stiffness of the neck muscles; to exert certain effect on the patients accompanied by cervical spondylopathy; and to improve cerebral blood circulation.

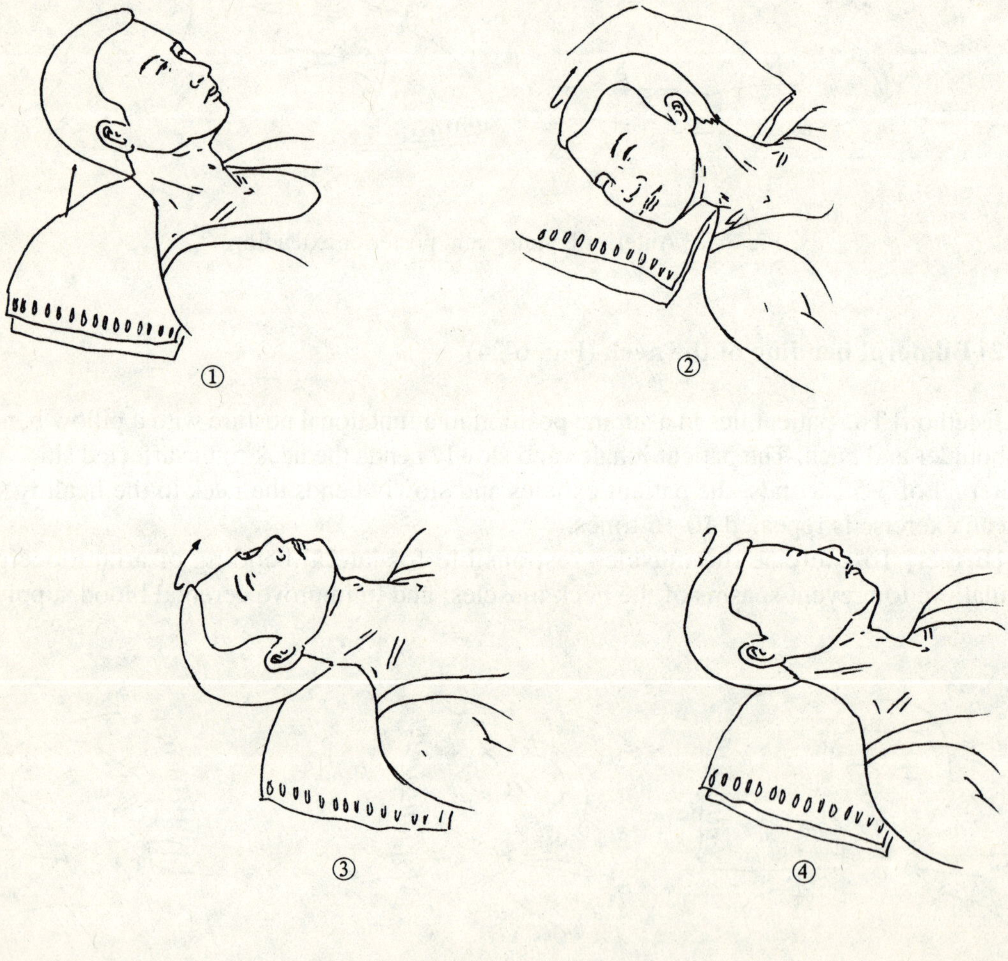

Fig. 6-25 Anterior and posterior rotation

(2) Upper limbs (lying position)

1) Anterior bending and lifting of the shoulder joint (Fig. 6-26)

[Method] The patient lies in a supine position in a functional posture with both upper limbs put beside the body, the elbows extended straight and the palm turned upward. The patient inhales and slowly bends the shoulder on the affected side in an anterior direction above the head. After an interval of 3-5 seconds, the patient exhales and slowly bends the elbow, touches the shoulder on the healthy side with the dorsum of the hand, slowly extends downward and then returns to the original position. Such an exercise is repeated 10-15 times.

[Effect] To exercise bending and extending of the shoulder and elbow joints and muscles responsible for pronation and a supine position of the forearm; and to prevent adhesion of the shoulder joint and spasms of the elbow joint.

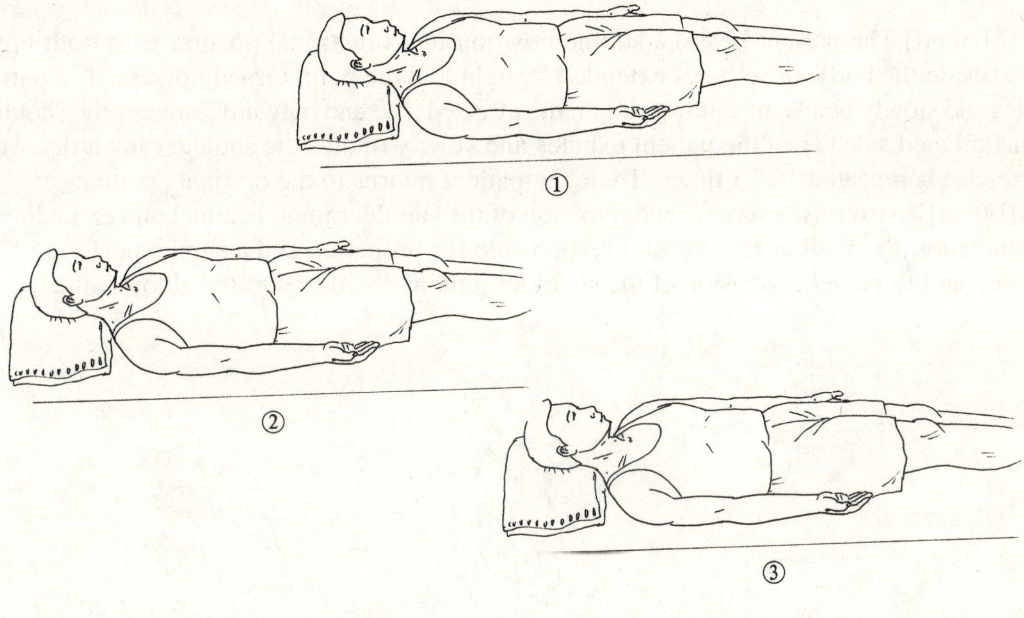

Fig. 6-26 Anterior bending and lifting

2) Abducting and adducting the shoulder joint (Fig. 6-27)

[Method] The patient lies in a supine position in a functional posture with both upper limbs beside the body, the elbows extended straight and the palm turned upward. The patient inhales and slowly abducts the shoulder on the affected side above the head as much as possible. After an interval of 3-5 seconds, the patient exhales and slowly adducts the shoulder. Such an exercise is repeated 10-15 times. Then the patient returns to the original position.

[Effect] To exercise abduction and adduction of the shoulder joint as well as the muscles responsible for extending the elbow joint; to prevent semiluxation of the shoulder joint and spasm of the elbow joint.

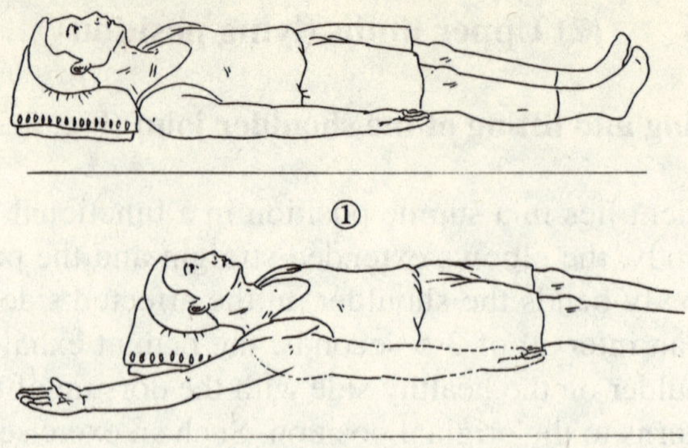

① ②

Fig. 6-27 Abduction and adduction

3) Eversion and intorsion of the shoulder joint (Fig. 6-28)

[Method] The patient lies in a supine position in a functional posture with both upper limbs beside the body, the elbows extended straight and the palm turned upward. The patient inhales and slowly bends the elbow joint on the affected side and outwardly rotates the shoulder on the affected side. Then the patient exhales and slowly rotates the shoulder inwardly. Such an exercise is repeated 10-15 times. Then, the patient returns to the original position.

[Effect] To exercise eversion and intorsion of the shoulder joint, bending and extending of the elbow joint as well as the muscles responsible for pronation and a supine position of the forearm; and to prevent adhesion of the shoulder joint and stiffness of the elbow joint.

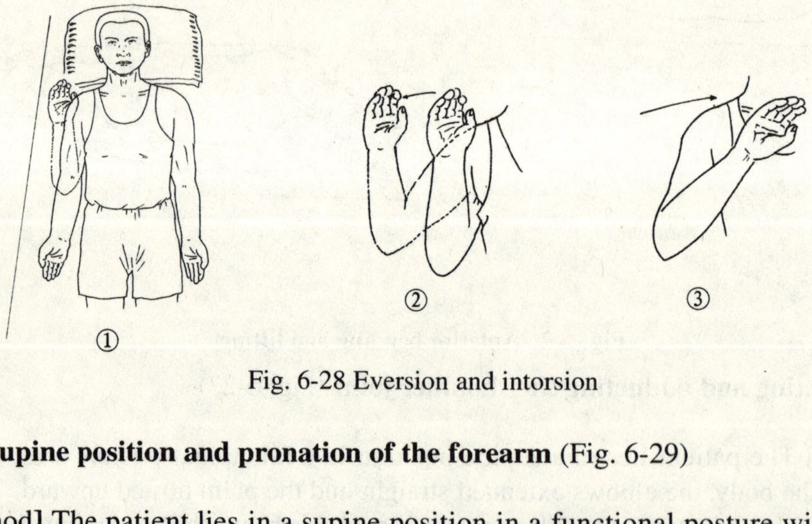

① ② ③

Fig. 6-28 Eversion and intorsion

4) A supine position and pronation of the forearm (Fig. 6-29)

[Method] The patient lies in a supine position in a functional posture with both upper limbs beside the body, the elbows extended straight and the palm turned upward. The patient inhales and slowly abducts the shoulder on the affected side through 90°; rotates the forearm as much as possible; bends the elbow and turns the palm outward. Then, the patient exhales and slowly rotates the shoulder in a posterior direction, extends the elbow and turns the palm upward. Such an exercise is repeated 10-15 times. Then the patient returns to the original position.

[Effect] To exercise the muscles responsible for pronation and a supine position of the forearm as well as bending and extending the elbow joint; to separate common bending and extending of the elbow joint and the forearm to reduce spasm; and to prevent semiluxation of the shoulder joint.

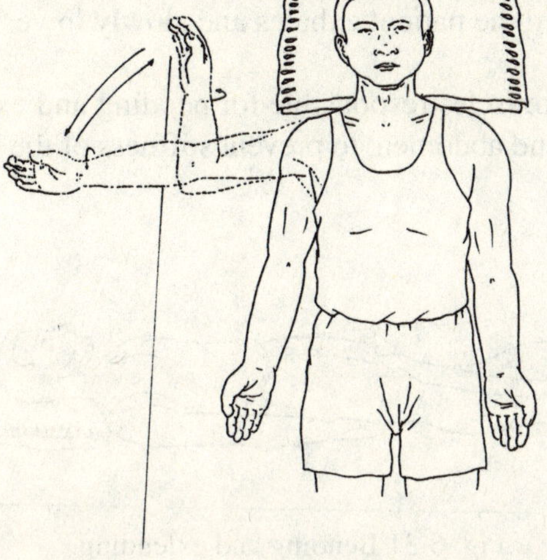

Fig. 6-29 A supine position and pronation

5) Dorsal and palmar bending of the wrist joint (Fig. 6-30)

[Method] The patient lies in a supine position in a functional posture with both upper limbs put beside the body. The patient inhales and slowly bends the elbow on the affected side to 90°, extends the wrist dorsally as much as possible, turns the palm upward and bends the fingers with the dorsal parts of the fingers facing the foot. Then the patient exhales and slowly bends the wrist, turns the palm downward and extends the fingers with the tips of the four fingers facing the foot. Such an exercise is repeated 10-20 times. Then the patient returns to the original position.

[Effect] To exercise the muscles responsible for bending and extending of the wrist and fingers as well as pronation and a supine position of the forearm; to separate common bending and extending of the elbow and the forearm as well as the wrist and fingers to reduce spasm.

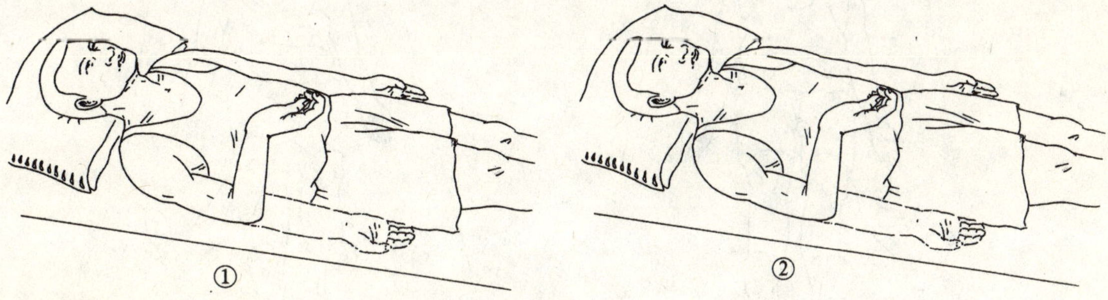

Fig. 6-30 Dorsal and palmar bending

(3) Lower limbs (lying position)

1) Bending and extending the hip joint (Fig. 6-31)

[Method] The patient lies in a supine position in a functional posture with both lower limbs extended naturally. The patient inhales and slowly bends the hip joint on the affected side as much as possible. Then the patient exhales and slowly lowers the hip. Such an exercise is repeated 10-15 times.

[Effect] To exercise the muscles responsible for bending and extending of the hip joint as well as muscles on the waist and abdomen; to prevent stiffness of the hip joint; and to strengthen the stability of the hip joint.

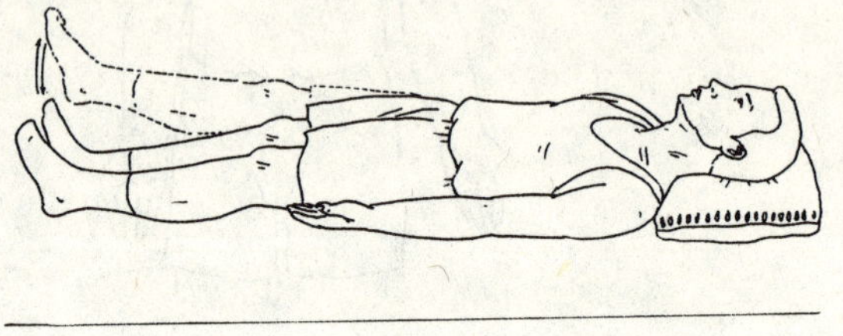

Fig. 6-31 Bending and extending

2) Abducting and adducting the hip joint (Fig. 6-32)

[Method] The patient lies in a supine position in a functional posture with both lower limbs extended naturally. The patient inhales and slowly abducts the hip joint on the affected side as much as possible. Then the patient exhales and slowly adducts the hip joint as much as possible. Such an exercise is repeated 10-15 times. And then the patient returns to the original position.

[Effect] To exercise the muscles responsible for abduction and adduction of the hip joint; and to strengthen the stability of the hip joint to prevent swinging of the hip in walking.

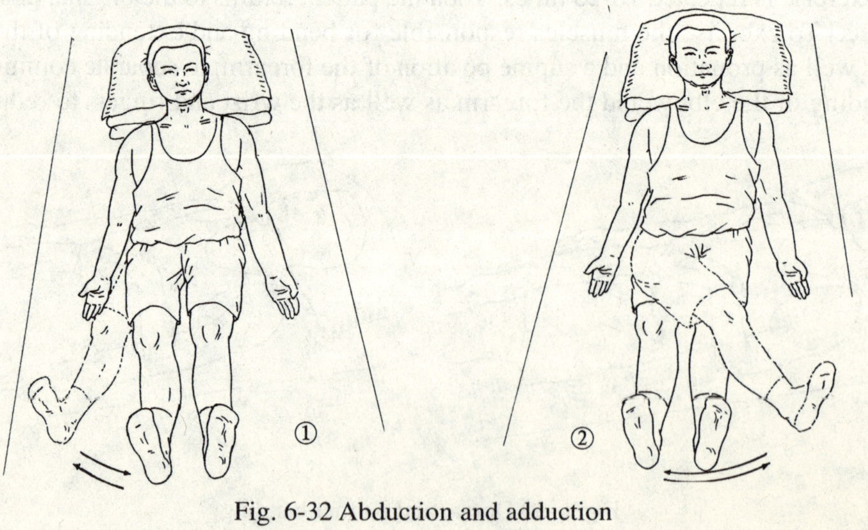

Fig. 6-32 Abduction and adduction

3) Bending the hip and extending the knee (Fig. 6-33)

[Method] The patient lies in a supine position in a functional posture with both knees put beside the bed in a bending position. The patient inhales and slowly bends and the hip on the affected side and extends the knee as much as possible. Then the patient exhales and slowly extends, lowers and bends the knee. Such an exercise is repeated 10-15 times. Then the patient returns to the original position.

[Effect] To exercise the muscles responsible for bending and extending the hip and knee joints as well as muscles on the waist and abdomen; and to separate the common bending and extending of the hip and knee joints to reduce spasm.

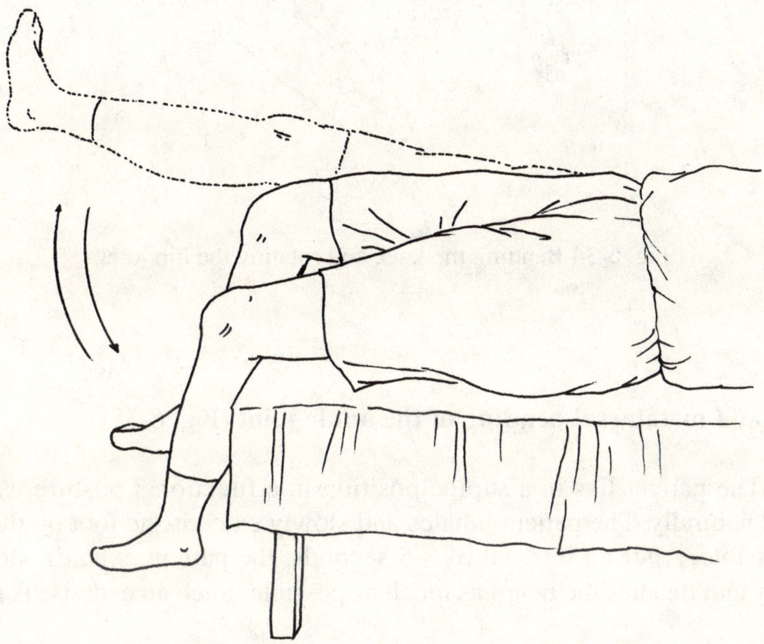

Fig. 6-33 Bending the hip and extending the knee

4) Bending the knee and rotating the hip joint (Fig. 6-34)

[Method] The patient lies in a supine position in a functional posture with both lower limbs extended naturally. The patient inhales and slowly bends the knee on the affected side and puts the sole in a stable position on the bed as much as possible. In the early period, the foot on the healthy side is fixated and the hip is inwardly rotated as much as possible. After an interval of 3-5 seconds, the patient exhales and slowly relaxes. Such an exercise is repeated 10-30 times. And then the patient returns to the original position

[Effect] To exercise the muscles responsible for bending the knee joint and internal rotation of the hip joint; and to prevent "lifting the hip" in walking.

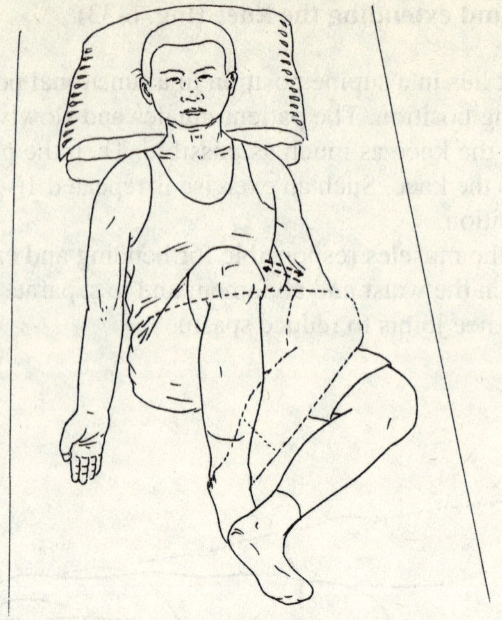

Fig. 6-34 Bending the knee and rotating the hip joint

5) Dorsal and metatarsal bending of the ankle joint (Fig. 6-35)

[Method] The patient lies in a supine position in a functional posture with both lower limbs extended naturally. The patient inhales and slowly extends the foot on the affected side as much as possible. After an interval of 3-5 seconds, the patient exhales, slowly performs bending activity and treadles the board as much as possible. Such an exercise is repeated 10-30 times.

[Effect] To exercise the muscles responsible for dorsal and metatarsal bending of the ankle joint; and to prevent foot droop and strephenopodia.

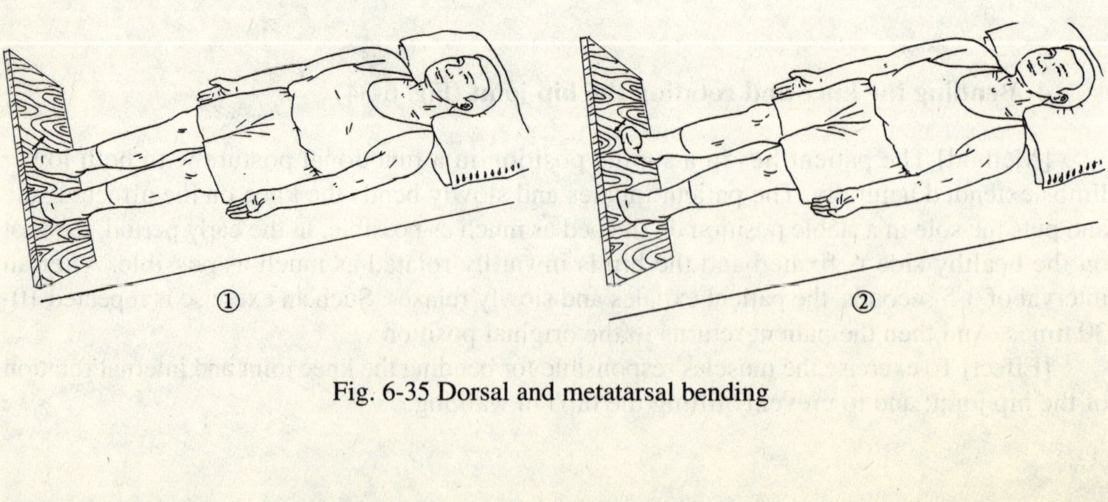

Fig. 6-35 Dorsal and metatarsal bending

6) Bending the knee and suspending the waist (Fig. 6-36)

[Method] The patient lies in a supine position in a functional posture with both lower limbs extended naturally. The patient inhales and slowly bends the lower limbs, puts and fixates the sole in a stable position on the bed, slowly extends the hip joint on the affected side as much as possible, lifts the buttocks off the bed and suspends the waist for 3-5 seconds. Then the patient exhales and slowly lowers the knee. Such an exercise is repeated 10-15 times. The patient then returns to the original position.

[Effect] To exercise the muscles responsible for bending and extending the hip joint and the spine as well as the muscles for bending the knee joints; and to strengthen the stability of the hip, knee and ankle joints to prevent deformity of the spine.

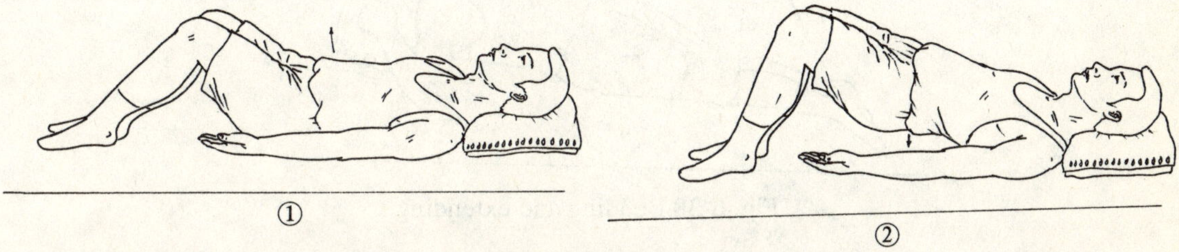

Fig. 6-36 Bending the knee and suspending the waist

7) Sit-ups (Fig. 6-37)

[Method] The patient lies in a supine position in a functional posture with both lower limbs extended naturally. The patient inhales, contracts the abdomen, and slowly bends the hip, bending the spine in an anterior direction to enable the upper part of the body to move away from the bed and sit up. Then, the patient exhales, extends the hip and spine and lies down slowly from the waist to the back and the head. Such an exercise is repeated 10-15 times (the upper part of the body should not lean toward the healthy side).

[Effect] To exercise the muscles responsible for bending and extending the hip joint and the spine; to prevent deformity of the spine and reduce the heaviness of the upper part of the body in standing; and to improve visceral functions.

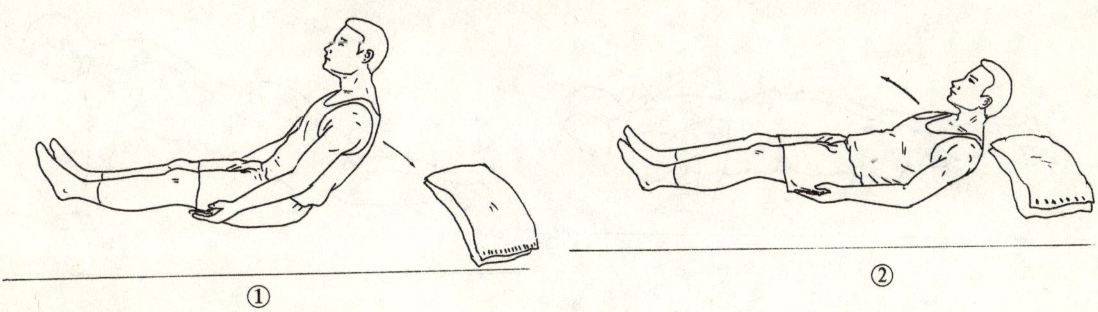

Fig. 6-37 Sit-ups

8) Bending and extending the knee joint (Fig. 6-38)

[Method] The patient lies in pronation in a functional posture with both lower limbs extended naturally. The patient inhales and slowly bends the affected knee as much as possible. After an interval of 3-5 seconds, the patient exhales and slowly extends the knee. Such an exercise is repeated 10-20 times (the hip should not be bent and the buttocks should not stick up).

[Effect] To exercise the muscles responsible for bending and extending the knee joints; to separate common bending and extending of the hip and knee joints to reduce spasms; and to prevent “external swinging ” of the shank in walking.

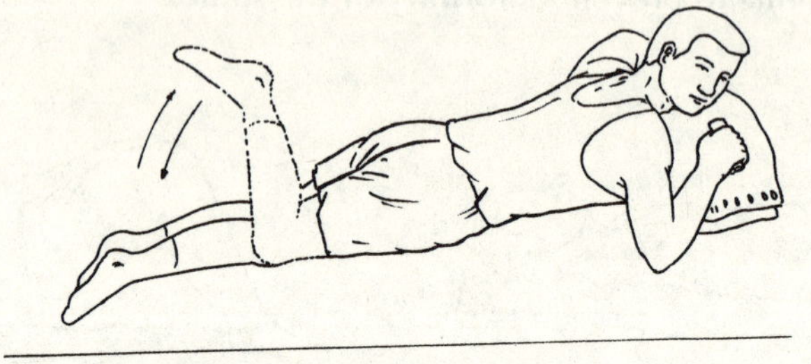

Fig. 6-38 Bending and extending

9) Half push-up (Fig. 6-39)

[Method] The patient lies in pronation in a functional posture with both lower limbs extended naturally, both hands pressing beside the body and the tips of the four fingers turned toward the head. The patient inhales, props himself or herself up with both hands and slowly extends the elbow and bends the shoulder to enable the upper part of the body to slowly move away from the bed. Then, the patient exhales and slowly lowers the hands. Such an exercise is repeated 10-15 times (at the beginning, the upper part of the body can get slightly away from the bed and the patient should not hold the breath).

[Effect] To exercise the muscles responsible for bending and extending the shoulder and elbow joints and dorsal bending of the wrist joint as well as the muscles on the waist and back; to separate common bending and extending of the shoulder and elbow joints to alleviate spasms; and to prevent semiluxation of the shoulder joint and stiffness of the elbow joint.

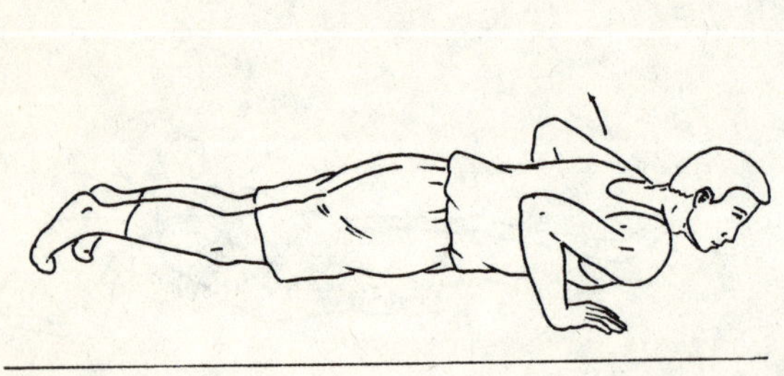

①

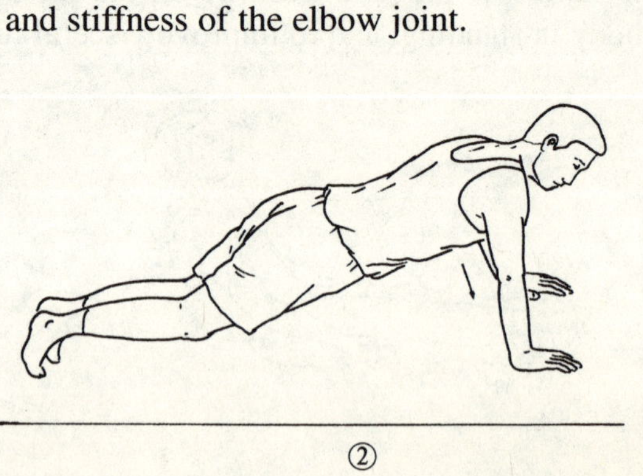

②

Fig. 6-39 Half push-up

(4) Head and neck (sitting position)

1) Anterior bending and posterior extending of the neck (Fig. 6-40)

[Method] The patient sits straight in a functional posture. The patient inhales and slowly bends the neck in an anterior direction as much as possible. Then, the patient exhales, contracts the abdomen, throws out the chest and slowly performs posterior extension activity. Such an exercise is repeated 10-20 times.

[Effect] To exercise the muscles responsible for bending and extending atlantooccipital articulation, as well as the muscles on the chest and abdomen; to prevent spasm and stiffness of the cervical muscles; to improve cerebral balance and blood circulation; and to exert a certain effect on the patient with cervical vertebral straightening.

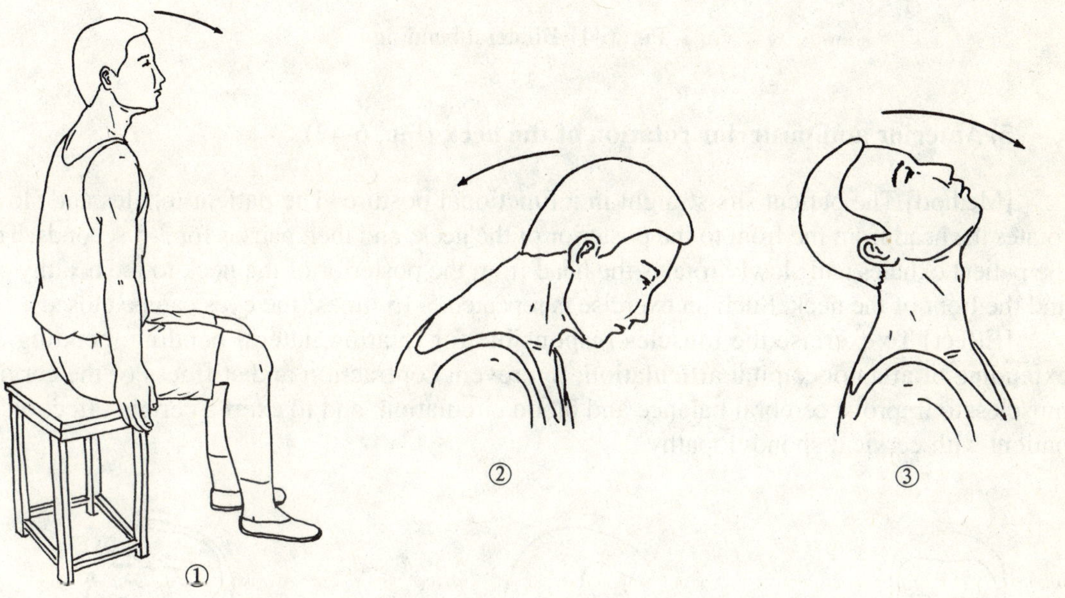

Fig. 6-40 Anterior bending and posterior extending

2) Bilateral bending of the neck (Fig. 6-41)

[Method] The patient sits straight in a functional posture. The patient inhales and slowly bends the neck to the affected side and then pauses for 3-5 seconds. Then, the patient exhales and slowly bends to the healthy side. Such an exercise is repeated 10-15 times.

[Effect] To exercise the muscles responsible for lateral bending of atlantooccipital articulation; to prevent contraction of the cervical muscles and deviation of the head and neck; to improve the cerebral blood supply; and to exert a certain effect on the patient with cervical spondylopathy.

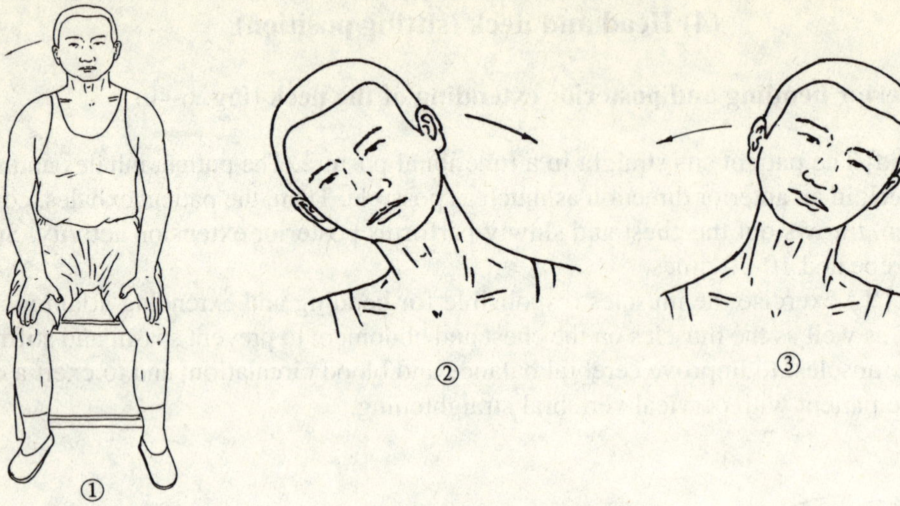

Fig. 6-41 Bilateral bending

3) Anterior and posterior rotation of the neck (Fig. 6-42)

[Method] The patient sits straight in a functional posture. The patient inhales and slowly rotates the head from the front to the posterior of the neck, and then pauses for 3-5 seconds. Then the patient exhales and slowly rotates the head from the posterior of the neck to the healthy side and the front of the neck. Such an exercise is repeated 5-15 times (the eyes can be closed).

[Effect] To exercise the muscles responsible for rotating, lateral bending, bending and extending of atlantooccipital articulation; to prevent contraction and stiffness of the cervical muscles; to improve cerebral balance and blood circulation; and to exert a certain effect on the patient with cervical spondylopathy

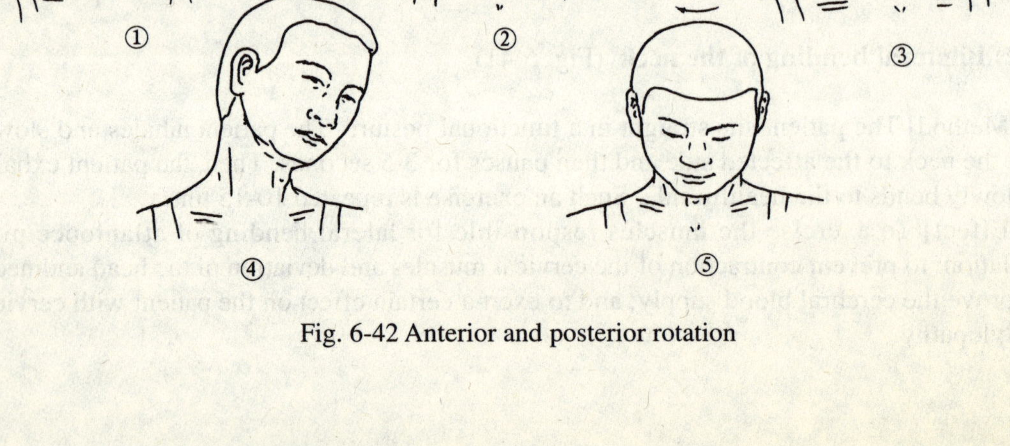

Fig. 6-42 Anterior and posterior rotation

(5) Upper limbs (sitting position)

1) Anterior bending and lifting of the shoulder joint (Fig. 6-43)

[Method] The patient sits straight in a functional posture with both upper limbs put down naturally and the palms turned in an anterior direction. The patient inhales, contracts the abdomen, throws out the chest, extends the elbows and slowly bends in an anterior direction and lifts the shoulders as much as possible. Then, the patient exhales and slowly lowers the upper limbs (the healthy hand can help the affected upper limb to prevent sudden drop). Such an exercise is repeated 10-20 times.

[Effect] To exercise the muscles responsible for bending and extending the shoulder joint, extending the elbow joint, pronation and a supine position of the forearms as well as chest and abdominal muscles; to prevent adhesion of the shoulder joint; and to strengthen the functions of the heart and lungs.

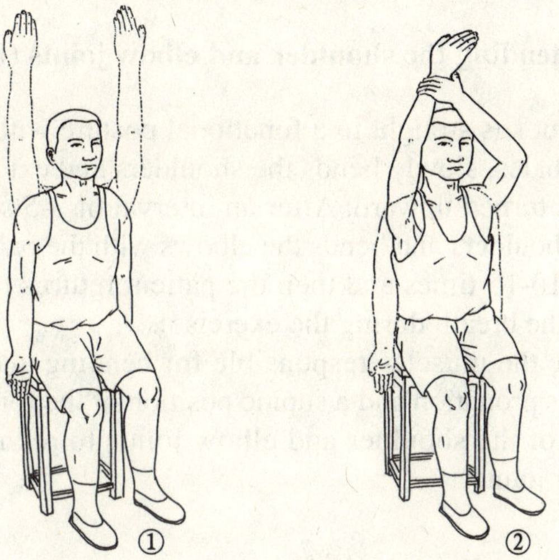

Fig. 6-43 Anterior bending and lifting

2). Abducting and lifting the shoulder joint (Fig. 6-44)

[Method] The patient sits straight in a functional posture with both upper limbs laid naturally beside the body, the palms turned outward. The patient inhales, contracts the abdomen, throws out the chest, extends the elbows and slowly abducts and lifts the shoulders as much as possible. Then, the patient exhales and slowly adducts and lowers the upper limbs. Such an exercise is repeated 10-20 times.

[Effect] To exercise the muscles responsible for abduction and adduction of the shoulder joint, extending the elbow joint, pronation and a supine position of the forearms as well as the muscles on the chest and abdomen; and to prevent semiluxation of the shoulder joint and spasms of the elbow joint.

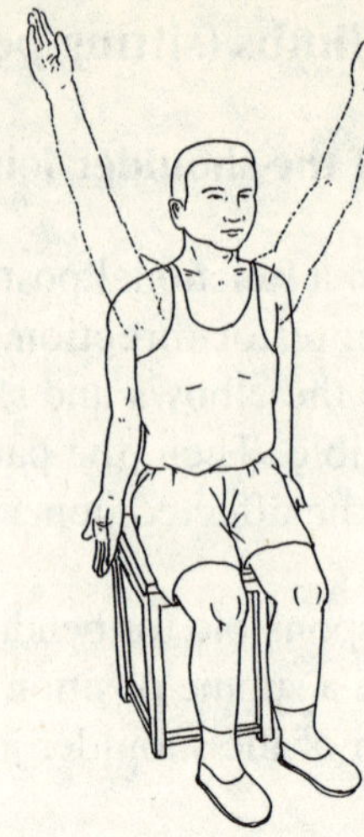

Fig. 6-44 Abducting and lifting

3) Bending and extending the shoulder and elbow joints (Fig. 6-45)

[Method] The patient sits straight in a functional posture with both upper limbs hanging naturally. The patient inhales, slowly bends the shoulders and extends the elbows as much as possible, with the palms turned upward. After an interval of 3-5 seconds, the patient exhales and slowly extends the shoulders and bends the elbows with the palms turned downward. Such an exercise is repeated 10-15 times and then the patient returns to the original position (the patient should not hold the breath during the exercise).

[Effect] To exercise the muscles responsible for bending and extending the elbow and shoulder joints, as well as pronation and a supine position of the forearms; to separate common bending and extending of the shoulder and elbow joints to reduce spasms; and to prevent adhesion of the shoulder joint.

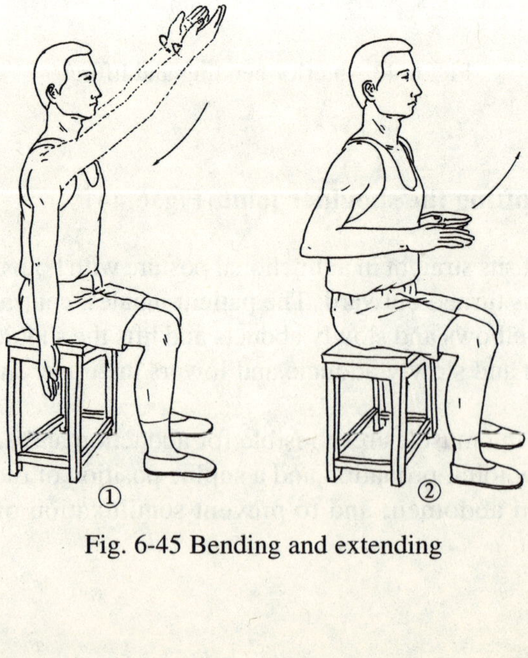

Fig. 6-45 Bending and extending

4) Dorsal and palmar bending of the wrist joint (Fig. 6-46)

[Method] The patient sits straight in a functional posture with the affected upper limb on the table and the shoulder and elbow bent. The elbow is cushioned with a pillow and fixated with the healthy hand. The patient inhales and slowly extends the wrist as much as possible with the palm upward. The fingers are bent with the dorsal parts turned in an anterior direction. Then, the patient exhales, slowly bends the palm, turns the palm downward, extends the fingers and turns the tips of the four fingers in an anterior direction. Such an exercise is repeated 10-20 times.

[Effect] To exercise the muscles responsible for bending and extending the wrist and finger joints as well as pronation and a supine position of the forearms; and to separate common bending and extending of the forearms and wrist as well as the wrist and fingers to reduce spasm.

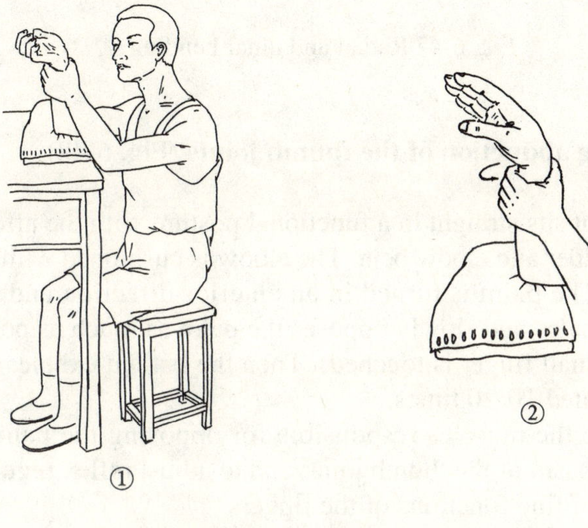

①　②

Fig. 6-46 Dorsal and palmar bending

5) Radial and ulnar bending of the wrist (Fig. 6-47)

[Method] The patient sits straight in a functional posture with the affected upper limb put on the table and the shoulder and elbow bent. The elbow is cushioned with a pillow with the palm turned in an anterior direction and the wrist slightly extended. The healthy hand is used to fixate the affected wrist. The patient inhales and slowly abducts the wrist as much as possible. After an interval of 3-5 seconds, the patient exhales and slowly adducts the writst. Such an exercise is repeated 10-20 times.

[Effect] To exercise the muscles responsible for radial and ulnar bending of the radial-wrist joints; and to prevent suspension of the wrist and spasm of the thumb.

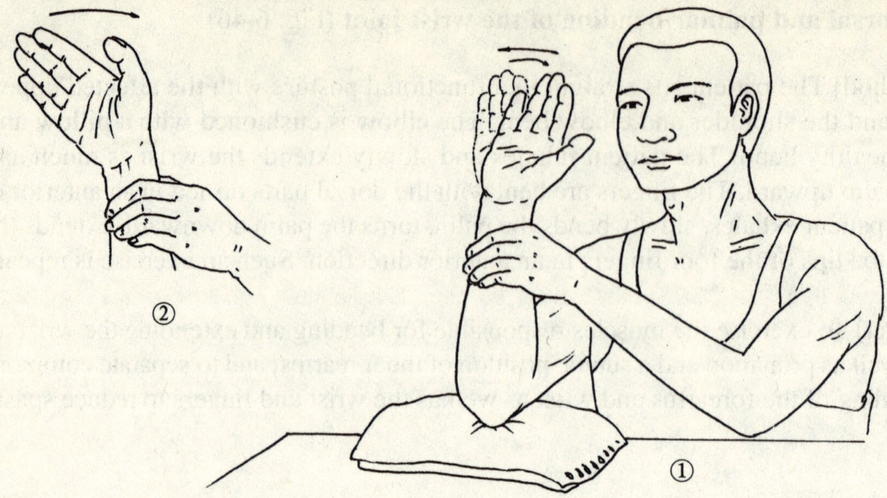

Fig. 6-47 Radial and ulnar bending

6) Palmar opposing abduction of the thumb joints (Fig. 6-48)

[Method] The patient sits straight in a functional posture with the affected upper limb put on the table and the shoulder and elbow bent. The elbow is cushioned with a pillow and fixated with the healthy hand. The palm is turned in an anterior direction and the wrist is slightly extended. The patient inhales and slowly opposes the palm as much as possible with the palm turned upward (till the small finger is touched). Then the patient exhales and slowly abducts. Such an exercise is repeated 10-20 times.

[Effect] To exercise the muscles responsible for opposing the palm and abducting the thumb joint; to prevent spasm of the thumb joint; and to adjust reflex regulation of the brain to promote the restoration of fine functions of the fingers.

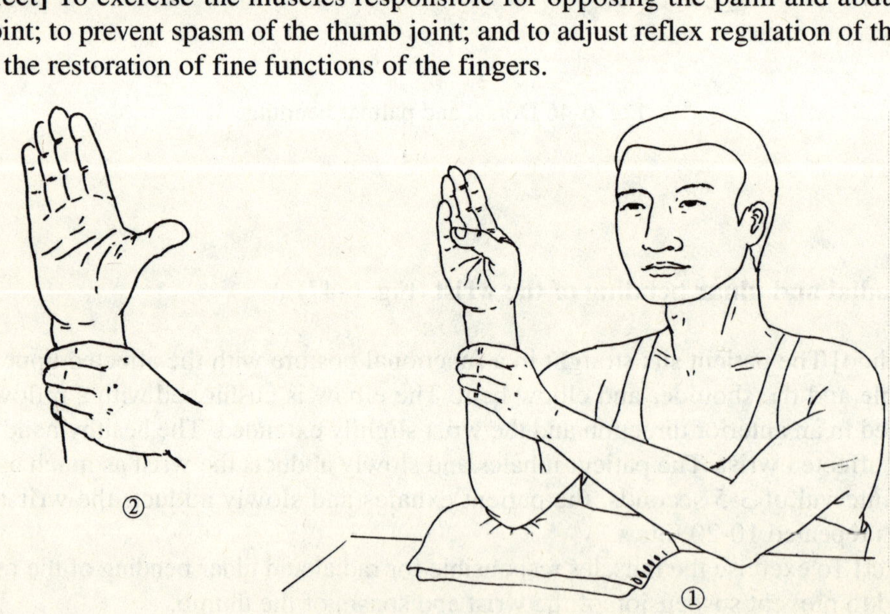

Fig. 6-48 Palmar opposing abduction

7) Bending and extending the finger joints (Fig. 6-49)

[Method] The patient sits straight in a functional posture with the affected upper limb put on the table and the shoulder and elbow bent. The elbow is cushioned with a pillow and fixated with the healthy hand. The palm is turned in an anterior direction and the writst is slightly extended. The patient inhales and slowly bends the 2nd-5th fingers as much as possible. Then the patient exhales, slowly extends the fingers, then pausing for 3-5 seconds. Such an exercise is repeated 20-30 times.

[Effect] To exercise the muscles responsible for bending and extending finger joints; to prevent spasm of the fingers; and to adjust reflex regulation of the brain to promote restoration of the functions of the fingers.

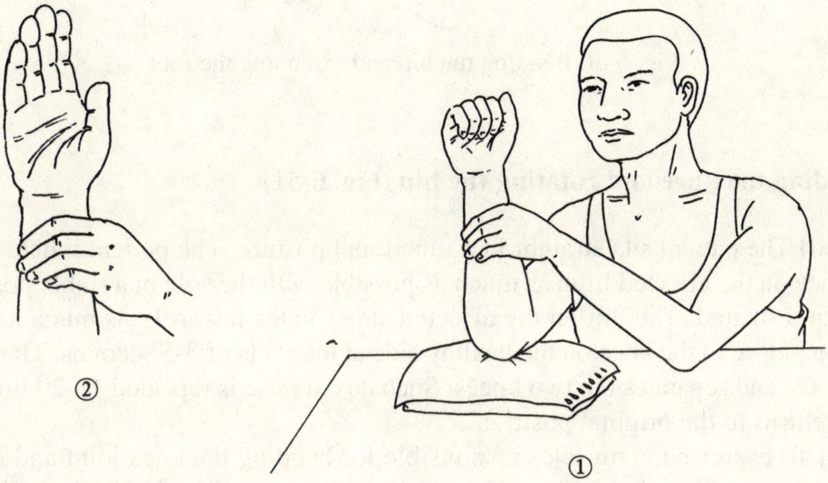

Fig. 6-49 Bending and extending

(6) Lower limbs (sitting position)

1) Bending the hip and extending the foot (Fig. 6-50)

[Method] The patient sits straight in a functional posture. The patient inhales and slowly bends the hip and extends the foot as much as possible with the affected lower limb at intervals of 3-5 seconds. Then the patient exhales and slowly lowers the lower limb with the sole in a stable position put on the ground. Such an exercise is repeated 10-15 times and then the patient returns to the original position.

[Effect] To exercise the muscles responsible for bending of the hip joint and dorsal bending of the ankle joint; and to prevent spasm and stiffness of the hip joint as well as foot droop and strephenopodia.

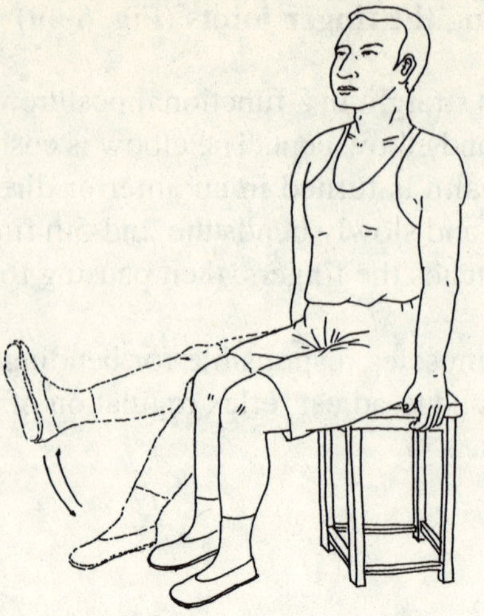

Fig. 6-50 Bending the hip and extending the foot

2) Bending the knee and rotating the hip (Fig. 6-51)

[Method] The patient sits straight in a functional posture. The patient inhales and slowly bends the knee on the affected limb as much as possible with the sole in a stable position put on the ground and fixated. The hip on the affected side rotates inwardly as much as possible to enable it to get close to the knee on the healthy side at intervals of 3-5 seconds. Then the patient exhales, relaxes and separates the two knees. Such an exercise is repeated 10-20 times and then the patient returns to the original position.

[Effect] To exercise the muscles responsible for bending the knee joint and intorting the hip joint; and to strengthen the stability of the hip joint to prevent "swinging the hip" in walking.

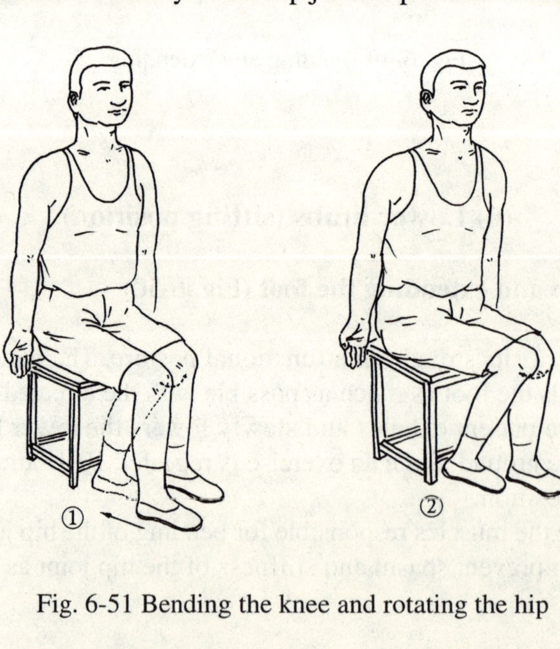

Fig. 6-51 Bending the knee and rotating the hip

3) Bending and extending the knee joint (Fig. 6-52)

[Method] The patient sits straight in a functional posture. The patient inhales and slowly bends the knee on the affected side as much as possible with the foot on the affected lower limb extended and raised above the ground. After an interval of 3-5 seconds, the patient exhales, slowly extends the knee and bends the affected foot. Such an exercise is repeated 10-20 times and then the patient returns to the original position.

[Effect] To exercise the muscles responsible for bending and extending the knee joint as well as dorsal bending and metatarsal bending of the ankle joint; to separate common bending and extending of the knee and ankle joints to reduce spasm; and to prevent spasm of knee joints.

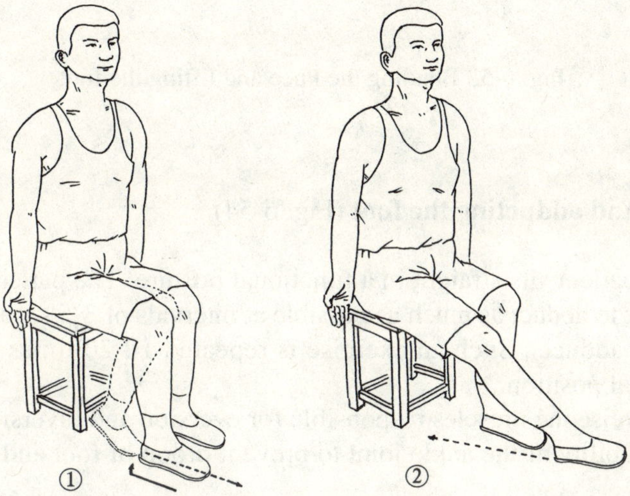

Fig. 6-52 Bending and extending

4) Bending the knee and lifting the foot (Fig. 6-53)

[Method] The patient sits straight in a functional posture. The patient inhales and slowly bends the knee on the affected limb as much as possible with the foot on the affected lower limb bent and the heel lifted at intervals of 3-5 seconds. Then the patient exhales and slowly lowers the foot with the sole in a stable position put on the ground. Such an exercise is repeated 10-20 times and then the patient returns to the original position.

[Effect] To exercise the muscles responsible for bending of the knee joint and metatarsal bending of the ankle joint; and to strengthen stability of the ankle joint to prevent droop of foot and strephenopodia.

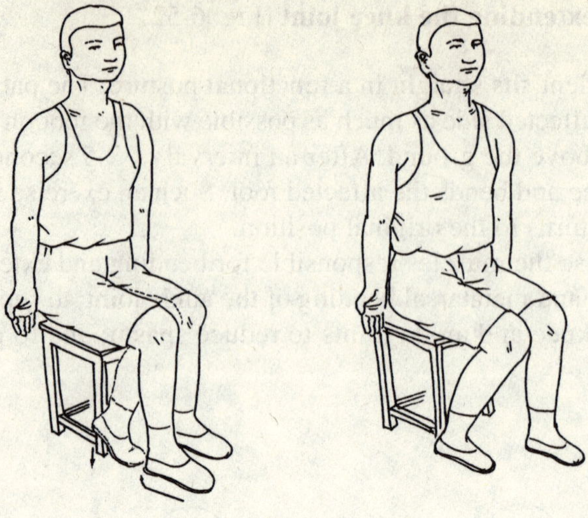

Fig. 6-53 Bending the knee and lifting the foot

5) Abducting and adducting the foot (Fig. 6-54)

[Method] The patient sits straight in a functional posture. The patient inhales and slowly lifts the affected foot to abduct as much as possible at intervals of 3-5 seconds. Then the patient exhales and slowly adducts. Such an exercise is repeated 10-20 times and then the patient returns to the original position.

[Effect] To exercise the muscles responsible for eversion and inversion of the ankle joint; and to strengthen stability of the ankle joint to prevent droop of foot and strephenopodia.

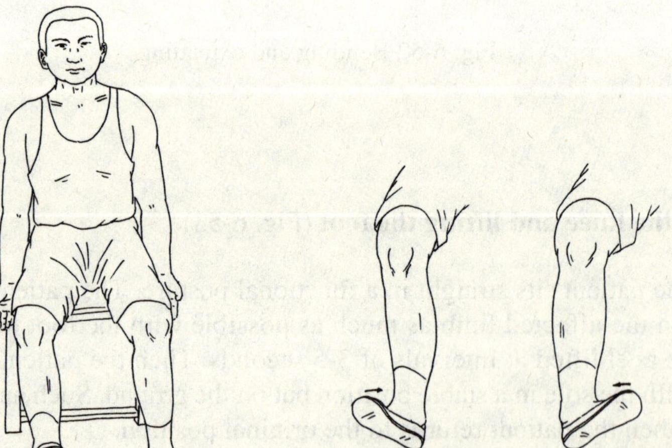

Fig. 6-54 Abduction and adduction

(7) Left and right rotation of the waist (sitting position)

[Method] The patient sits straight in a functional posture. The patient inhales and slowly turns the upper part of the body to the affected side at intervals of 3-5 seconds. Then the patient exhales and slowly turns to the healthy side. Such an exercise is repeated 10-20 times and then the patient returns to the original position.

[Effect] To exercise the muscles responsible for rotating the waist and spine; to prevent deformity of the spine; and to improve functions of the viscera in the chest and abdomen.

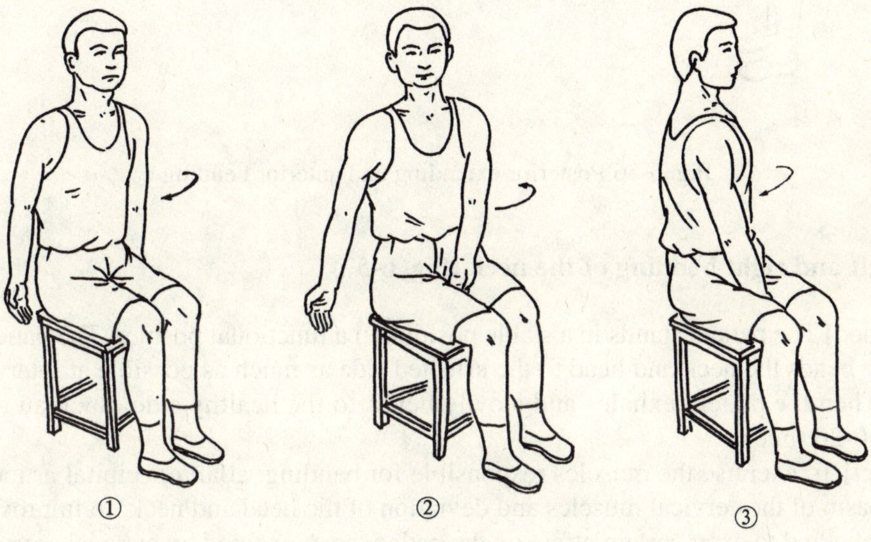

Fig. 6-55 Left and right rotation

(8) Head and neck (standing position)

1) Posterior extending and anterior bending of the neck (Fig. 6-56)

[Method] The patient stands in a stable position in a functional posture. The patient inhales, contracts the abdomen, throws out the chest and slowly extends the neck in a posterior direction as much as possible at intervals of 3-5 seconds. Then the patient exhales and slowly bends in an anterior direction. Such an exercise is repeated 10-20 times (the doctor or nurse should take care of the patient to prevent falling).

[Effect] To exercise the muscles responsible for bending and extending atlantooccipital articulation and the muscles on the chest and abdomen; to prevent spasm and stiffness of the cervical muscles; to improve cerebral balance and blood circulation; and to exert certain effect on the patient accompanied by cervical spondylopathy.

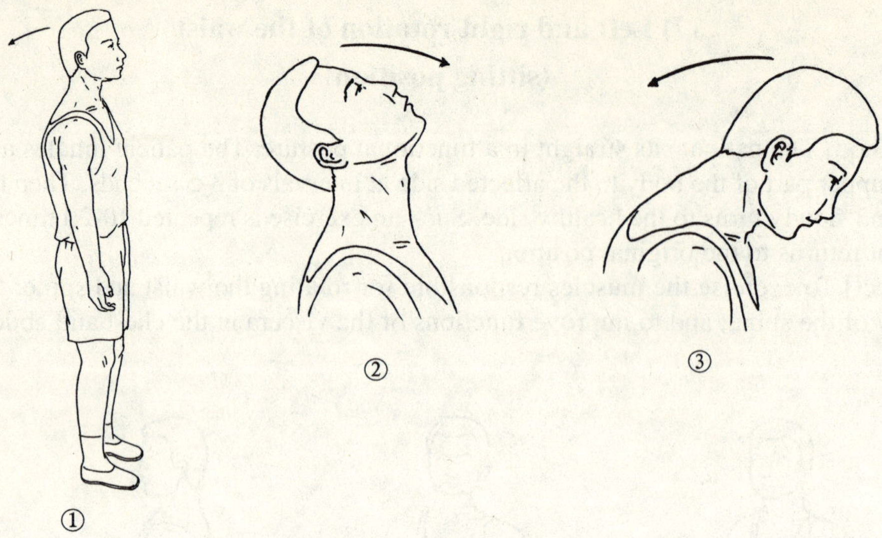

Fig. 6-56 Posterior extending and anterior bending

2) Left and right bending of the neck (Fig. 6-57)

[Method] The patient stands in a stable position in a functional posture. The patient inhales and slowly bends the neck and head to the affected side as much as possible at intervals of 3-5 seconds. Then the patient exhales and slowly bends to the healthy side. Such an exercise is repeated 10-20 times.

[Effect] To exercise the muscles responsible for bending atlantooccipital articulation; to prevent spasm of the cervical muscles and deviation of the head and neck; to improve cerebral blood supply; and to exert certain effect on the patient accompanied by cervical spondylopathy.

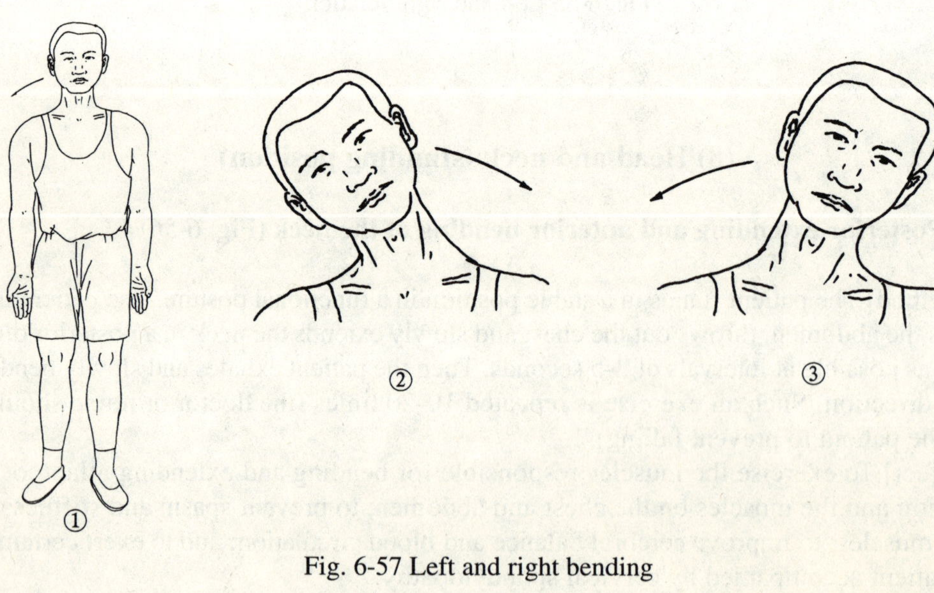

Fig. 6-57 Left and right bending

(9) Upper limbs (standing position)

1) Abducting and lifting the shoulder joint (Fig. 6-58)

[Method] The patient stands in a stable position in a functional posture with both upper limbs hanging naturally at the sides, and the palms turned outward. The patient inhales, contracts the abdomen, throws out the chest, extends the elbows and slowly abducts and lifts the shoulders as much as possible. Then the patient exhales and slowly adducts and lowers the upper limbs. Such an exercise is repeated 10-20 times.

[Effect] To exercise the muscles responsible for abduction and adduction of the shoulder joints, extension of the elbow joints, pronation and a supine position of the forearm as well as the muscles on the chest and abdomen; and to prevent semiluxation of the shoulder joints and spasm of the elbow joints.

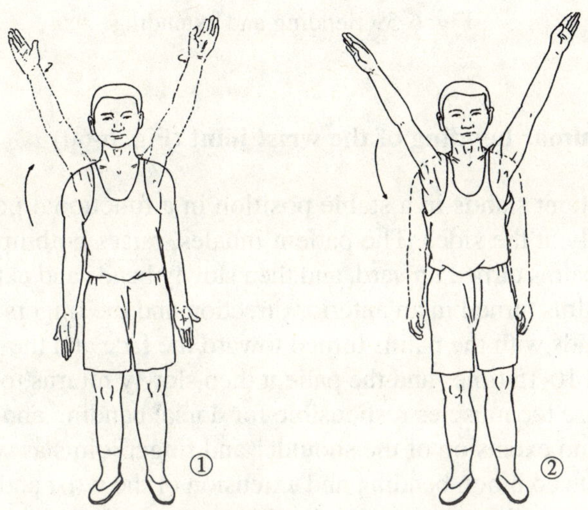

Fig. 6-58 Abducting and lifting

2) Bending and extending the shoulder and elbow joints (Fig. 6-59)

[Method] The patient stands in a stable position in a functional posture with both upper limbs hanging naturally at the sides. The patient inhales and slowly bends the shoulders and extends the elbows as much as possible with the palms turned in an anterior direction. After an interval of 3-5 seconds, the patient exhales, slowly extends the shoulders and bends the elbows with the palms turned downward. Such an exercise is repeated 10-15 times and the patient then returns to the original position (no holding of breath during the exercise).

[Effect] To exercise the muscles responsible for bending and extending the shoulder and elbow joints as well as pronation and a supine position of the forearm; to separate common bending and extending of the shoulder and elbow joints to reduce spasms; and to prevent adhesion of the shoulder joints.

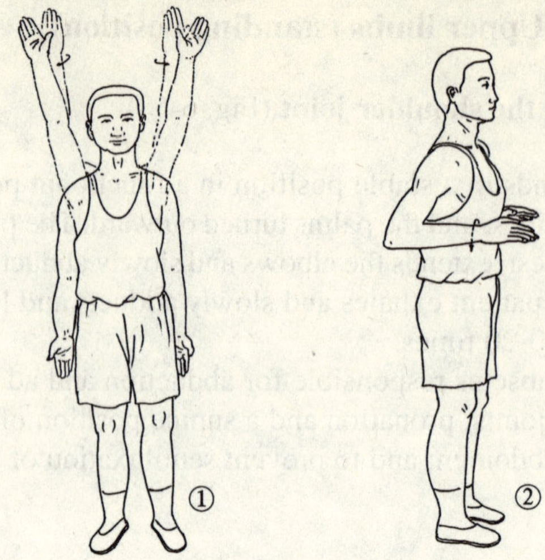

Fig. 6-59 Bending and extending

3) Dorsal and palmar bending of the wrist joint (Fig. 6-60)

[Method] The patient stands in a stable position in a functional posture with both upper limbs hanging naturally at the sides. The patient inhales, raises both upper limbs straight and horizontally, with the palms turned upward, and then slowly bends and extends the wrist as much as possible with the palms turned in an anterior direction and the fingers bent. Then, the patient exhales and slowly bends with the palms turned toward the face and the fingers extended. Such an exercise is repeated 10-15 times and the patient then slowly returns to the original position.

[Effect] To exercise the muscles responsible for dorsal bending and palmar bending of the wrist joints, bending and extension of the shoulder and finger joints as well as extension of the elbow joints; to separate common bending and extension of the wrist and finger joints to reduce spasms; and to prevent semiluxation of the shoulder joints and suspension of the wrist.

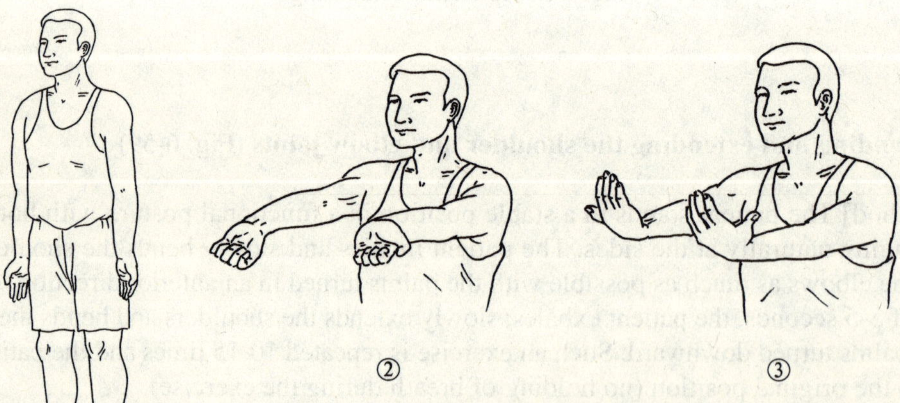

Fig. 6-60 Dorsal and palmar bending

4) Extending and bending the finger joints (Fig. 6-61)

[Method] The patient stands in a stable position in a functional posture with both upper limbs hanging naturally at the sides. The patient inhales, raises both upper limbs straight and horizontally with the palms turned upward, and slowly extends the fingers as much as possible. Then the patient exhales and slowly bends as much as possible. Such an exercise is repeated 10-20 times and the patient then slowly returns to the original position.

[Effect] To exercise the muscles responsible for bending and extending the finger and shoulder joints, as well as extending the elbow joints; to prevent semiluxation of the shoulder joint and spasms of the elbow joints; and to adjust the reflex regulation of the brain to promote restoration of the fine functions of the fingers.

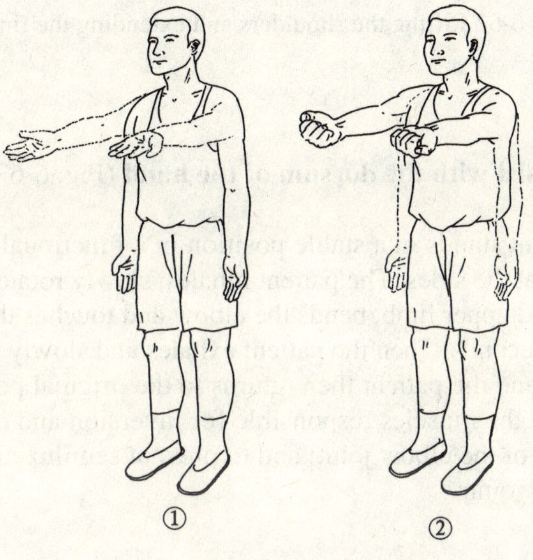

Fig. 6-61 Extending and bending

5) Lifting the shoulders and extending the fingers (Fig. 6-62)

[Method] The patient stands in a stable position in a functional posture with both upper limbs hanging naturally at the sides, with the palms turned in an anterior direction. The patient inhales and slowly lifts the shoulders and extends the fingers as much as possible at intervals of 3-5 seconds. Then the patient exhales and slowly lowers the upper limbs. Such an exercise is repeated 10-20 times and the patient then returns to the original position.

[Effect] To exercise the muscles responsible for bending and extending the shoulder joints, and extending the elbow and finger joints; and to prevent adhesion of the shoulder joints and spasms of the fingers.

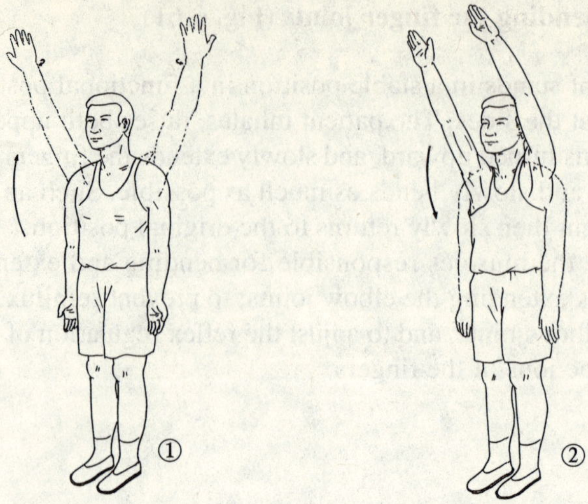

Fig. 6-62 Lifting the shoulders and extending the fingers

6) Touching the waist with the dorsum of the hand (Fig. 6-63)

[Method] The patient stands in a stable position in a functional posture with both upper limbs hanging naturally at the sides. The patient inhales, slowly rotates inward and extends the shoulder with the affected upper limb, bends the elbow and touches the waist with the affected hand at intervals of 3-5 seconds. Then the patient exhales and slowly relaxes. Such an exercise is repeated 10-15 times and the patient then returns to the original position.

[Effect] To exercise the muscles responsible for inversion and extension of the shoulder joint, as well as bending of the elbow joint; and to prevent semiluxation of the shoulder joints and spasms of the elbow joints.

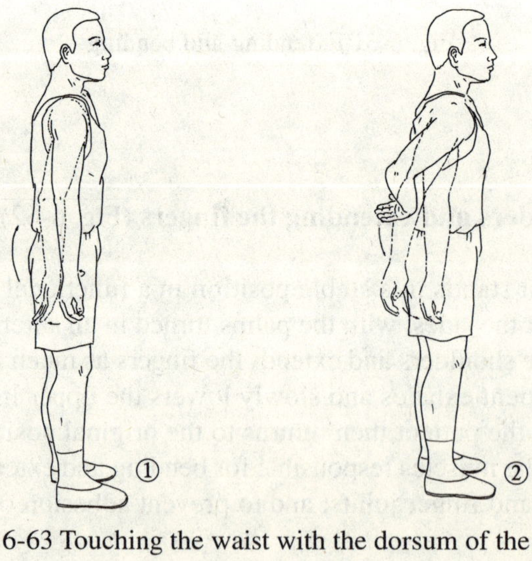

Fig. 6-63 Touching the waist with the dorsum of the hand

(10) Waist and abdomen (standing position)

1) Posterior extending and anterior bending of the waist (Fig. 6-64)

[Method] The patient stands in a stable position in a functional posture with both upper limbs hanging naturally at the sides. The patient inhales and slowly extends the upper part of the body in a posterior direction at intervals of 3-5 seconds. Then the patient exhales and slowly bends the body in an anterior direction. Such an exercise is repeated 10-20 times. The doctor or nurse should take care of the patient, who should not over-extend and bend the waist.

[Effect] To exercise the muscles responsible for bending and extending the spine; to prevent deviation or twisting of the body; and to improve visceral functions.

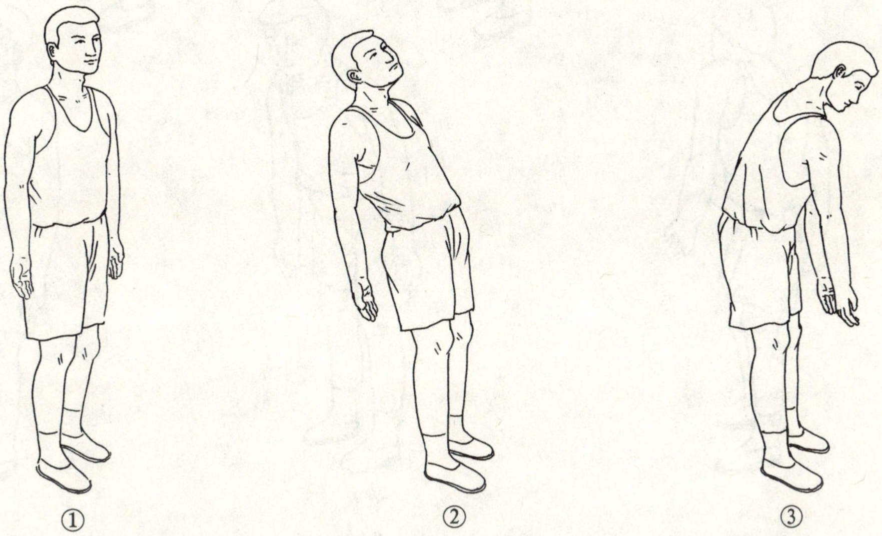

Fig. 6-64 Posterior extending and anterior bending

2) Left and right rotation of the waist (Fig. 6-65)

[Method] The patient stands in a stable position in a functional posture with both upper limbs hanging naturally at the sides. The patient inhales, keeps both lower limbs still and slowly turns the upper part of the body to the affected side as much as possible at intervals of 3-5 seconds. Then the patient exhales and slowly turns to the healthy side. Such an exercise is repeated 10-20 times and the patient then returns to the original position.

[Effect] To exercise the muscles responsible for bending, extending, laterally bending and rotating the spine as well as musculi pectoralis majoris and intercostal muscles; to intensify the activity of the spine; to improve the functions of the heart and lung; and to exert certain curative effect on the patients with cervical spondylopathy.

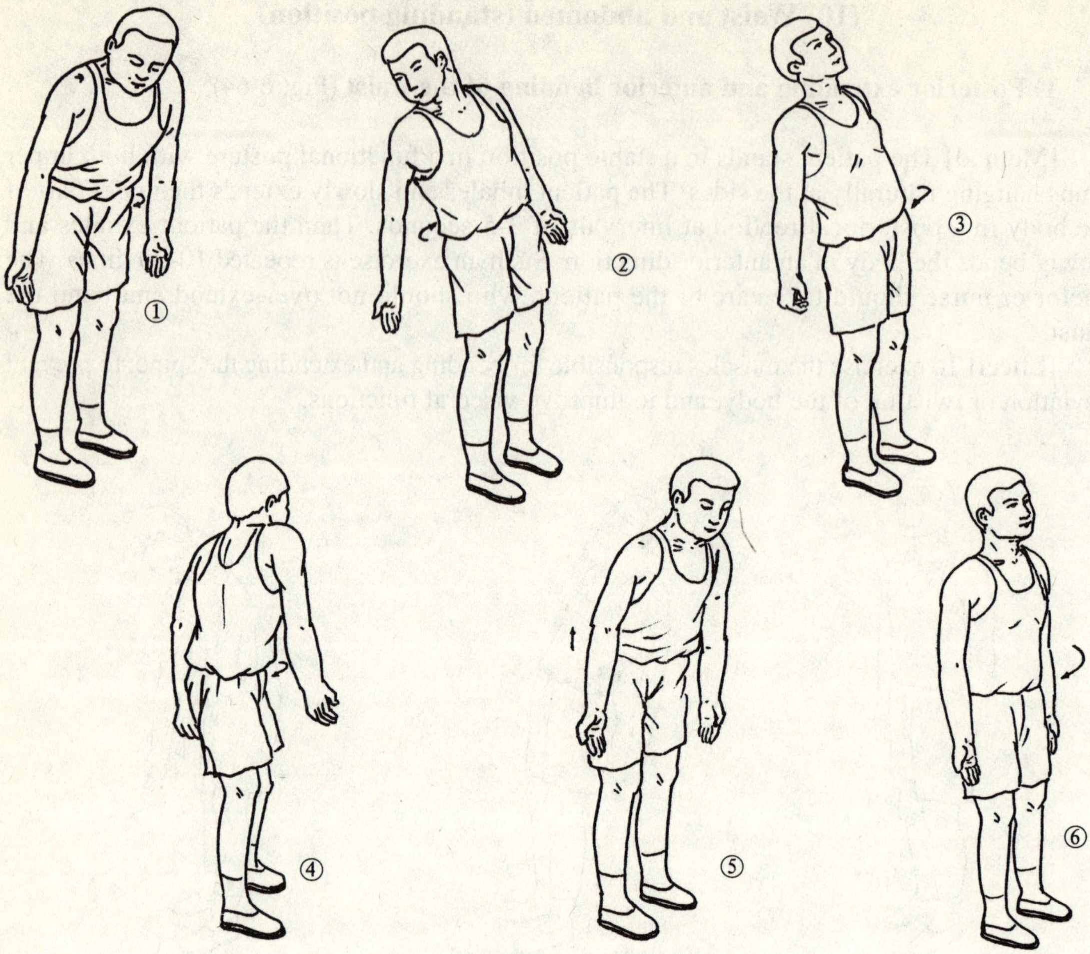

Fig. 6-65 Left and right rotation

(11) Lower limbs (standing position)

1) Bending and extending the hip and knee joints (Fig. 6-66)

[Method] The patient stands in a stable position in a functional posture with both upper limbs hanging naturally at the sides. The patient inhales, shifts the center of the body to the healthy side and slowly extends the hip and bends the knee as much as possible with the affected lower limb at intervals of 3-5 seconds. Then the patient exhales, slowly bends the hip and extends the knee, returns to the original position and puts the sole in a stable position on the ground. Such an exercise is repeated 10-20 times.

[Effect] To exercise the muscles responsible for bending and extending the hip and knee joints; to separate common bending and extending of the hip and knee joints to reduce spasms; and to prevent lifting of the hip and swinging of the leg in walking.

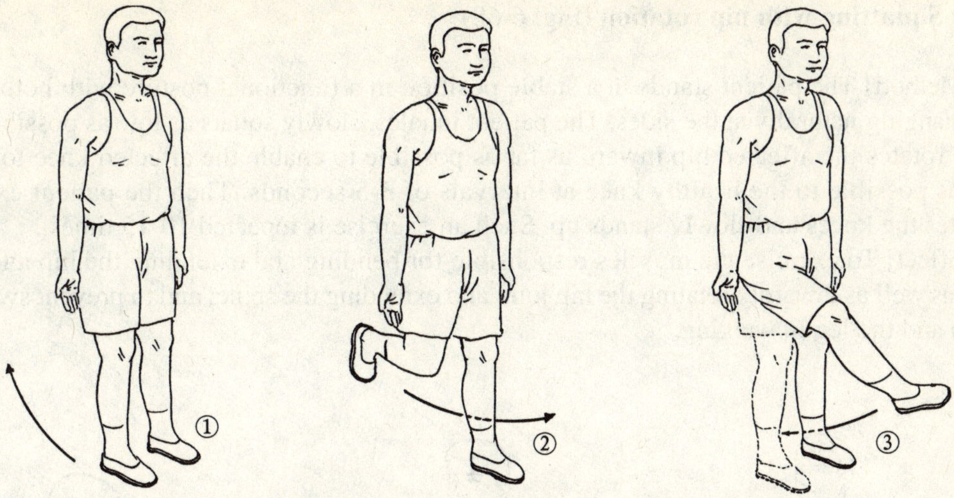

Fig. 6-66 Bending and extending the hip and knee joints

2) Bending and extending the knee joint (Fig. 6-67)

[Method] The patient stands in a stable position in a functional posture with both upper limbs hanging naturally at the sides. The patient inhales, shifts the center of the body to the healthy side and slowly bends the affected knee as much as possible at intervals of 3-5 seconds. Then the patient exhales, slowly extends and puts the sole in a stable position on the ground. Such an exercise is repeated 10-20 times.

[Effect] To exercise the muscles responsible for bending and extending the knee joints; and to prevent lifting the hip and dragging the leg in walking.

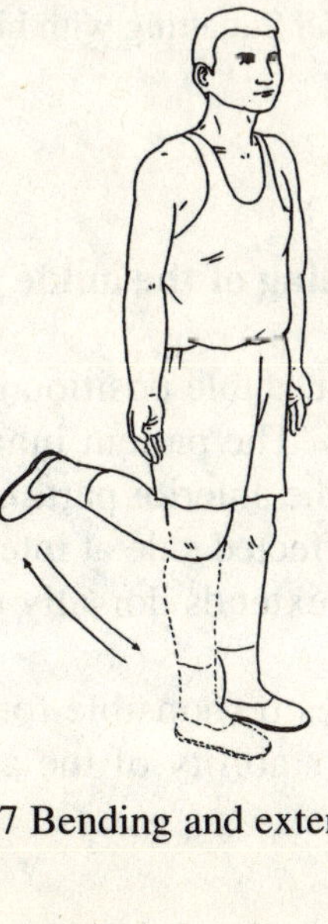

Fig. 6-67 Bending and extending

3) Squatting with hip rotation (Fig. 6-68)

[Method] The patient stands in a stable position in a functional posture with both upper limbs hanging naturally at the sides. The patient inhales, slowly squats as low as possible, and slowly rotates the affected hip inward as far as possible to enable the affected knee to get as close as possible to the healthy knee at intervals of 3-5 seconds. Then the patient exhales, separates the knees and slowly stands up. Such an exercise is repeated 10-15 times.

[Effect] To exercise the muscles responsible for bending and extending the hip and knee joints, as well as inwardly rotating the hip joint and extending the spine; and to prevent swinging the hip and the leg in walking.

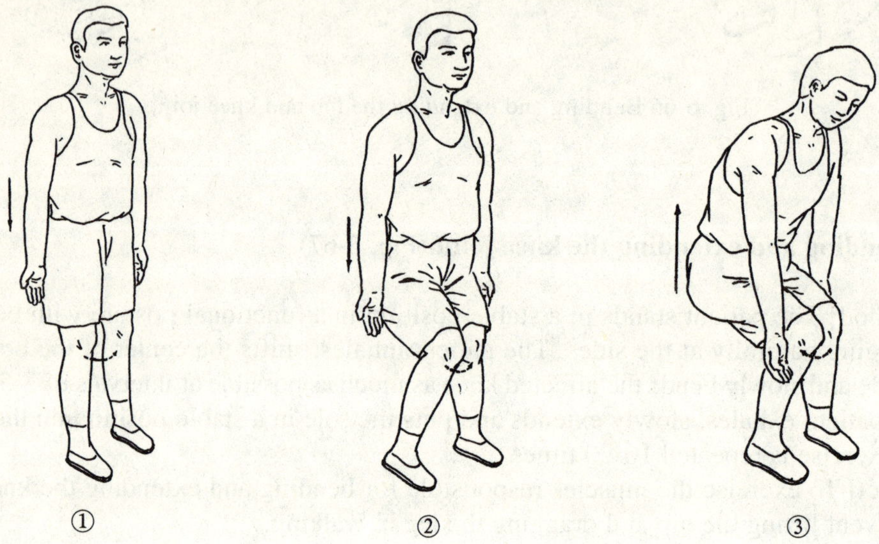

Fig. 6-68 Squatting with hip rotation

4) Metatarsal and dorsal bending of the ankle joint (Fig. 6-69)

[Method] The patient stands in a stable position in a functional posture with both upper limbs hanging naturally at the sides. The patient inhales, slowly lifts both heels as high as possible, bends the ankle joint, puts the anterior parts of the soles on the ground and gradually shifts the center of the body to the affected side at intervals of 3-10 seconds. Then the patient exhales, slowly lowers the feet and extends dorsally to 0°. Such an exercise is repeated 10-20 times.

[Effect] To exercise the muscles responsible for metatarsal and dorsal bending of the ankle joints; and to strengthen the stability of the ankle joints to prevent foot droop and strephenopodia.

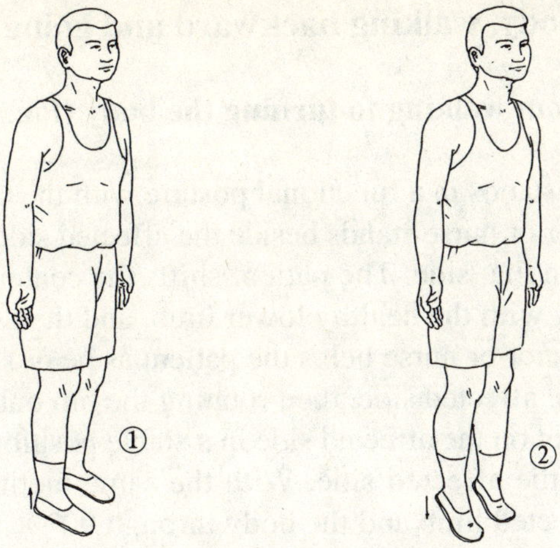

Fig. 6-69 Metatarsal and dorsal bending

(12) Raising the arm and foot, squatting with hip rotation

[Method] The patient stands in a stable position in a functional posture with both upper limbs hanging naturally at the sides. The patient inhales, contracts the abdomen, throws out the chest, extends the upper limbs straight, turns the palms in an anterior direction, slowly raises the hands and heels as much as possible at intervals of 3-10 seconds. Then the patient exhales, slowly lowers the lower limbs and heels, and squats as low as possible, rotates the affected hip inward to enable the affected knee to get close to the healthy knee. Such an exercise is repeated 10-15 times and then the patient returns to the original position.

[Effect] To exercise the muscles responsible for bending and extending the shoulder, hip, knee and ankle joints as well as extending the elbow joints and the chest and abdominal muscles; to strengthen the stability of the joints on the lower limbs and the constitution; and to improve blood circulation.

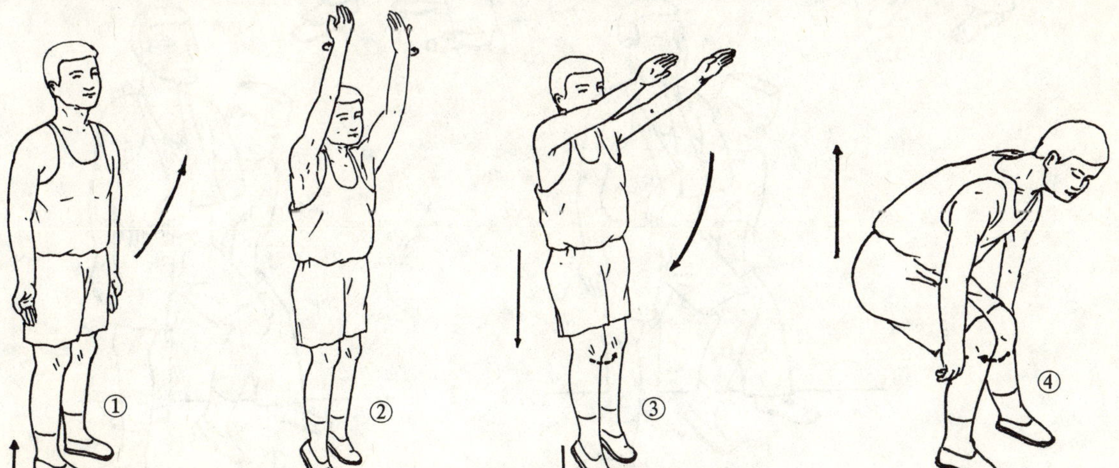

Fig. 6-70 Raising the arm and foot, squatting with hip rotation

(13) Turning the body, walking backward and going up and down stairs

1) Passive change from walking to turning the body (Fig. 6-71)

[Method] The patient stands in a functional posture with the affected upper limb dangling before the chest. The doctor or nurse stands beside the affected side of the patient and holds the patient's knee and waist on that side. The patient shifts the center of the body to the affected side, walks a step medially with the healthy lower limb, and then shifts the center of the body to the healthy side. The doctor or nurse helps the patient as he or she slowly bends the hip and knee, lifting the foot on the affected side, then rotating the hip outwards and turning the body through 90°, putting the foot on the affected side in a stable position on the ground and shifting the center of the body to the affected side. With the same method, the patient extends the healthy limb, turns the affected limb and the body through 90°.

[Effect] To exercise the muscles responsible for bending and extending the hip, knee and ankle joints as well as everting the hip joint; to strengthen the coordination of the lower limbs; and to improve cerebral balance.

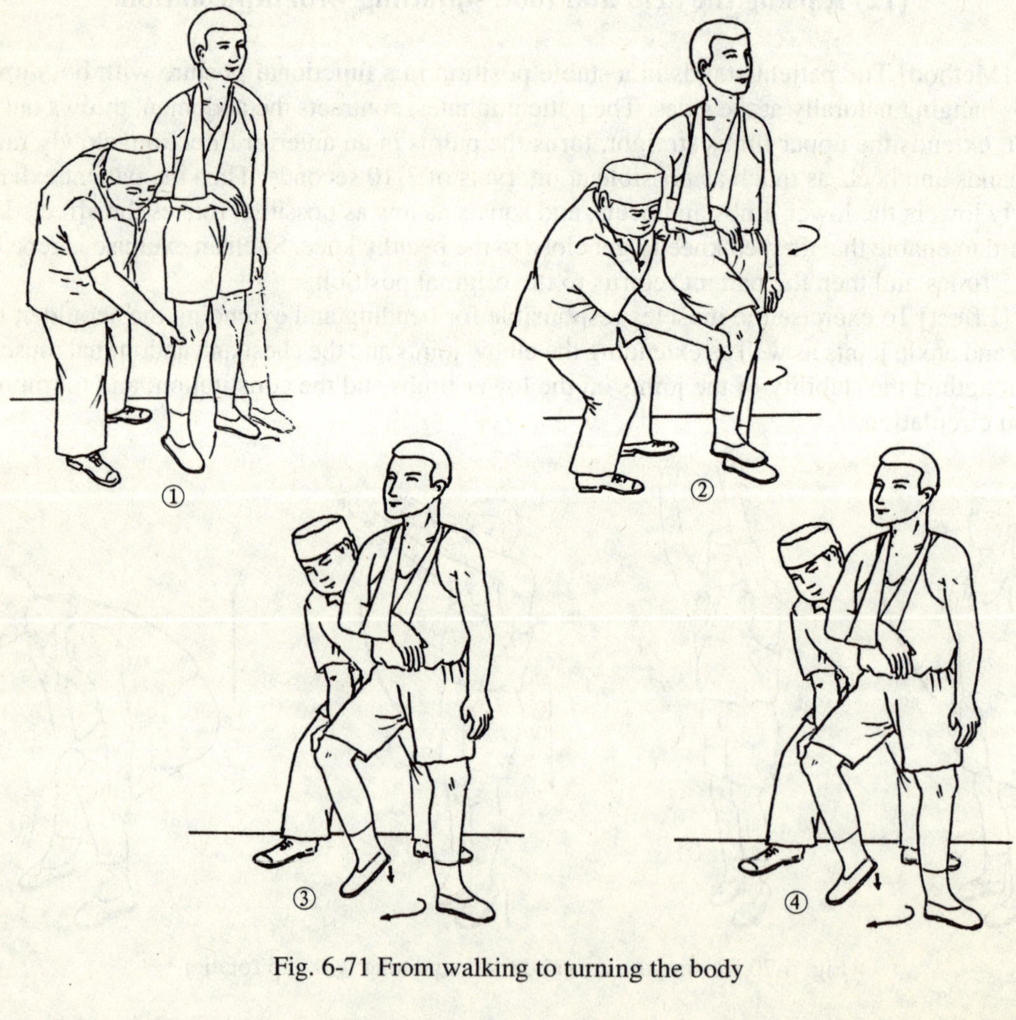

Fig. 6-71 From walking to turning the body

2) Active change from walking to turning the body (Fig. 6-72)

[Method] The patient stands in a functional posture with the affected upper limb dangling before the chest. The doctor stands beside the affected side and holds the patient's knee and waist on that side. The patient shifts the center of the body to the affected side, walks a small step medially with the healthy lower limb, and then, raising the anterior part of the affected foot, abducts the foot and rotates the hip outwardly, turning the body through 90° and shifting the center of the body to the affected side with the posterior part of the affected foot as the fixing point. With the same method the patient extends the healthy limb, rotating the affected hip, and turns the body through 90°. Gradually, the patient may walk without help (but the doctor or nurse should still stand beside the affected side).

[Effect] To exercise the muscles responsible for abduction of the talocalcanean articulation, dorsal bending of the ankle joint and eversion of the hip joint; and to improve cerebral balance and the locating function.

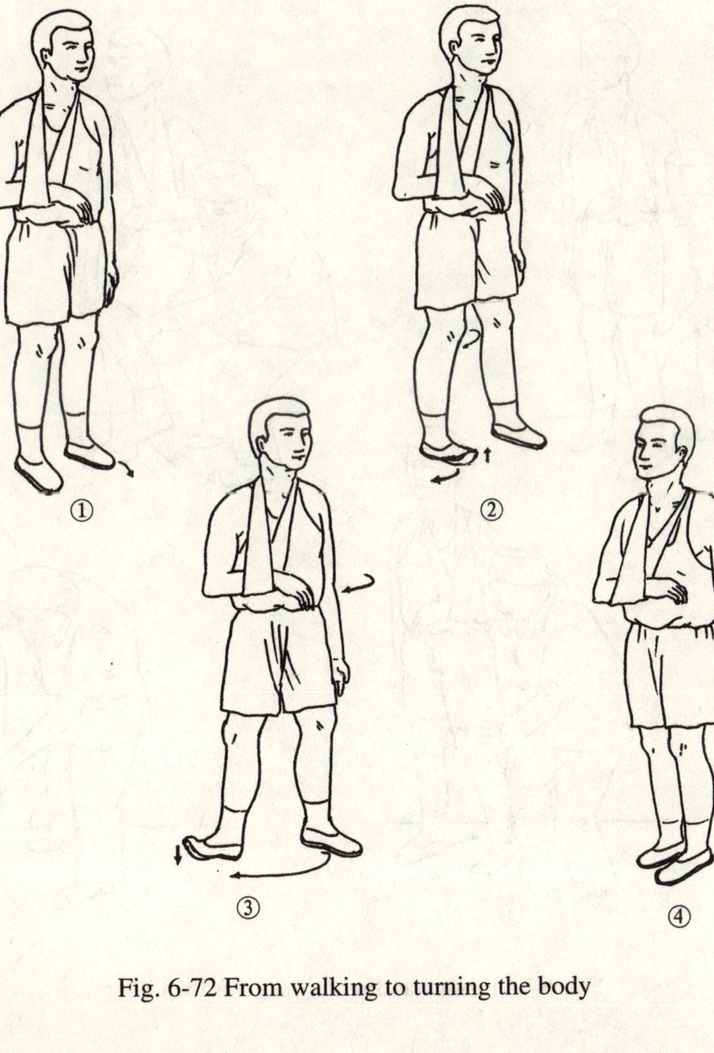

Fig. 6-72 From walking to turning the body

3) Passive change from standing to backward walking (Fig. 6-73)

[Method] The patient stands in a functional posture with the affected upper limb dangling before the chest. The doctor or nurse stands beside the affected side and holds the patient's knee and waist on that side. The patient shifts the center of the body to the healthy side. The doctor or nurse helps the patient to slowly bend the hip and knee and lift the foot on the affected side. The patient takes a small step backward with the affected lower limb, extending the hip and knee, touching the ground with the anterior part of the sole, slowly putting the entire sole in a stable position on the ground and then shifting the center of the body to the affected side. With the same method, the patient takes a small step backward, keeping the healthy foot and affected foot parallel to each other and maintaining an upright stance. The lower limbs walk backward alternatively with the same method.

[Effect] To exercise the muscles responsible for bending and extending the hip, knee and ankle joints, as well as the waist and back muscles; to prevent leaning forward with the upper part of the body while walking; and to improve cerebral balance.

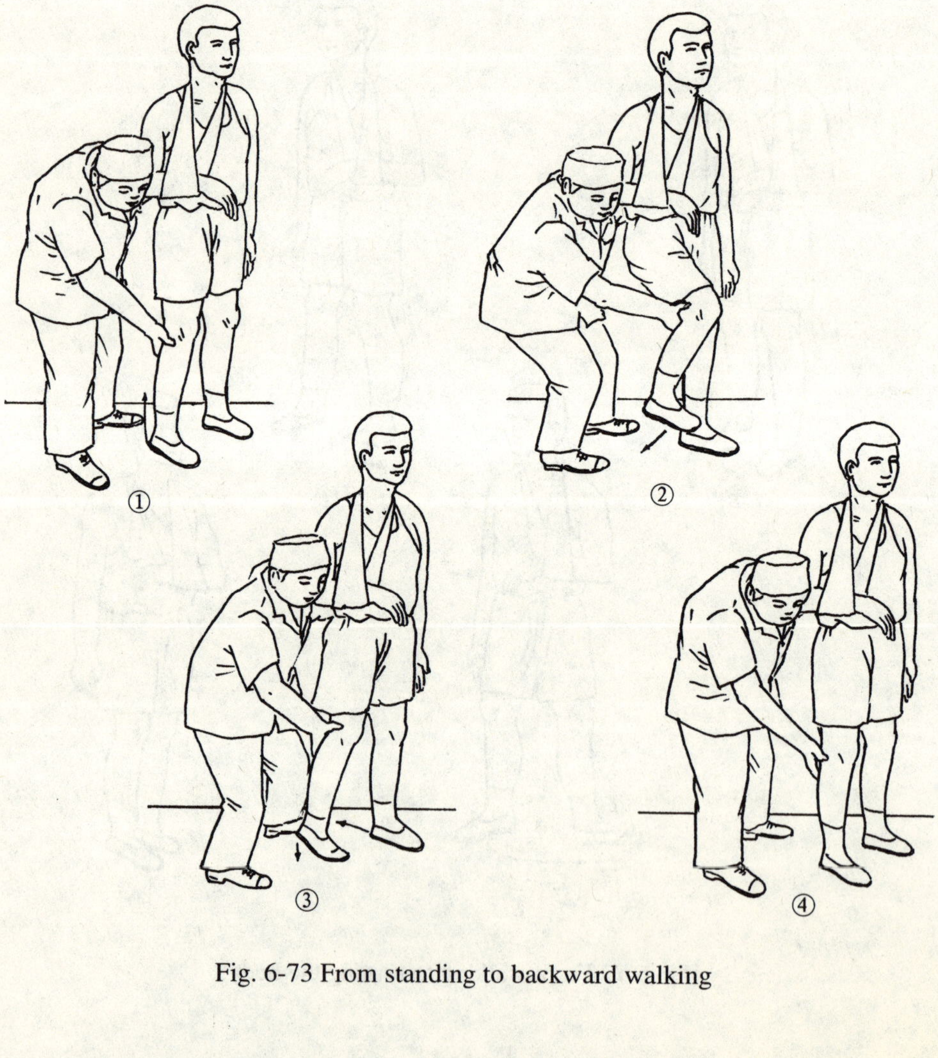

Fig. 6-73 From standing to backward walking

4) Active change from standing to backward walking (Fig. 6-74)

[Method] The patient stands in a functional posture with the affected upper limb dangling before the chest. The patient shifts the center of the body to the healthy side, slowly bends the hip and knee and lifts the foot as much as possible with the affected lower limb, takes a step straight backward, extends the hip and knee with the anterior part of the foot touching the ground first, slowly puts the whole foot in a stable position on the ground, and then shifts the center of the body to the affected side. With the same method, the healthy limb takes a step backward, and this should continue alternately (the doctor or nurse stands behind the patient for protection).

[Effect] To exercise the muscles responsible for bending and extending the hip, knee and ankle joints as well as the waist and back muscles; to prevent "humpback"; and to improve cerebral functions and strengthen the balance, coordination and skill ability.

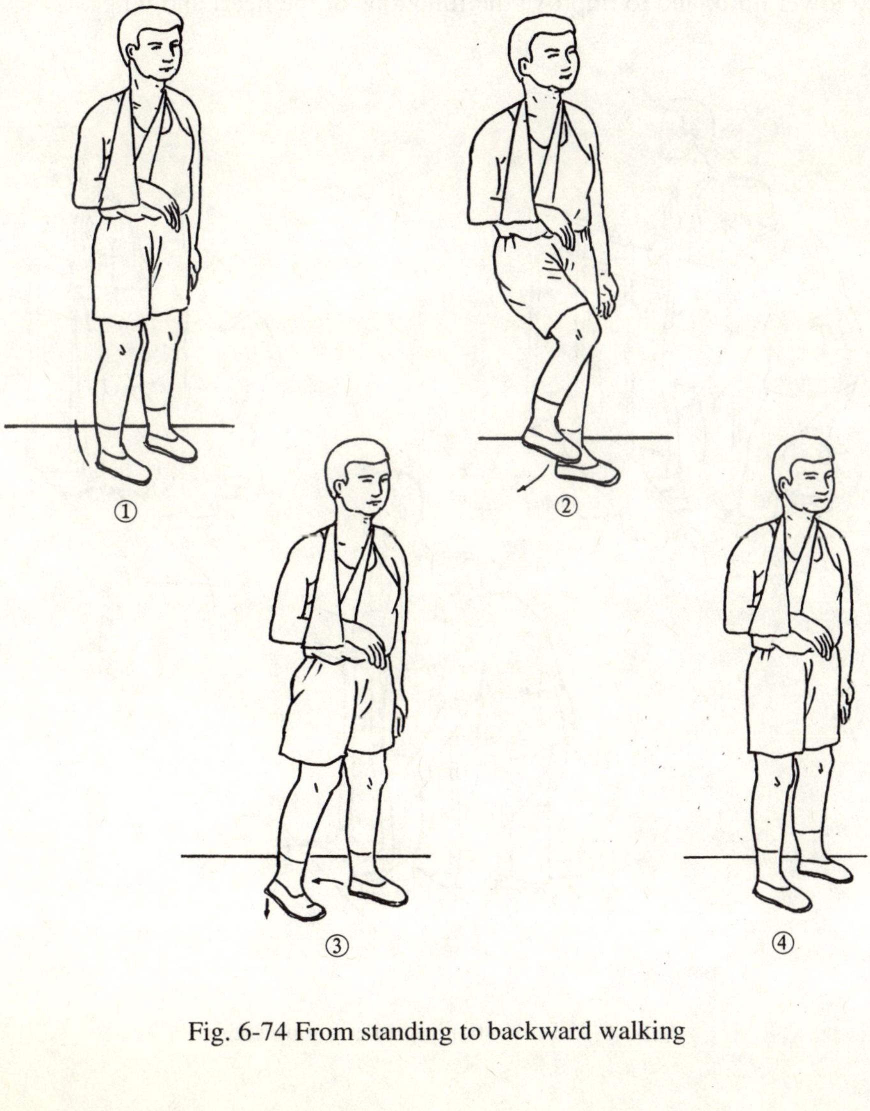

Fig. 6-74 From standing to backward walking

5) Passive change from standing to going up stairs (Fig. 6-75)

[Method] The patient stands in a functional posture with the affected upper limb dangling in front of the chest. The doctor or nurse stands beside the affected side and holds the patient's knee and waist on that side. The patient shifts the center of the body to the affected side, bends the hip and knee on the healthy limb, quickly steps onto the stair and then shifts the center of the body to the healthy side. The patient inhales and the doctor or nurse helps the patient slowly bend the hip and knee and lift the foot on the affected side. At the same time, the healthy lower limb is used to extend the hip and knee as much as possible, and the patient lifts the body as the affected lower limb slowly steps onto the stair. Then the patient exhales, stretches out the hip and knee on the affected limb, puts the whole foot in a stable position on the ground and stands in a stable position.

[Effect] To exercise the muscles responsible for bending and extending the hip, knee and ankle joints as well as the waist and abdominal muscles; to strengthen the myodynamia of the muscles responsible for extending the healthy lower limb; to prevent stiffness of the joints on the affected lower limb; and to improve the functions of the heart and lungs.

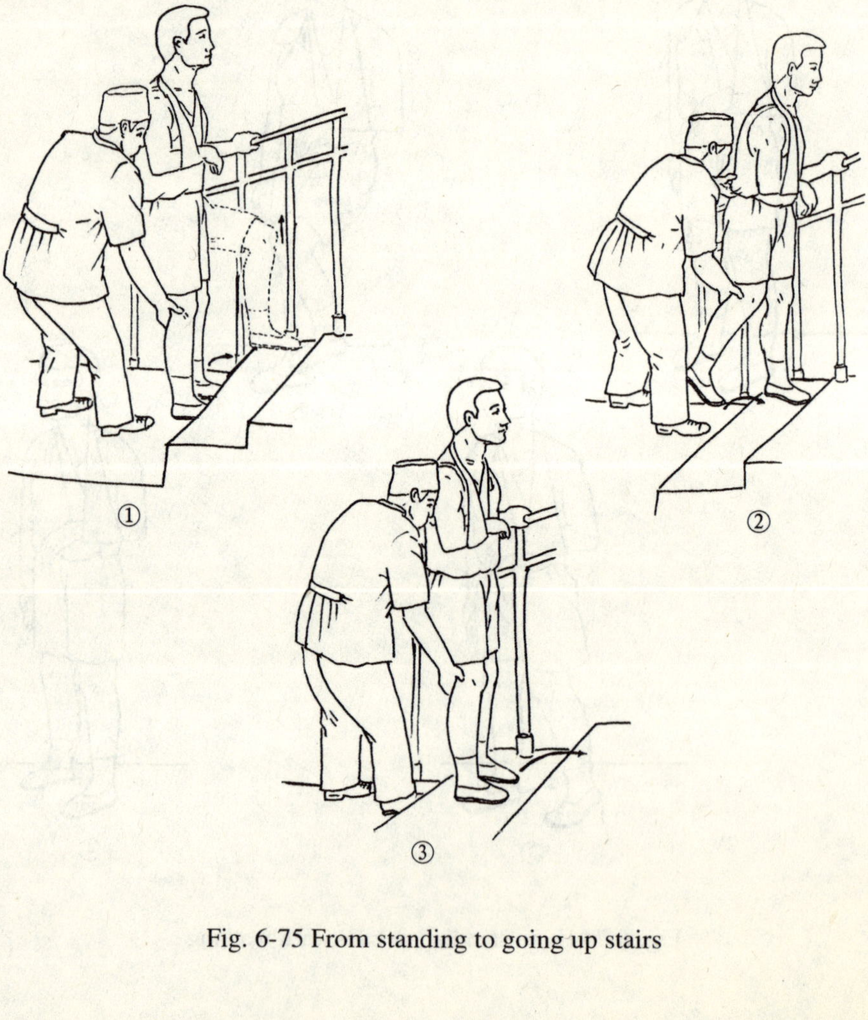

Fig. 6-75 From standing to going up stairs

6) Passive change from standing to going down stairs (Fig. 6-76)

[Method] The patient stands in a stable position in a functional posture with the affected upper limb hanging in front of the chest. The doctor or nurse stands beside the affected side and holds the patient's knee and waist. The patient shifts the center of the body to the healthy side, bends the hip and knee on the healthy lower limb, and lowers the body. The patient inhales and the doctor or nurse helps the patient slowly bend the hip and knee and lift the foot as much as possible on the affected side. The patient steps onto the next stair, puts the sole in a stable position and shifts the center of the body to the affected side. Then the patient exhales, quickly brings the healthy lower limb into line and stands in a stable position.

[Effect] To exercise the muscles responsible for bending and extending the hip, knee and ankle joints, as well as the waist and abdominal muscles; to strengthen the myodynamia of the muscles responsible for bending the healthy lower limb and stability of the joints on the affected lower limb; to reduce spasms of the hip and knee joints, as well as the cerebrovascular functions.

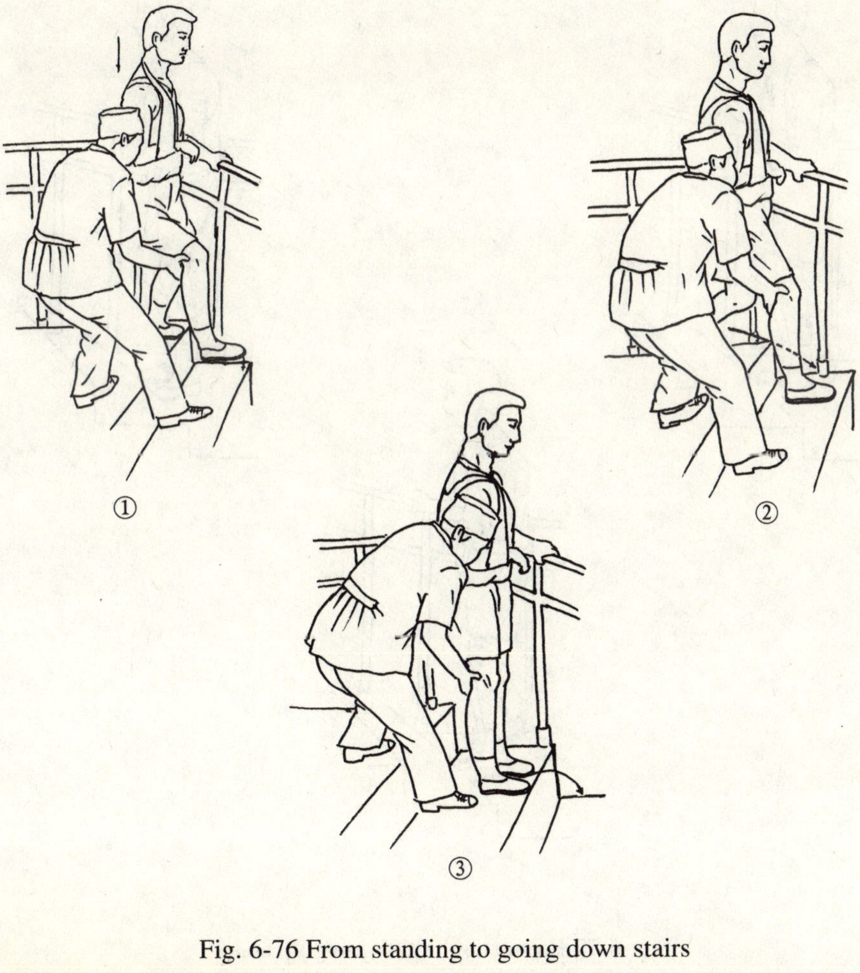

Fig. 6-76 From standing to going down stairs

7) Active change from standing to going up stairs (Fig. 6-77)

[Method] The patient stands in a functional posture with the affected upper limb hanging before the chest and the center of the body shifting to the healthy side. The patient inhales, slowly bends the hip and knee and lifts the foot as much as possible on the affected side, slowly stepping onto the next stair and gradually shifting the center of the body to the affected side. Then the patient exhales, treads the stair with the healthy lower limb, lifts the foot, extends the hip and knee with the affected limb, and raises the body to step into line. Gradually, the patient walks up stairs alternately with the healthy and affected lower limbs (the doctor or nurse walks behind and keeps his hands beside the waist to prevent the patient from leaning forward).

[Effect] To exercise the muscles responsible for bending and extending the hip, knee and ankle joints, as well as the waist and abdominal muscles; to strengthen the myodynamia of the muscles responsible for extending the healthy lower limb and stability of the joints on the affected lower limb; and to improve the functions of the heart and lungs as well as the cerebral balance.

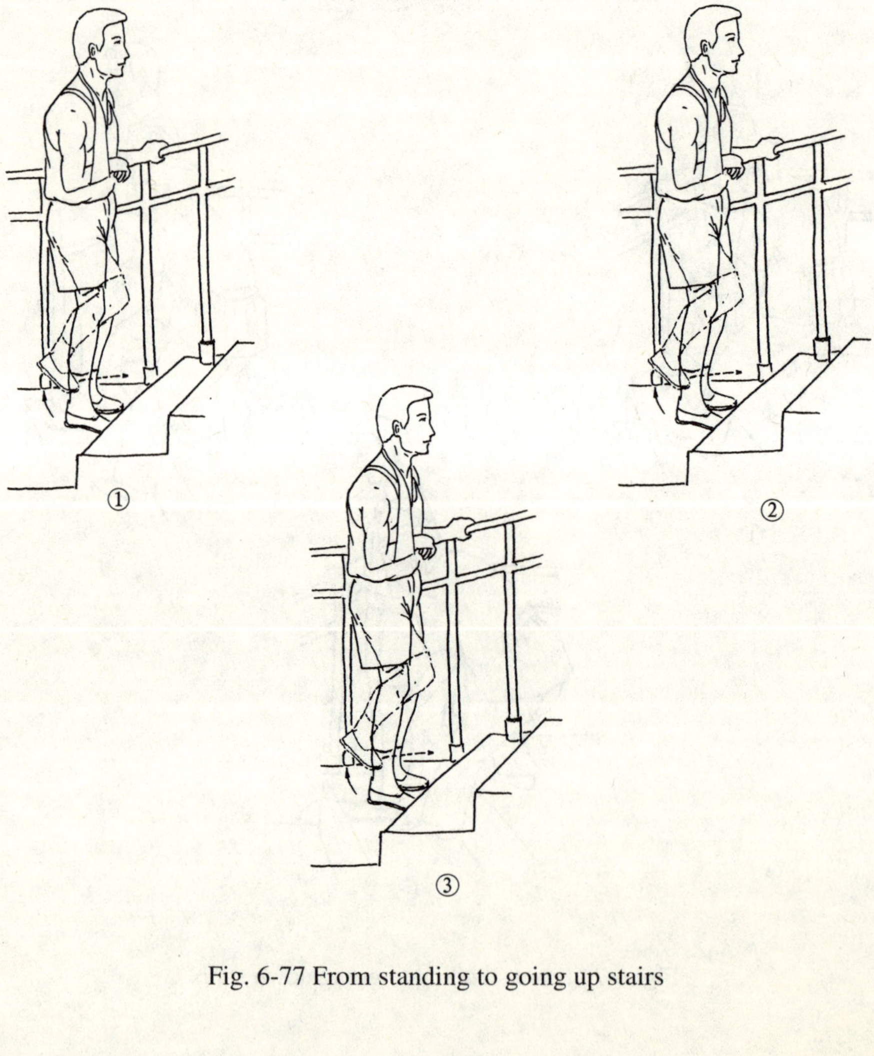

Fig. 6-77 From standing to going up stairs

8) Active change from standing to going down stairs (Fig. 6-78)

[Method] The patient stands in a functional posture with the affected upper limb hanging before the chest and with the center of the body shifting to the affected side. The patient inhales, slowly bends the hip and knee on the affected side, lowers the body, slowly stepping onto the next lower stair and quickly shifting the center of the body to the healthy side. Then the patient exhales, lifts the affected lower limb to step onto the same stair with the sole in a stable position. Gradually the patient walks down stairs alternately with the healthy and affected lower limbs (the doctor or nurse stands in front to prevent the patient from leaning forward).

[Effect] To exercise the muscles responsible for bending and extending the hip, knee and ankle joints as well as the muscles on the waist and abdomen; to strengthen the myodynamia of the muscles responsible for bending the affected lower limb; and to improve the cardio and cerebrovascular functions.

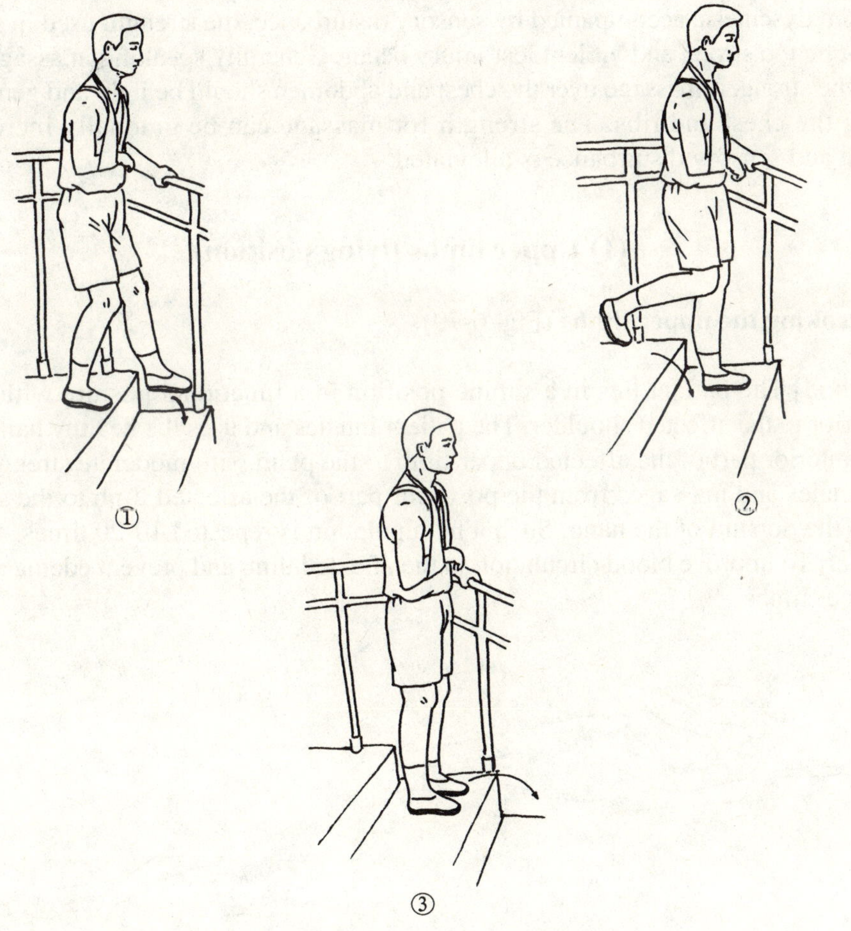

Fig. 6-78 From standing to going down stairs

3. SELF-MASSAGE

If the patient is conscious and has no dysfunction of the heart and lungs, he/she may massage himself/herself. Self-massage not only supplements treatment, but also exercises the healthy limb and promotes blood circulation in the affected limb to improve the cardio and cerebrovascular functions, as well as strengthening the constitution and ensuring early rehabilitation.

Before performing self-massage, the patient should get familiar with acupoints and their locations and effects by reading relevant books under the guidance and instruction of the doctor. It is advisable to cut and polish the nails on the healthy hand to avoid scratching the skin. To massage with toes on the healthy foot, the patient should wear a clean sock to prevent cross infection.

In doing self-massage, the manipulation at the beginning should be light and done sequentially and systematically according to the illustrations in this part. Self-massage should be done once a day for 30-50 minutes each time. Since the patient with hemiplegia usually suffers from dyscinesia accompanied by sensory disturbance, the strength used in self-massage should not be too strong and violent lest injury occur. Generally speaking, massage around the joints can be stronger; massage over the chest and abdomen should be light and gentle, avoiding damaging the chest and ribs. The strength for massage can be gradually increased as the dyscinesia and sensory disturbance is alleviated.

(1) Upper limbs (lying position)

1) Stroking the upper limbs (Fig. 6-79)

[Method] The patient lies in a supine position in a functional posture with the healthy hand anterior to the affected shoulder. The patient inhales and uses the healthy hand massaging from the anterior part of the affected upper limb to the palm with moderate strength. Then the patient exhales and massages from the posterior part of the affected limb to the shoulder and back with the dorsum of the hand. Such a manipulation is repeated 10-20 times.

[Effect] To improve blood circulation in the affected limb and prevent edema and bedsores on the upper limbs

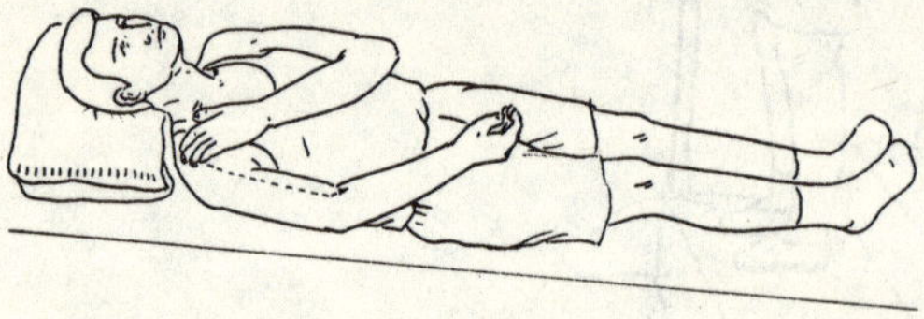

①

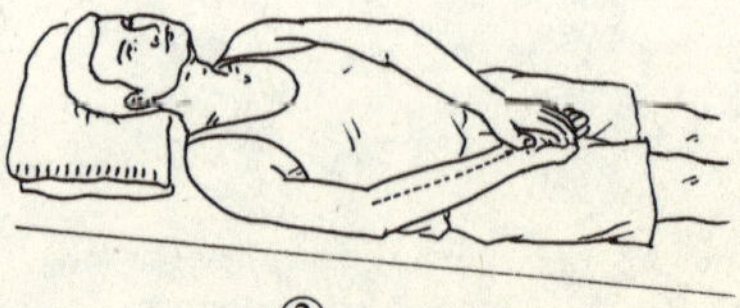

②

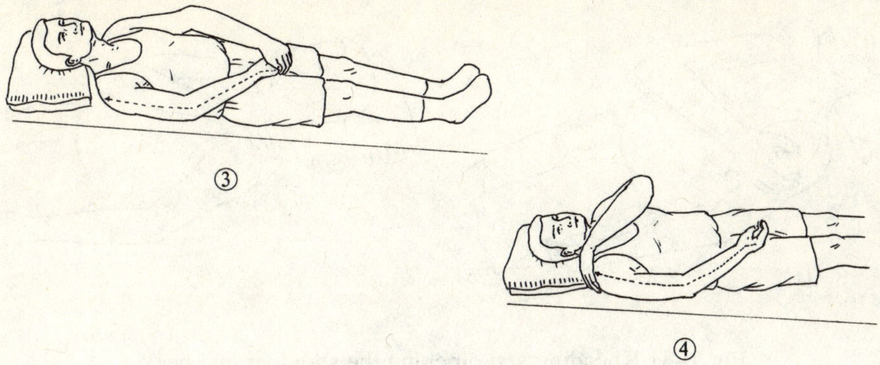

Fig. 6-79 Stroking the upper limbs

2) Kneading and pinching the upper limbs (Fig. 6-80)

[Method] The patient lies in a supine position in a functional posture with the fingers of the healthy hand placed anterior and medial to the affected shoulder. The patient kneads and pinches from the anterior and medial part of the affected upper limb to the wrist with moderate strength. Then the patient kneads and pinches from the dorsal side of the fingers on the affected side to the posterior side of the affected limb and shoulder. Such a manipulation is repeated 10-20 times.

[Effect] To improve blood circulation in the affected limb and prevent shoulder-hand syndrome; and to help eliminate fatigue of the affected limb after exercise.

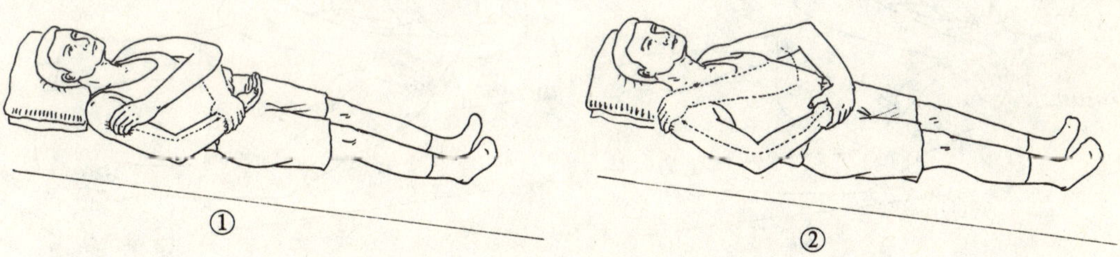

Fig. 6-80 Kneading and pinching the upper limbs

3) Kneading and pinching the shoulder and neck (Fig. 6-81)

[Method] The patient lies in a supine position in a functional posture with the finger pads of the healthy hand beside the affected acromion. The patient kneads and pinches from the upper part of the shoulder to the shoulder and neck with moderate strength. Such a manipulation is repeated 10-15 times.

[Effect] To prevent deviation of the head and neck and relieve pain in the shoulder and back; and to relieve accompanied cervical spondylopathy to a certain extent.

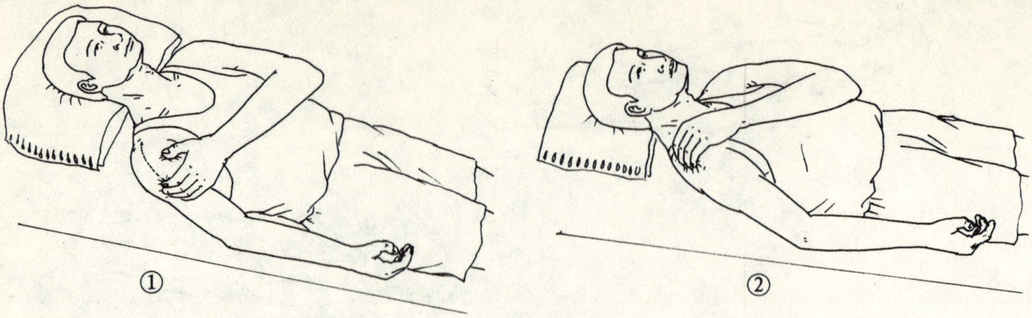

Fig. 6-81 Kneading and pinching the shoulder and neck

4) Kneading and pressing Jianjing point (Fig. 6-82)

[Method] The patient lies in a supine position in a functional posture with the finger bellies of the healthy hand beside the trapezium muscle. The patient kneads and pinches 10-20 times with moderate strength. Then the middle finger is used to press and knead Jianjing (GB 21) 3-5 times, 10-15 seconds each time.

[Acupoint] Jianjing: Located on the middle point of the line connecting the acromion with the point below the seventh cervical vertebral process.

[Effect] To prevent deviation of the head and neck; to refresh the mind and achieve certain effects in relieving mental fatigue and somnolence after falling ill.

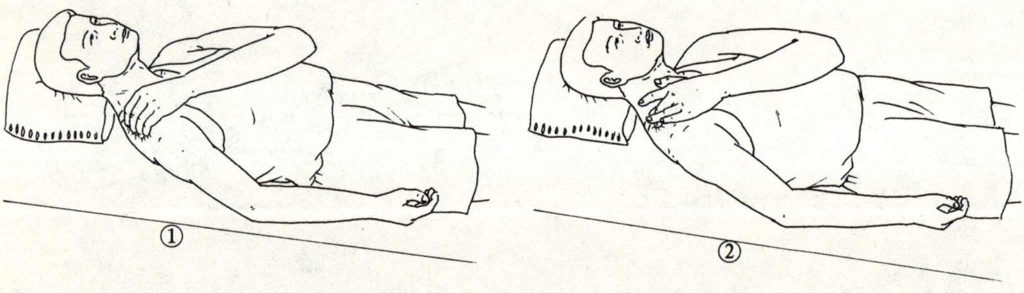

Fig. 6-82 Kneading and pressing Jianjing point

5) Kneading and pinching the shoulder and arm (Fig. 6-83)

[Method] The patient lies in a supine position in a functional posture with the finger pads of the healthy hand above the deltoid muscle. The patient kneads and pinches from the lateral part to the lower border of the deltoid muscle with moderate strength. Such a manipulation is repeated 10-15 times.

[Effect] To promote the restoration of the shoulder and arm myodynamia to prevent semiluxation of the shoulder joint.

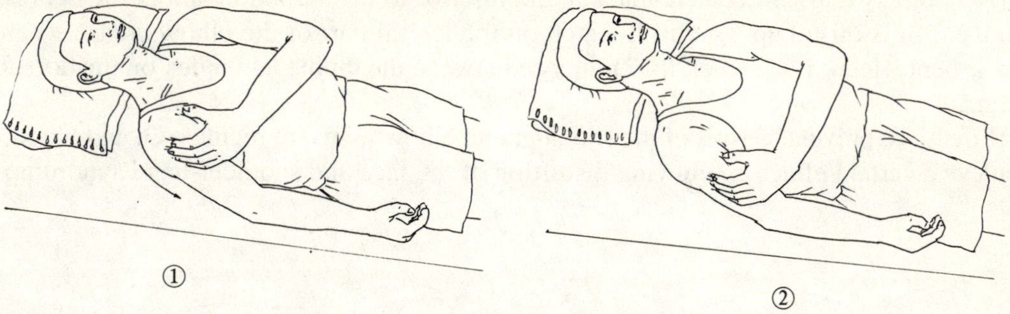

Fig. 6-83 Kneading and pinching the shoulder and arm

6) Kneading and pinching shoulder acupoints (Fig. 6-84)

[Method] The patient lies in a supine position in a functional posture. The thumb and index finger of the healthy hand are put on Jianyu (LI 15) and Jianliao (TE 14), kneading for 1-2 minutes with moderate strength. Then the palm is used to rub around 10-15 times.

[Acupoints] Jianyu: Located anterior and inferior to the acromion and in the depression when the arm is raised up. Jianliao: Located posterior and inferior to the acromion and in the depression behind Jianyu.

[Effect] To promote the restoration of the functions of the deltoid muscle to prevent semiluxation of the shoulder joint; to relieve convulsion and pain; and to alleviate pain in the shoulder and arm.

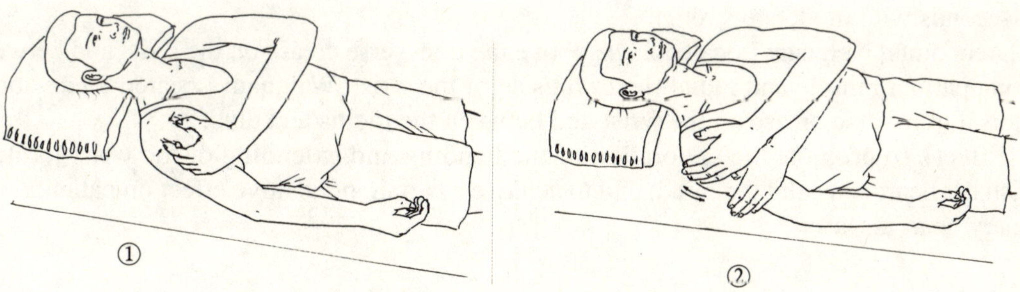

Fig. 6-84 Kneading and pinching shoulder acupoints

7) Pressing and kneading three acupoints on the arm (Fig. 6-85)

[Method] The patient lies in a supine position in a functional posture. The thumb and index finger of the healthy hand are put on the Jianyu (LI 15), Hegu (BL 55) and Quchi (LI 11) on the affected hand and arm and knead for 3-5 seconds respectively with moderate strength. Such a manipulation is repeated 3-5 times.

[Acupoints] Jianyu: Located anterior and inferior to the acromion and in the depression when the arm is raised up. Quchi: Located on the lateral part of the elbow crease when the elbow is bent. Hegu: Located on the eminence between the thumb and index on the dorsum of the hand.

[Effect] To prevent spasms of the shoulder and elbow joints; to regulate Qi and blood; and to achieve a certain effect in relieving distortion of the face and shoulder-hand syndrome.

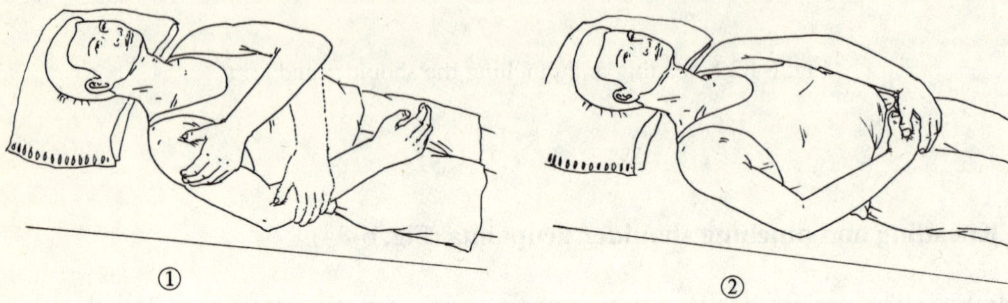

Fig. 6-85 Pressing and kneading three acupoints on the arm

8) Kneading and pressing the forearm (Fig. 6-86)

[Method] The patient lies in a supine position in a functional posture with the finger pads of the healthy hand beside the wrist on the affected side. The patient kneads and pinches from the anterior and posterior parts of the forearm to the elbow 5-15 times with moderate strength. The thumb and index finger are put on the Neiguan (PC 6) and Waiguan (TE 15) and knead for 5-15 seconds with moderate strength.

[Acupoints] Neiguan: Located 2 *cun* above the transverse crease on the wrist and between the long palmar muscle and radial flexor muscle of the wrist. Waiguan: Located 2 *cun* above the dorsal transverse crease on the wrist and between the radius and ulna.

[Effect] To promote the restoration of the bending and extending of the wrist joint; to nourish the heart and calm the mind; and to achieve a certain preventive effect on patients with coronary heart disease.

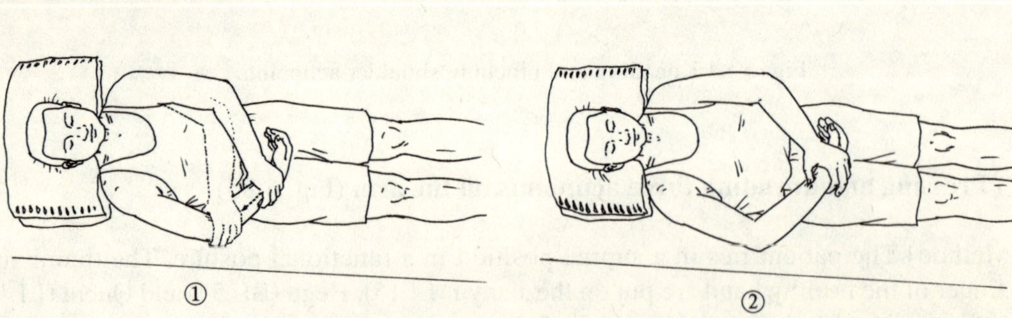

Fig. 6-86 Kneading and pressing the forearm

9) Flicking Xiaohai (Fig. 6-87)

[Method] The patient lies in a supine position in a functional posture. The tips of the four fingers of the healthy hand are put on Xiaohai (SI 8) located posterior and medial to the affected elbow to flick with moderate strength until an aching and numb sensation are felt on the fourth finger and the small finger on the affected limb. Such a flicking manipulation is repeated 5-10 times

[Acupoint] Xiaohai: Located in the depression between the olecranon and medial epicondyle.

[Effect] To prevent spasm of the elbow joint and help restore the functions of fingers; to dredge the meridians and activate the collaterals; and to achieve a certain effect in relieving accompanied headache and cervical pain.

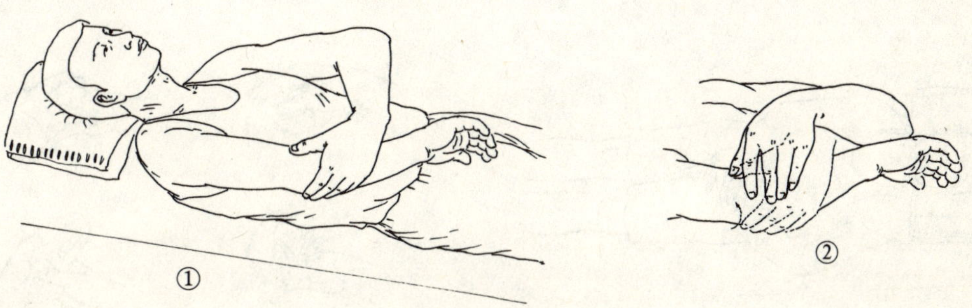

Fig. 6-87 Flicking Xiaohai

10) Kneading and pressing Hegu (Fig. 6-88)

[Method] The patient lies in a supine position in a functional posture. The palm of the healthy hand is put on the dorsal side of the fingers on the affected hand. Then the patient kneads and presses from the dorsal transverse crease on the wrist upward with moderate strength 10-20 times. Then the thumb is used to press Hegu for 30-60 seconds with moderate strength.

[Acupoint] Hegu: Located on the eminence between the thumb and index on the dorsum of the hand.

[Effect] To restore the bending and extending function of the finger joints as well as the abduction and adduction of the thumb; to disperse wind and dredge the collaterals; and to achieve a certain curative effect in relieving a distorted face and dysphasia.

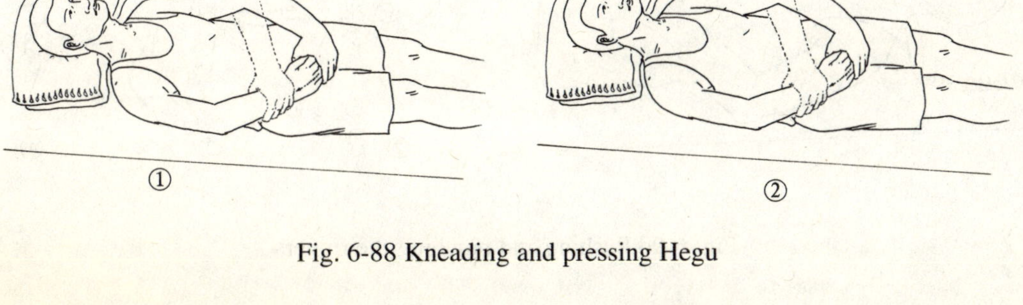

Fig. 6-88 Kneading and pressing Hegu

11) Kneading and pressing the palm (Fig. 6-89)

[Method] The patient lies in a supine position in a functional posture. The thumb and index finger of the healthy hand are put in an anterior and posterior direction to the major and minor thenar of the affected hand. The patient kneads upward to the wrist crease 10-15 times respectively with moderate strength. Then the thumb is used to press and knead Laogong for 1-2 minutes with moderate strength.

[Acupoint] Laogong (PC 8): Located between the second and third metatarsal bones and on the tip of the middle finger when the fingers are bent to form a fist.

[Effect] To help restore fine functions of the fingers; to ease fear and tranquilize the mind; and to achieve a certain effect in relieving insomnia and palpitation.

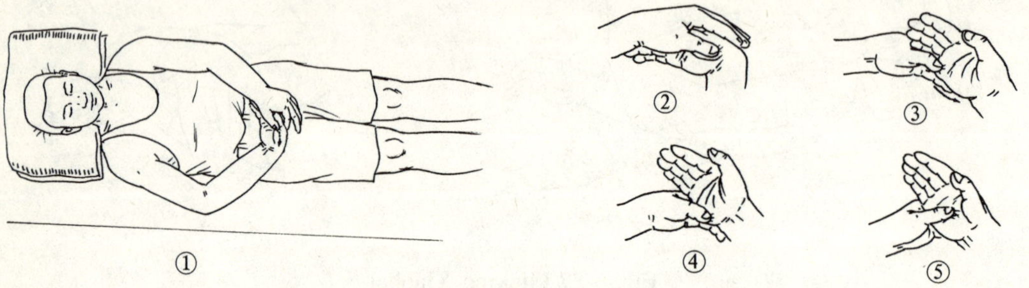

Fig. 6-89 Kneading and pressing the palm

12) Pushing and pinching the fingers (Fig. 6-90)

[Method] The patient lies in a supine position in a functional posture. The thumb and index finger of the healthy hand are put in an anterior and posterior direction as well as laterally and medially to the affected hand. The patient pushes and pinches upward to the palmar side of the wrist crease 3-5 times, respectively, with moderate strength.

[Effect] To help restore bending and extending functions of the finger joints; and to prevent edema of the fingers.

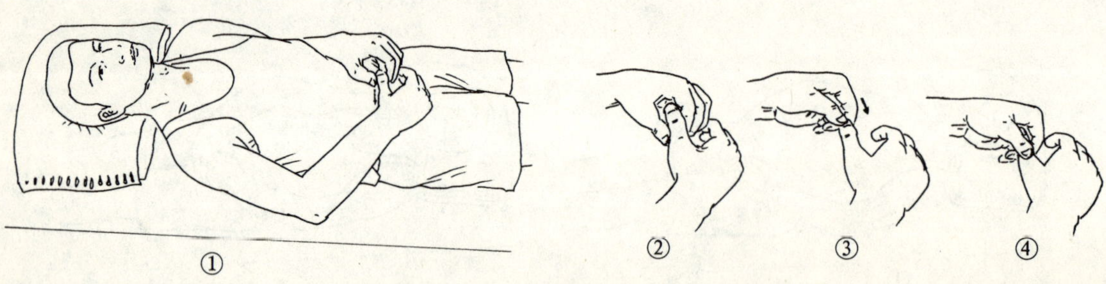

Fig. 6-90 Pushing and pinching the fingers

(2) Chest and abdomen (lying position)

1) Holding and pinching thoracic muscles (Fig. 6-91)

[Method] The patient lies in a supine position in a functional posture. The fingers of the healthy hand are put in an anterior direction and laterally to the armpit on the affected side. The patient pinches from the lateral border to the lower border of the greater pectoral muscle 3-5 times with moderate strength, until an aching and numb sensation is felt.

[Effect] To alleviate spasms of the greater pectoral muscle and promote restoration of the functions of the shoulder joint; and to relieve chest distress.

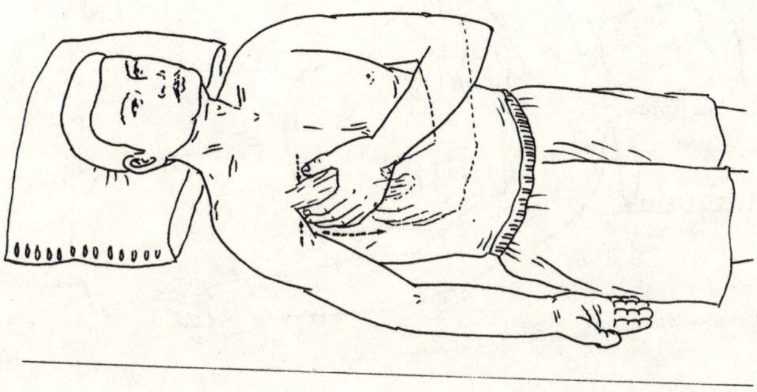

Fig. 6-91 Holding and pinching thoracic muscles

2) Patting the chest and rib-side (Fig. 6-92)

[Method] The patient lies in a supine position in a functional posture with the palm of the healthy hand bent into a soft fist. The patient pats from the lateral border to the lower border of the greater pectoral muscle 3-5 times with moderate strength. The patient shouts "Hei, Hei" while patting.

[Effect] To eliminate chest and rib pain due to long-term lying on the bed; to improve the functions of the heart and lungs; and to promote discharge of phlegm and prevent inhalation pneumonia.

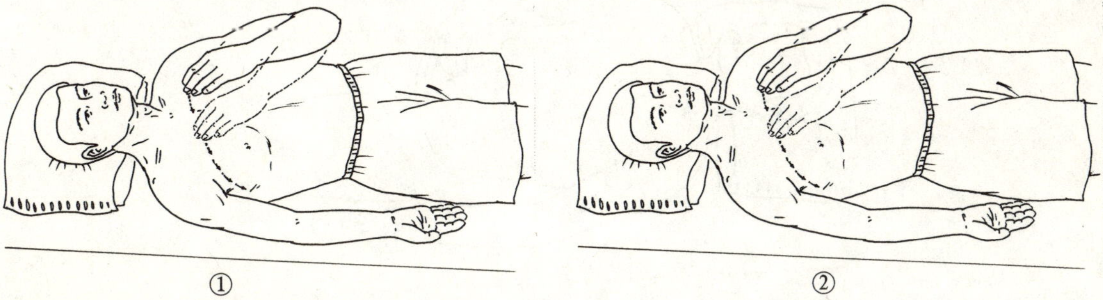

① ②

Fig. 6-92 Patting the chest and rib-side

3) Stroking the chest and rib-side (Fig. 6-93)

[Method] The patient lies in a supine position in a functional posture with the palm of the healthy hand put above the middle point of the chest. The patient strokes obliquely from the lateral part to the lower border of the costal arch with moderate strength. Such manipulation is repeated 5-10 times.

[Effect] To eliminate aching pain in the chest and rib, prevent common cold and relieve chest distress.

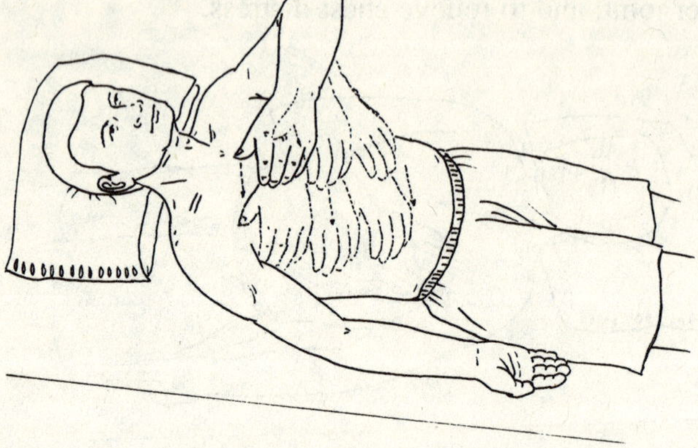

Fig. 6-93 Stroking the chest and rib-side

4) Patting the abdomen (Fig. 6-94)

[Method] The patient lies in a supine position in a functional posture with the palm of the healthy hand bent into a soft fist. The patient pats the abdomen clockwise and counterclockwise with moderate strength (only clockwise patting for constipation, and for diarrhea, only counterclockwise patting) for 20 rounds respectively.

[Effect] To improve visceral functions and prevent constipation and indigestion; and to achieve a certain effect in relieving accompanied prostate disorder and visceral prolapse.

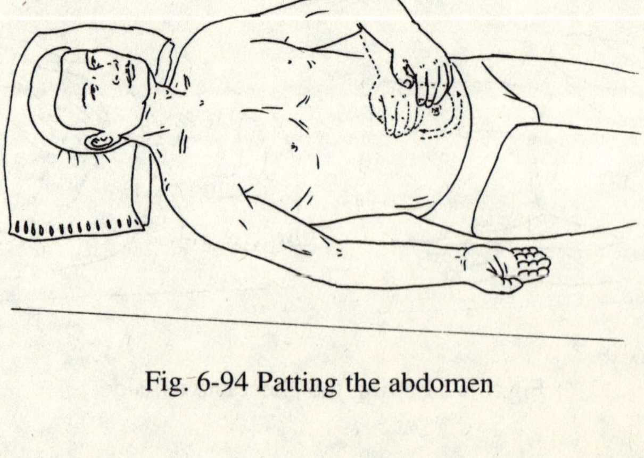

Fig. 6-94 Patting the abdomen

(3) Lower limbs (lying position)

1) Percussing Zusanli (Fig. 6-95)

[Method] The patient lies in a supine position in a functional posture with the heel of the healthy foot put at the lower border of the affected knee. The patient percusses from the anterior medial border to the crease on the dorsum of the foot 3-5 times with moderate strength. Then Zusanli (ST 36) on the affected limb is percussed 10-20 times.

[Acupoint] Zusanli: Located one transverse finger to the tibial crest.

[Effect] To eliminate aching and flaccidity of the lower limbs; to strengthen the spleen and tendons; and to reinforce the constitution and improve digestion.

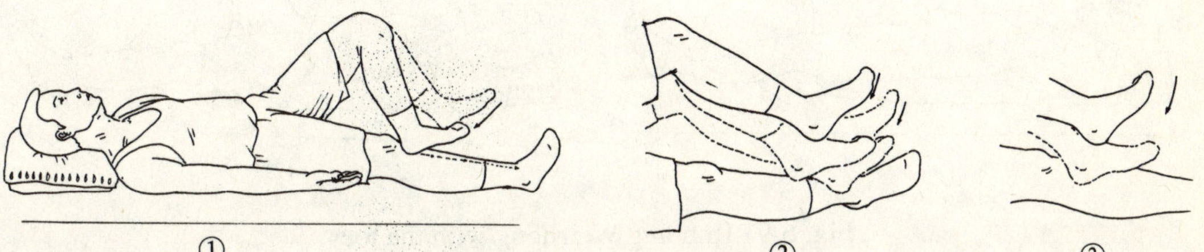

① ② ③

Fig. 6-95 Percussing Zusanli

2) Percussing Yanglingquan (Fig. 6-96)

[Method] The patient lies in a supine position in a functional posture with the heel of the healthy foot put at the lateral and lower border of the affected knee. The patient percusses from the anterior medial border to the lateral malleolus 3-5 times with moderate strength. Then, Yanglingquan (GB 34) on the affected limb is percussed 10-20 times.

[Acupoint]Yanglingquan: Located in the depression below the small head of the fibula.

[Effect] To alleviate spasms and stiffness of the lower limbs and prevent foot droop and strephenopodia; to clear the gall bladder and dredge dampness; and to achieve a certain effect in relieving bitterness and greasiness in the mouth.

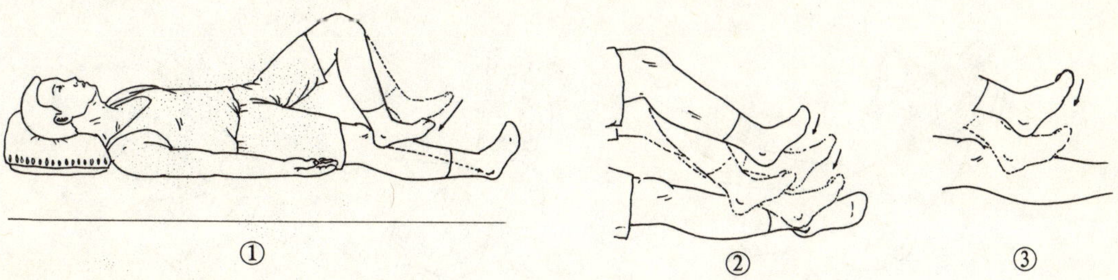

① ② ③

Fig. 6-96 Percussing Yanglingquan

3) Rubbing Weizhong with the toes (Fig. 6-97)

[Method] The patient lies in a supine position in a functional posture with the big toe of the healthy foot put at Weizhong (BL 40). The patient rubs with moderate strength for 1-2 minutes. Then, the dorsum of the healthy foot is used to rub downward to the Achilles tendon 5-10 times.

[Acupoint] Weizhong: Located on the center of the popliteal fossa.

[Effect] To alleviate spasms and stiffness of the knee joint and prevent foot droop; to dredge the meridians and collaterals; and to achieve a certain effect in relieving spasms of the shank and lumbago.

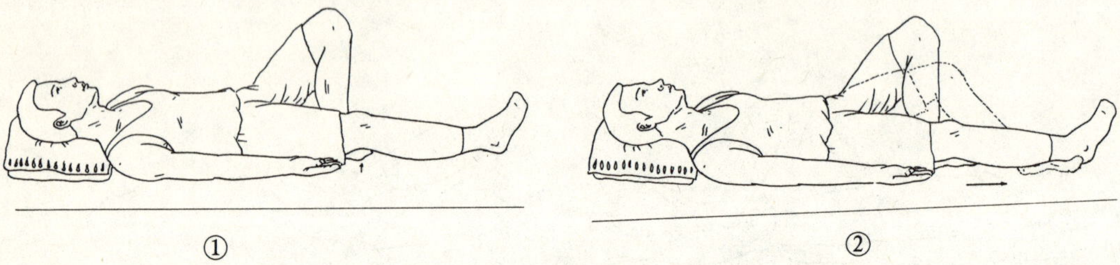

Fig. 6-97 Rubbing Weizhong with the toes

4) Rubbing and massaging the toes (Fig. 6-98)

[Method] The patient lies in a supine position in a functional posture with the dorsum of the healthy foot put anterior to the sole of the affected foot. The patient rubs upward and downward for 1-2 minutes with moderate strength. Then the tip of the big toe on the healthy foot is used to rub Yongquan (KI 1) for 30-60 seconds. The heel of the healthy foot is used to rub from the dorsal side of the toes on the affected foot upward to the crease on the dorsum of the foot with moderate strength 20-30 times.

[Acupoint] Yongquan: Located 1/3 to the anterior part of the sole and in the depression when the toes are bent.

[Effect] To help restore the bending functions of the toes and prevent foot droop; to nourish Yin and open orifices; and to achieve a certain effect in relieving tongue dryness, loss of voice and feverish sensation over the five centers (the chest, palms and soles).

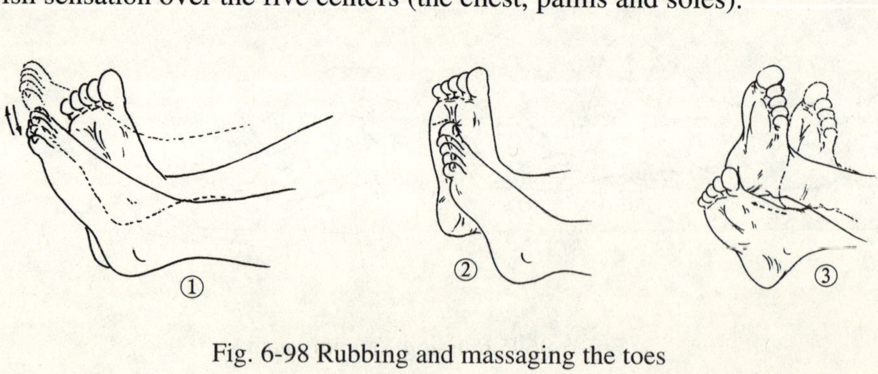

Fig. 6-98 Rubbing and massaging the toes

(4) Upper limbs, waist and back (sitting position)

1) Kneading and pinching the hand and neck (Fig. 6-99)

[Method] The patient sits straight in a functional posture with the palm of the healthy hand put at the dorsal side of the affected fingers. The patient rubs and pinches along the posterior side of the affected upper limb upward to the arm, shoulder, neck and posterior hairline with moderate strength. This manipulation is repeated 3-5 times.

[Effect] To prevent shoulder-hand syndrome and deviation of the head and neck.

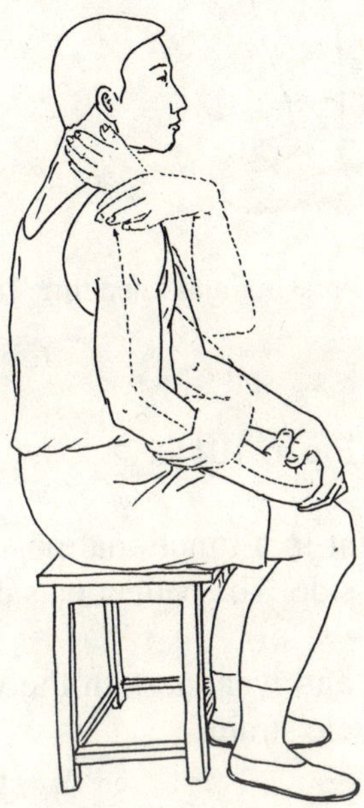

Fig. 6-99 Kneading and pinching the hand and neck

2) Pressing and kneading Tianzong (Fig. 6-100)

[Method] The patient sits straight in a functional posture with the palm of the healthy hand on the scapula on the affected side. The patient uses the tip of the middle finger to rub Tianzong (SI 11) with moderate strength for 30-60 seconds. Then, the healthy palm strokes from the shoulder and back on the affected side to the head and neck. This manipulation is repeated 3-5 times.

[Acupoint] Tianzong: Located in the lower fossa of the spine of the scapula parallel to the fourth thoracic vertebral process.

[Effect] To help restore abduction and adduction of the shoulder joint and eliminate pain in the shoulder and back; to relieve convulsion and asthma; and to achieve a certain effect in relieving asthma due to long-term lying on the bed.

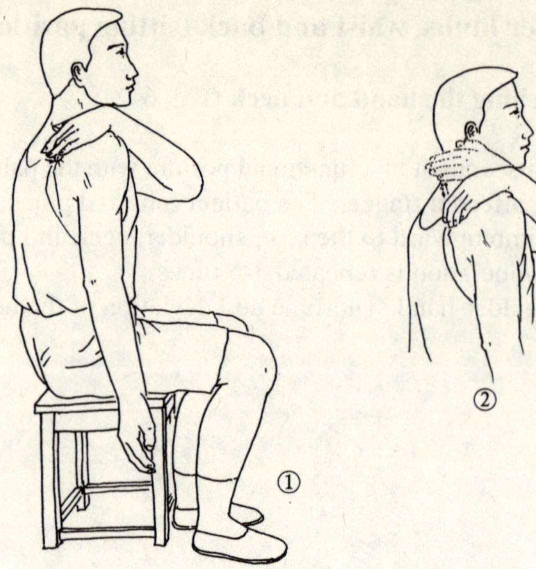

Fig. 6-100 Pressing and kneading Tianzong

3) Patting the back and waist (Fig. 6-101)

[Method] The patient sits straight in a functional posture with the healthy hand on the upper part of the back on the affected side. The patient pats downward to the waist and sacrum with moderate strength 5-10 times.

[Effect] To help eliminate pain and weakness in the waist and back; and to achieve a certain effect in relieving lumbar muscle strain.

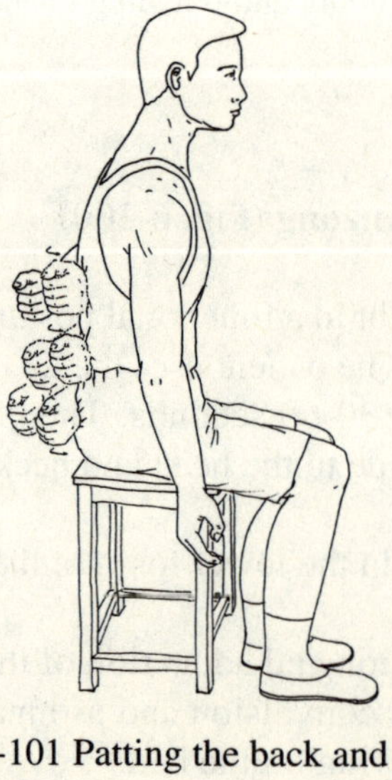

Fig. 6-101 Patting the back and waist

4) Stroking the waist (Fig. 6-102)

[Method] The patient sits straight in a functional posture with the palm of the healthy hand on the affected side of the waist. The patient strokes the waist back and forth 30-60 times with moderate strength till the waist is warm.

[Effect] To improve the bending and extending functions of the waist; to warm Yang, expel wind and prevent seminal emission; and to achieve a certain effect in relieving frequent urination, polyuria in the night and cold pain in the waist and knee.

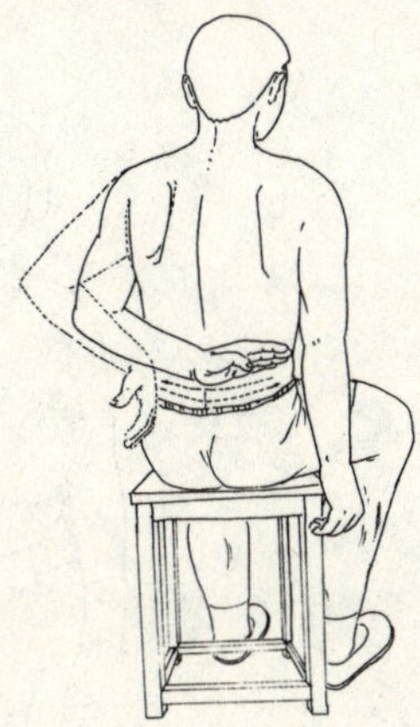

Fig. 6-102 Stroking the waist

(5) Shaking the scrotum with the palm

[Method] The patient sits straight in a functional posture. The healthy palm rubs till warm on the thigh, and is then put beneath the scrotum to shake it rhythmically 99 times until a light ache and distended sensation are felt in the lower abdomen.

[Effect] To improve the sexual function through reflex regulation of the central nervous system; to consolidate and warm the scrotum; and to achieve a certain effect in relieving accompanied prostate disease.

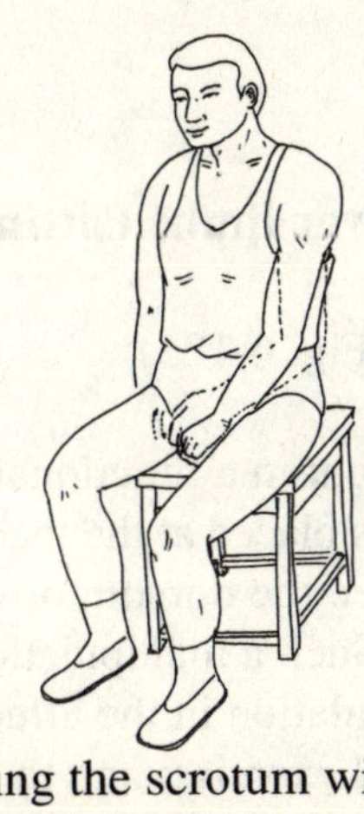

Fig. 6-103 Shaking the scrotum with the palm

(6) Shaking and rubbing both breasts

[Method] The patient sits straight in a functional posture. The healthy palm is placed below the breast and shakes the breast rhythmically with moderate strength, 36 times on the healthy side and then 99 times on the affected side. Then the thumb and index finger are used to rub the nipple, 30 seconds for the healthy side and 60 seconds for the affected side.

[Effect] To improve the sexual function through reflex regulation of the central nervous system; to relieve chest distress and discomfort.

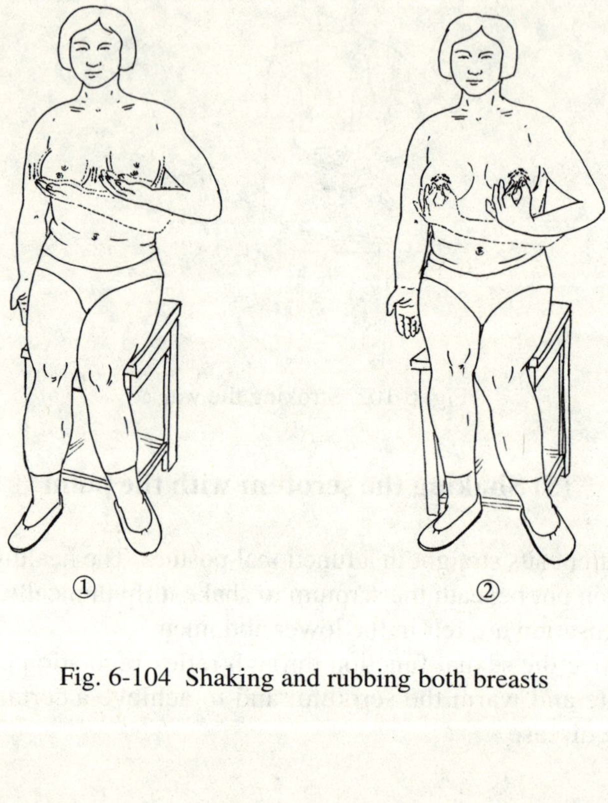

①　②

Fig. 6-104 Shaking and rubbing both breasts

(7) Lower limbs (sitting position)

1) Stroking the lower limbs (Fig. 6-105)

[Method] The patient sits straight in a functional posture. The affected lower limb is put on a small stool. The healthy palm is placed at the medial side of the affected thigh and strokes from there to the medial ankle. Then the dorsum of the affected foot is used to stroke to the lateral and upper part of the thigh. Such a manipulation is repeated 10-20 times.

[Effect] To improve blood circulation in the affected limb and relieve aching and fatigue due to prolonged lying or functional exercise; and to prevent edema of the lower limb.

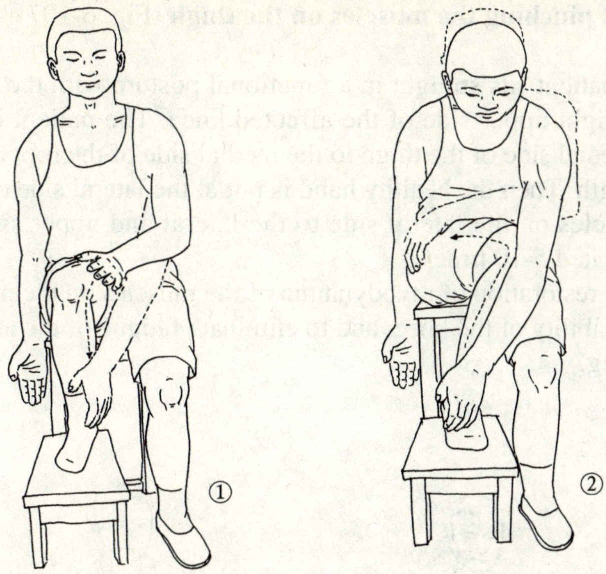

Fig. 6-105 Stroking the lower limbs

2) Holding the muscles on the medial side of the thigh (Fig. 6-106)

[Method] The patient sits straight in a functional posture with the fingers on the healthy hand placed at the medial side of the affected knee. The patient holds and pinches the muscles from there to the medial side of the root of the thigh with moderate strength. Such a manipulation is repeated 5-10 times until an aching and distended sensation is felt.

[Effect] To help restoration of myodynamia of the muscles on the medial side of the thigh and prevent external deviation of the thigh; to prevent seminal emission; and to achieve a certain effect in relieving irregular urination.

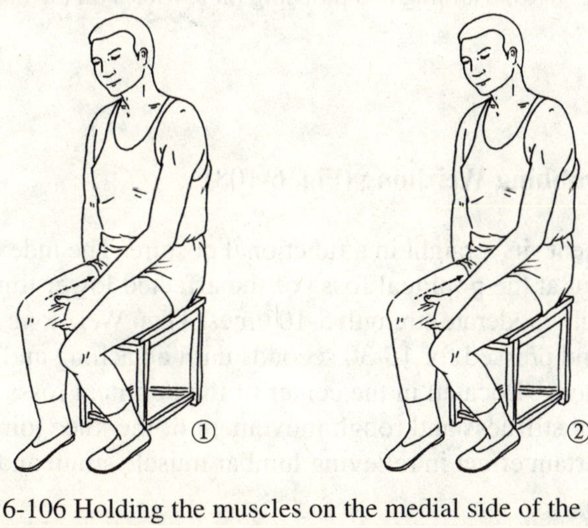

Fig. 6-106 Holding the muscles on the medial side of the thigh

3) Holding and pinching the muscles on the thigh (Fig. 6-107)

[Method] The patient sits straight in a functional posture with the fingers on the healthy hand placed at the right upper side of the affected knee. The patient holds and pinches the muscles from the medial side of the thigh to the medial side of the root of the thigh 5-10 times with moderate strength. Then the healthy hand is put at the lateral side of the knee to hold and pinch from the muscles on the lateral side to the lateral and upper sides of the thigh. This manipulation is repeated 5-10 times.

[Effect] To help restoration of myodynamia of the muscles on the medial side of the thigh and strengthen the stability of the knee; and to eliminate fatigue of the affected lower limb due to prolonged standing.

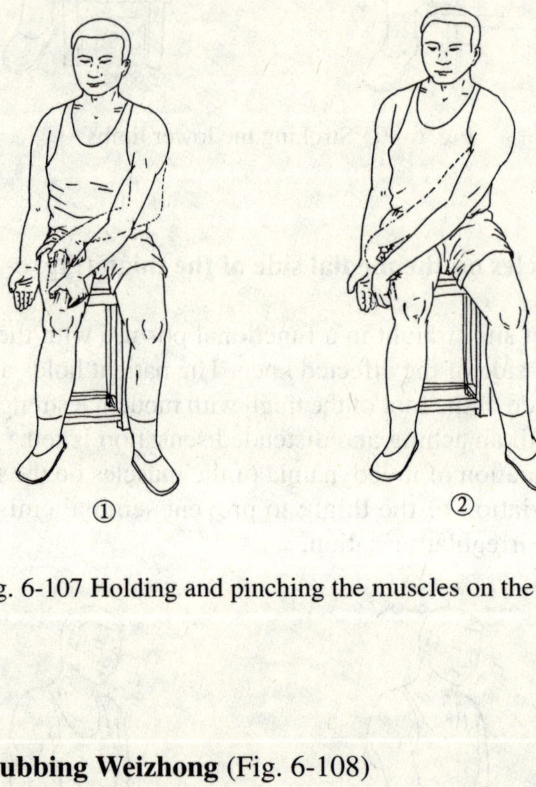

Fig. 6-107 Holding and pinching the muscles on the thigh

4) Flicking and rubbing Weizhong (Fig. 6-108)

[Method] The patient sits straight in a functional posture. The index and middle fingers on the healthy hand are put at the popliteal fossa of the affected lower limb to flick the popliteal tendons and muscles with moderate strength 5-10 times. Then Weizhong (BL 40) on the affected lower limb is rubbed and pressed for 15-30 seconds until an aching and numb sensation is felt.

[Acupoint] Weizhong: Located in the center of the popliteal fossa.

[Effect] To prevent stiffness and rough movement of the knee joint; to regulate meridian Qi; and to achieve a certain effect in relieving lumbar muscle strain and cold pain in the lower limbs.

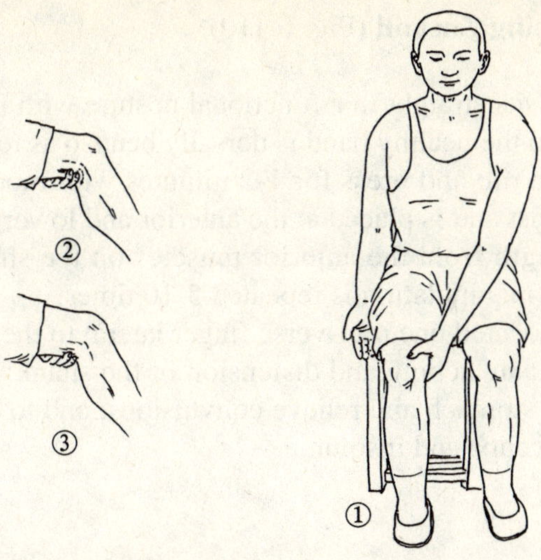

Fig. 6-108 Flicking and rubbing Weizhong

5) Flicking the shank (Fig. 6-109)

[Method] The patient sits straight in a functional posture with the affected lower limb on a small stool. The fingers on the healthy hand are placed at the anterior lower part of the affected shank to flick from the gastrocnemius muscle to the anterior and lower border of the knee with moderate strength. Such a manipulation is repeated 5-10 times until an aching and distended sensation is felt.

[Effect] To help restoration of myodynamia of the muscles on the foot and prevent foot droop and strephenopodia; to strengthen the spleen and improve appetite; and to achieve a certain effect in relieving anorexia, constipation or diarrhea and abdominal distension.

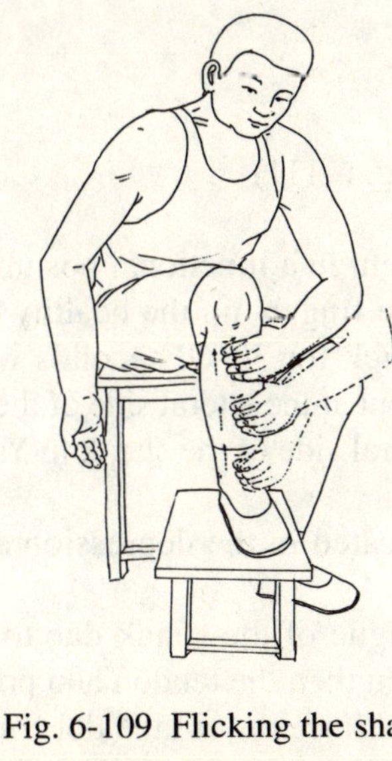

Fig. 6-109 Flicking the shank

6) Pressing and rubbing Zusanli (Fig. 6-110)

[Method] The patient sits straight in a functional posture with the affected lower limb on a small stool. The thumb on the healthy hand is dorsally bent so as to be placed on Zusanli (ST 36) on the affected limb to rub and press for 1-2 minutes with moderate strength. Then, the healthy hand forms a soft fist and is placed at the anterior and lower part of the affected shank to hit with moderate strength from the anterior muscles on the shank to the anterior lower border of the knee. Such a manipulation is repeated 5-10 times.

[Acupoint] Zusanli: Located one transverse finger lateral to the anterior crest of the tibia.

[Effect] To help eliminate aching and distension of the shank; to promote restoration of foot functions; to calm the stomach and relieve convulsions; and to achieve a certain effect in relieving stomach ache, hiccups and insomnia.

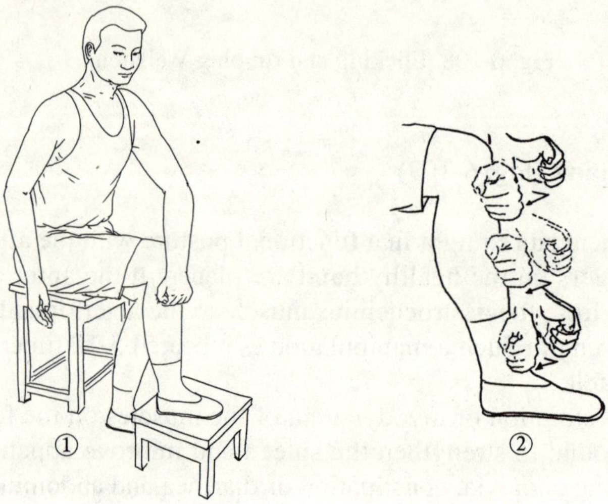

Fig. 6-110 Pressing and rubbing Zusanli

7) Flicking Yanglingquan (Fig. 6-111)

[Method] The patient sits straight in a functional posture with the affected lower limb on a small stool. The index and middle fingers on the healthy hand are placed at Yanglingquan (GB 34) on the affected limb to flick for 30-60 seconds with moderate strength. Then the healthy hand forms a soft fist ant is put at the lateral side of the lateral ankle to hit with moderate strength from the muscles at the lateral side of the shank to Yanglingquan. This manipulation is performed 10-20 times.

[Acupoint] Yanglingquan: Located in the depression anterior and inferior to the small head of the tibia.

[Effect] To help eliminate fatigue of the shank due to functional exercise; to promote restoration of foot functions; to strengthen the tendon and promote urination; and to achieve a certain effect in relieving edema and flaccidity of the dorsum of the foot.

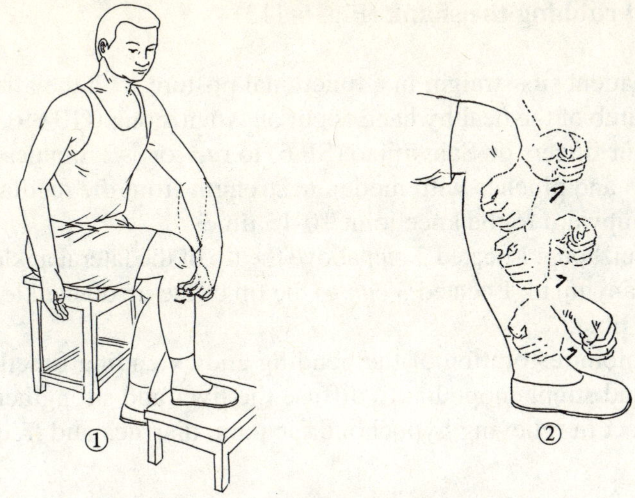

① ②

Fig. 6-111 Flicking Yanglingquan

8) Holding and pinching the shank (Fig. 6-112)

[Method] The patient sits straight in a functional posture with the affected limb on a small stool. The fingers on the healthy hand are put at the lower border of the calf on the affected lower limb to hold and pinch upward to the posterior fossa of the knee 5-10 times with moderate strength. Then the dorsum of the hand is used to pat from the lower part to the upper part with moderate strength 5-10 times.

[Effect] To help restore the myodynamia of the muscle responsible for bending the knee and strengthening knee stability.

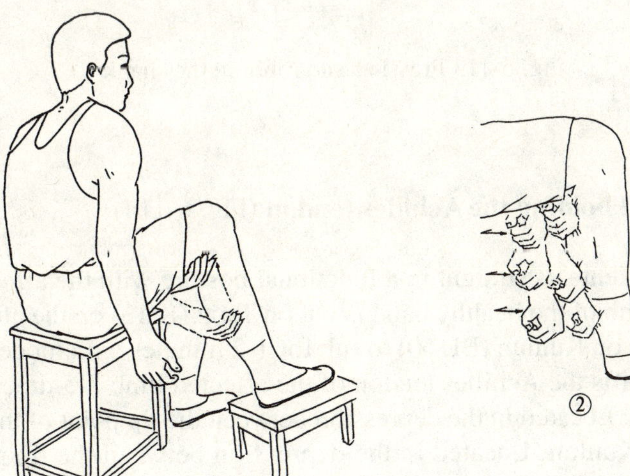

① ②

Fig. 6-112 Holding and pinching the shank

9) Pressing and rubbing the shank (Fig. 6-113)

[Method] The patient sits straight in a functional posture with the affected lower limb on a small stool. The thumb of the healthy hand is put on Xuanzhong (GB 39) on the affected limb and the remaining four fingers on Sanyinjiao (SP 6) to rub for 1-2 minutes with great strength. Then the patient rubs and pinches with moderate strength from the medial border of the tibia on the affected limb upward to the knee joint 10-15 times.

[Acupoints] Xuanzhong: Located 3 *cun* above the tip of the lateral ankle and on the anterior border of the fibia. Sanyinjiao: Located 3 *cun* to the tip of the medial ankle and posterior to the medial border of the tibia.

[Effect] To promote restoration of the bending and extending functions of the foot and prevent foot droop and strephenopodia; to diffuse the liver and strengthen the spleen; and to achieve a certain effect in relieving hypochondriac pain, diarrhea and frequent urination.

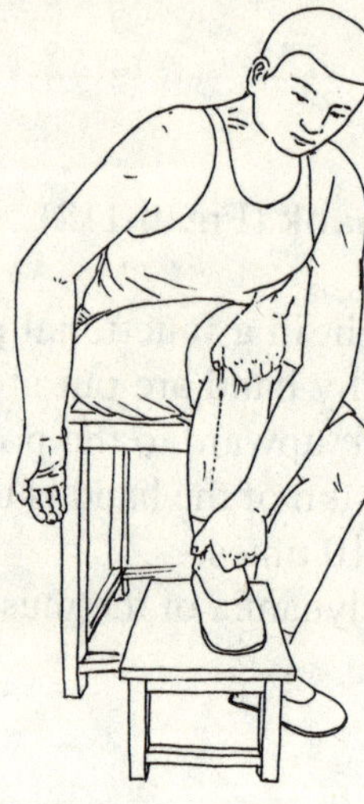

Fig. 6-113 Pressing and rubbing the shank

10) Pinching and holding the Achilles tendon (Fig. 6-114)

[Method] The patient sits straight in a functional posture with the affected lower limb on a small stool. The thumb of the healthy hand is put on Taixi (K 13) on the affected limb and the remaining four fingers on Kunlun (BL 60) to rub for 1-2 minutes with moderate strength. Then the patient holds and lifts the Achilles tendon of the affected limb 3-5 times.

[Acupoints] Taixi: Located in the depression between the tip point of the medial ankle and the Achilles tendon. Kunlun: Located in the depression between the tip point of the lateral ankle and the Achilles tendon.

[Effect] To promote restoration of the bending function of the foot; to nourish Yin and tranquilize the mind; and to achieve a certain effect in relieving enuresis, toothache and headache.

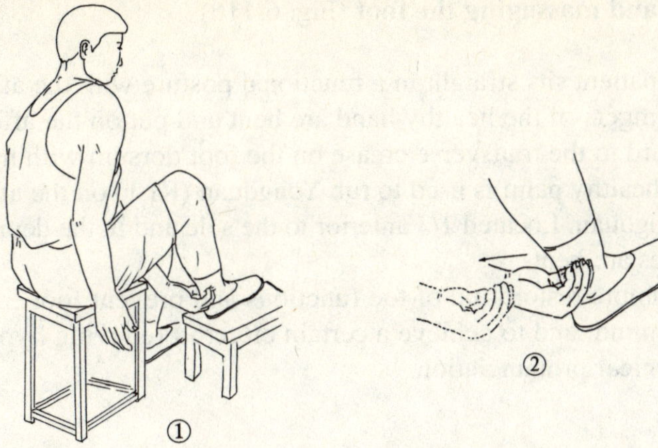

Fig. 6-114 Pinching and holding the Achilles tendon

11) Pressing and rubbing Taichong and Yongquan (Fig. 6-115)

[Method] The patient sits straight in a functional posture with the affected lower limb on a small stool. The thumb and index finger of the healthy hand are put on Taichong (LR3) and Yongquan (KI 1) on the affected foot to rub and press for 1-2 minutes with great strength. Then the patient holds the big toe and shakes it up and down 10-20 times.

[Acupoints] Taichong: Located on the dorsum of the foot and in the depression anterior to the juncture of the first and second metatarsal bones. Yongquan: Located 1/3 anterior to the sole and in the depression when the toes and metatarsal bones are bent.

[Effect] To promote restoration of the bending and extending functions of the big toe and prevent spasms of the toes; to eliminate depression and tranquilize the mind; and to achieve a certain effect in relieving hypertension, irritability and dizziness.

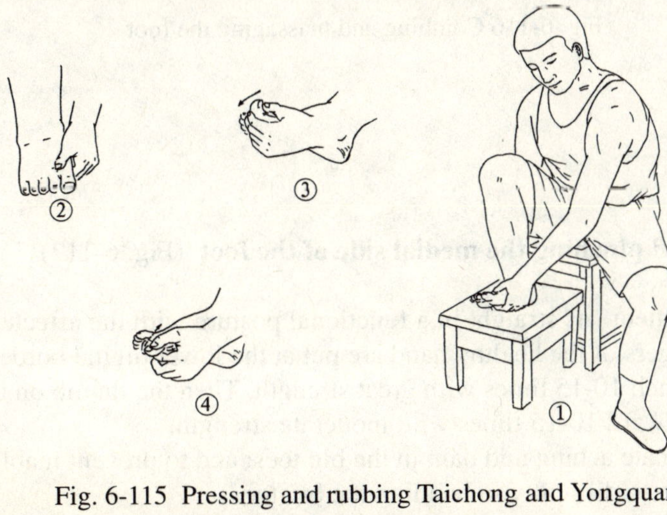

Fig. 6-115 Pressing and rubbing Taichong and Yongquan

12) Combing and massaging the foot (Fig. 6-116)

[Method] The patient sits straight in a functional posture with the affected lower limb on a small stool. The fingers of the healthy hand are bent and put on the affected foot dorsum to comb and rub upward to the transverse crease on the foot dorsum with moderate strength 20-30 times. Then the healthy palm is used to rub Yongquan (KI 1) on the affected foot 99 times.

[Acupoint] Yongquan: Located 1/3 anterior to the sole and in the depression when the toes and metatarsal bones are bent.

[Effect] To promote restoration of toe functions and prevent foot edema; to nourish Yin and tranquilize the mind; and to achieve a certain effect in relieving hypertension, insomnia, constipation and unclear pronunciation.

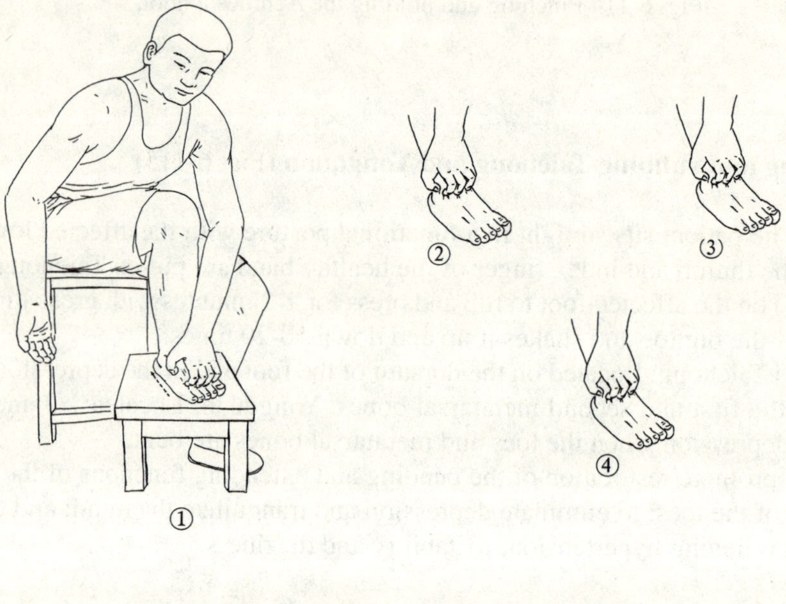

Fig. 6-116 Combing and massaging the foot

13) Rubbing and pinching the medial side of the foot (Fig. 6-117)

[Method] The patient sits straight in a functional posture with the affected lower limb on a small stool. The fingers of the healthy hand are put at the lower digital border of the affected foot arc to rub and pinch 10-15 times with great strength. Then the thumb on the healthy hand is used to punch backward 10-15 times with moderate strength.

[Effect] To eliminate aching and pain in the big toes; and to prevent inability to stand and instability to walk due to difficulty in bending the big toes.

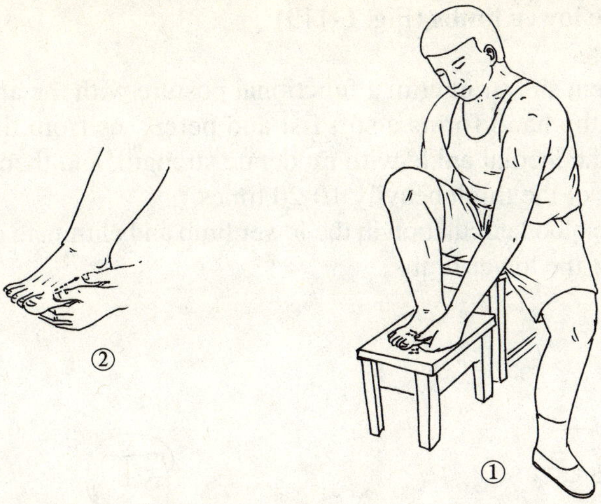

Fig. 6-117 Rubbing and pinching the medial side of the foot

14) Holding and pinching the toes (Fig. 6-118)

[Method] The patient sits straight in a functional posture with the affected lower limb on a small stool. The thumb and index finger of the healthy hand hold the toes on the affected foot to rub and pinch 10-20 times respectively with moderate strength and then shake heavily 10-20 times respectively.

[Effect] To promote restoration of the bending and extending functions of the toes; and to prevent spasms and stiffness of the toes.

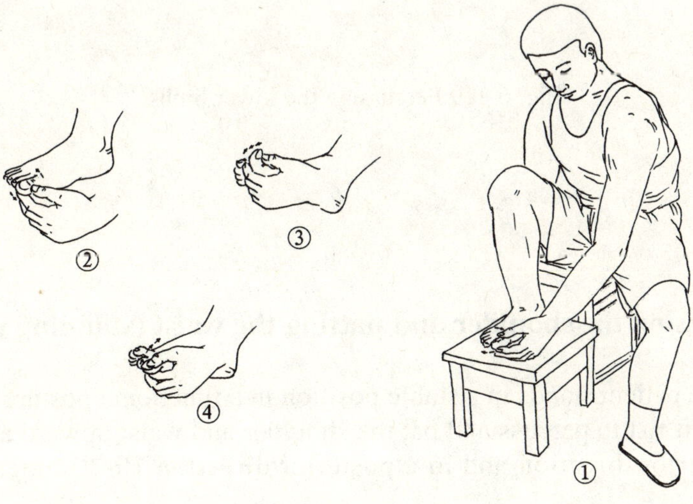

Fig. 6-118 Holding and pinching the toes

15) Percussing the lower limbs (Fig. 6-119)

[Method] The patient sits straight in a functional posture with the affected lower limb on a small stool. The healthy hand forms a soft fist and percusses from the medial side of the affected lower limb to the medial ankle with moderate strength, and then from the lateral side to the lateral upper side of the thigh heavily 10-20 times.

[Effect] To promote blood circulation in the lower limb and eliminate its aching and fatigue; and to prevent edema of the lower limbs.

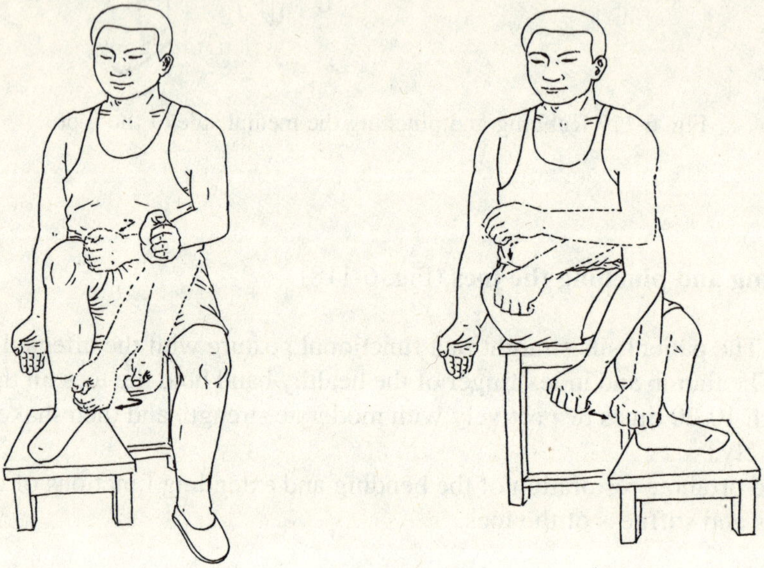

① ②

Fig. 6-119 Percussing the lower limbs

(8) Percussing the shoulder and patting the waist (standing position)

[Method] The patient stands in a stable position in a functional posture with the healthy hand forming a soft fist to percuss and pat the shoulder and waist upward and downward as well as in an anterior direction and in a posterior direction 10-20 times with moderate strength.

[Effect] To eliminate aching and fatigue in the shoulder, waist and back; and to improve the bending and extending functions of the shoulder joint, waist and spine.

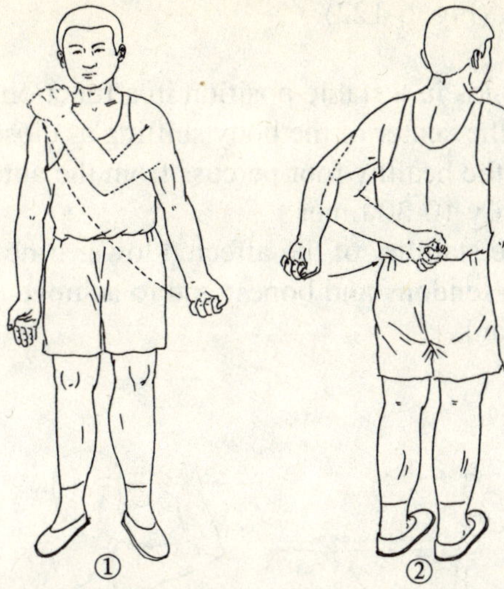

Fig. 6-120 Percussing the shoulder and patting the waist

(9) Lower limbs (standing position)

1) Percussing the popliteal fossa (Fig. 6-121)

[Method] The patient stands in a stable position in a functional posture with the healthy hand holding a supporter and the center of the body shifting as close as possible to the affected side. The dorsum of the healthy foot percusses the popliteal fossa on the affected lower limb lightly and then heavily 10-30 times until a numb and distending sensation is felt without bending the knee.

[Effect] To strengthen the stability of the affected lower limb; to dredge the meridians and activate the collaterals; and to achieve a certain effect in relieving lumbago and backache.

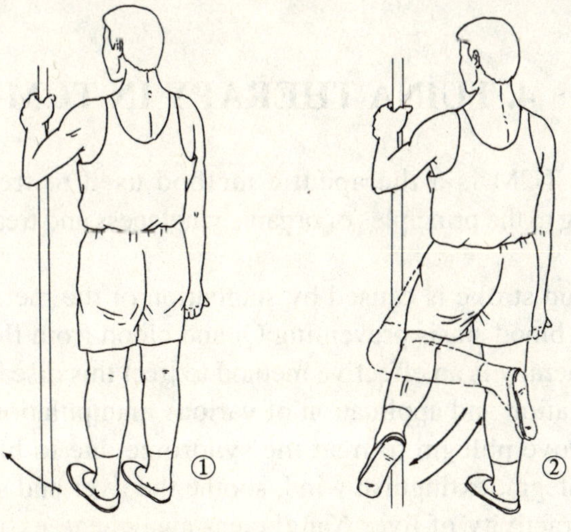

Fig. 6-121 Percussing the popliteal fossa

2) Percussing the shank (Fig. 6-122)

[Method] The patient stands in a stable position in a functional posture with the healthy hand holding a supporter and the center of the body shifting as close as possible to the affected side. The heel and dorsum of the healthy foot percuss from the anterior and posterior muscles on the shank to the knee heavily 10-30 times.

[Effect] To strengthen the stability of the affected lower limb; to prevent foot droop and strephenopodia; to strengthen tendons and bones; and to achieve a certain effect in relieving cold pain and spasm in the shank.

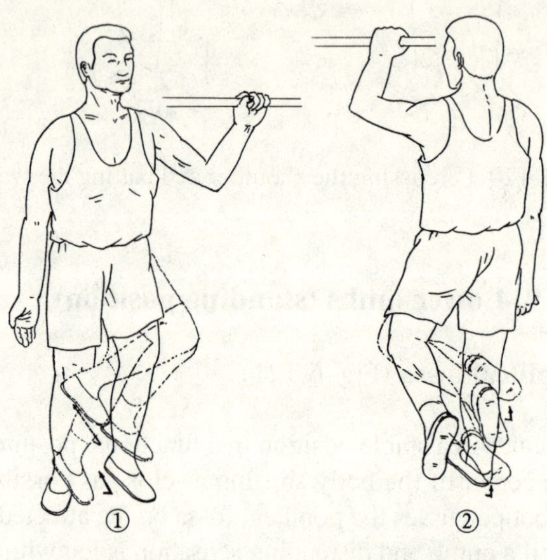

Fig. 6-122 Percussing the shank

4. TUINA THERAPY IN TCM

Tuina therapy in TCM is a therapeutic method used to treat disease with various manipulations according to the principles of organic wholeness and treatment based on syndrome differentiation.

Paralysis after wind stroke is caused by stagnation of the meridians and vessels due to wind, fire, phlegm and blood stasis preventing Qi and blood from flowing in the limbs.

Clinically Tuina therapy is an effective method to treat this disease. This is because, based on syndrome differentiation and application of various manipulations, it can eliminate wind, resolve stasis and remove phlegm to treat the syndrome due to blockage of the meridians caused by wind and phlegm; extinguish wind, soothe the liver and suppress Yang to treat the syndrome due to hyperactivity of liver-Yang; clear away heat, extinguish wind and resolve phlegm to treat the excess syndrome of Fu-organs due to phlegm-heat; benefit Qi, activate blood and resolve stasis to treat the syndrome due to Qi deficiency and blood stasis; nourish Yin and extinguish wind to treat the syndrome due to wind caused by Yin deficiency through smoothing the meridians, nourishing the limbs and lubricating the joints.

Modern medicine has discovered that Tuina therapy can cause local physical and chemical changes altering the local physiological reactions. By means of neural reflex regulation, it can regulate the body's functions, improve blood circulation and lymph circulation in the affected limbs, increase the number of white cells and phagocytes, strengthen the immune function of the body and benefit rehabilitation of the patients.

Paralysis due to wind stroke is characterized by stiffness, spasms, pain, and rough movement of the limbs. Tuina therapy can dilate the capillaries, increase skin temperature, promote sweating, enrich the blood (similar to resolving stasis) and provide the spastic tissues with sufficient blood, consequently relieving muscular strain, increasing elasticity of the skin, relieving adhesion, lubricating joints, improving nourishment for the joints and enlarging their movement range, benefiting the rehabilitation of the affected limbs, and preventing complications, and deformity and spasm of the limbs. Tuina therapy is also effective for regulating the gastrointestinal functions, promoting defecation (similar to elimination of phlegm-dampness), strengthening the absorptive functions of the stomach and intestines (similar to nourishing Qi and Yin) as well as relaxing tension and anxiety (similar to soothing the liver to suppress Yang). So, Tuina therapy is a very simple and effective method in TCM to treat paralysis due to wind stroke.

Clinically paralysis due to wind stroke is treated with different manipulations based on typing. The patient lies in a supine position and the treatment follows such an order: the head and face, chest, lower limb and upper limb. If the patient lies in pronation, the treatment follows the order: occiput, neck, back, waist and lower limb. So, in applying Tuina therapy, the practitioner should select manipulations according to the position of the patients.

If the relatives of the patients want to practice Tuina at home, they must follow the instructions of the practitioner and the requirements of the therapy, getting familiar with the acupoints, understanding the key points for each manipulative technique and memorizing the pithy formula for the performance of this therapy.

In performing this therapy, the practitioner should combine local manipulation with holistic manipulation according to the affected part and muscles. Generally speaking, local manipulation requires greater strength, 1-3 minutes for each manipulation; holistic manipulations are lighter, 15-30 seconds for each manipulation. Usually, this therapy is performed after functional exercise, or half an hour before or after a meal, taking medicine or other treatments, 1-1.5 hours each time. Prolonged performance of Tuina may lead to inhibited muscles and nerves, causing fatigue; short performance of Tuina may make it difficult to excite the muscles and nerves.

[Clinical manifestations] Hemiplegia, perhaps accompanied by distorted face, difficulty in speaking and half body numbness. It is usually divided into five types:

a. Wind-phlegm blocking the collaterals: Dizziness. This type is usually characterized by a bulgy tongue with tooth prints on the margins, grayish color, thin and whitish coating or whitish and greasy coating, swollen and purplish sublingual vein, taut and slippery pulse.

b. Extreme hyper function of liver-Yang: Dizziness, headache (involving the vertex and both sides of the head), reddish complexion and eyes, bitter taste in the mouth, restlessness, irritability, constipation, yellowish urine, reddish or purplish tongue with yellow coating, swollen and reddish sublingual vein, taut and forceful pulse.

c. Excess type of Fu-organ with phlegm-heat: Profuse sputum in the throat, vomiting of phlegm and dribbling, afternoon fever, abdominal distension, constipation, reddish tongue with yellow, greasy and thick coating, enlarged and distending sublingual vein, taut, slippery and large pulse.

d. Qi deficiency and blood stasis: Light whitish complexion, palpitation, shortness of breath, fatigue, frequent sweating, swelling and distension of hands and feet, grayish tongue or with petechia, thin, short and stagnant sublingual vein, thin and slow or thin and rough pulse.

e. Yin deficiency and wind-stirring: Dizziness, tinnitus, deafness, tremor of hands and feet, thin and reddish or grayish red of the tongue with scanty coating or without coating, thin, stagnant and reddish sublingual vein, thin and taut or rapid pulse.

[Therapeutic principles] Extinguishing wind and eliminating phlegm, nourishing Qi and Yin, resolving stasis and dredging meridians.

(1) Formulae of manipulations

1) Forked pushing before the forehead
2) Pressing Shangguan (GB 3) and Xiaguan (ST 7)
3) Pressing Wangu (GB 12)
4) Point-pressing the lateral sides of the chest and abdomen
5) Squeezing and pushing the lateral side of the abdomen
6) Rubbing and pinching the medial side of the thigh
7) Rubbing Zusanli (ST 36)
8) Rubbing and pinching the medial side of the shank
9) Pushing the lateral side of the foot
10) Dorsal bending of the ankle
11) Pushing Sanyang of the upper arm
12) Pushing Sanyang of the forearm
13) Pushing Sanyin of the upper arm
14) Pushing Sanyin of the forearm
15) Pressing Neiguan (PC 6) and Waiguan (TE 15)
16) Pinching neck muscles
17) Pushing Dazhui (GV 14) and Yangguan
18) Transverse stroking of the waist
19) Forking the waist with palms
20) Pressing Huantiao (GB 30)
21) Pushing the posterior side of the thigh
22) Holding Kunlun (BL 60)

(2) Combination of the manipulations

1) For wind-phlegm blocking the collaterals, add ① pressing Zhongfu (LU 1) and Yunmen (LU 2) ② stroking and pressing the upper abdomen ③ pressing the middle of the abdomen ④ holding and lifting the abdominal muscles ⑤ pressing the medial side of the skeleton ⑥ rubbing Xuanzhong (GB 39) ⑦ shaking the big toe ⑧ pressing Jiquan (HT 1) ⑨ forked pushing of the occipital region.

2) For sudden hyperactivity of liver-Yang, add ① forking the ribs ② forked stroking of the

hypochondriac region ③ minor Qi-dispersing method ④ pressing the medial side of the thigh ⑤rubbing Sanyinjiao (SP 6) ⑥ stroking and pressing the hypochondriac region ⑦ stroking the back ⑧ Qi-smoothing method ⑨ chest-expanding method.

3) For Sthenia-Fu syndrome due to phlegm-heat, add ① pressing the sternum ② pushing the upper abdomen ③ transverse stroking beside the navel ④ Stroking and pressing the lower abdomen ⑤ major Qi-dispersing method ⑥ rubbing around the knee ⑦ combing the dorsum of the foot ⑧ combing the dorsum of the hand ⑨ longitudinal stroking of the waist.

4) For blood stasis due to Qi deficiency, add ① binding the chest ② pressing Tianshu (ST 25) ③ binding the abdomen ④ stroking around the navel ⑤ pressing Qichong (ST 30) ⑥ pressing the medial side of the shank ⑦ rubbing Laogong (PC 8) ⑧ knocking the rib for supplementing Qi ⑨ perpendicular pushing of the waist for supplementing Qi.

5) For disturbance of wind due to Yin deficiency, add ① pressing the head from both sides ② pinching Sishencong (EX-HN 1) ③ expanding the chest ④ internal and external rotation of the ankle ⑤ rubbing Yongquan (KI 1) ⑥ rubbing Mingmen (GV 4) ⑦ pressing the waist with piled palms ⑧ forking the waist with fingers ⑨ rubbing the sides of the waist ⑩ rubbing Weizhong (BL 40).

(1) Formulae of manipulations

1) Forked pushing before the forehead (Fig. 6-123)

[Method] The doctor puts the palmar sides of the thumbs at the middle point of the patient's forehead and pushes toward the head laterally for 30-60 seconds. Then the palmar sides of the thumbs are placed on Touwei (ST 8) to transversely stroke toward the occiput and the Houding (GV 19) for 30-60 seconds.

[Acupoints] Touwei: Located 0.5 *cun* directly above the forehead angle. Houding: Located 5.5 *cun* above the middle point on the posterior hairline.

[Pithy formula] Forked pushing before the forehead stops dizziness; stroking is done from Touwei to Houding; such a manipulation is effective in treating rhinorrhea with turbid discharge and headache as well as improving eyesight.

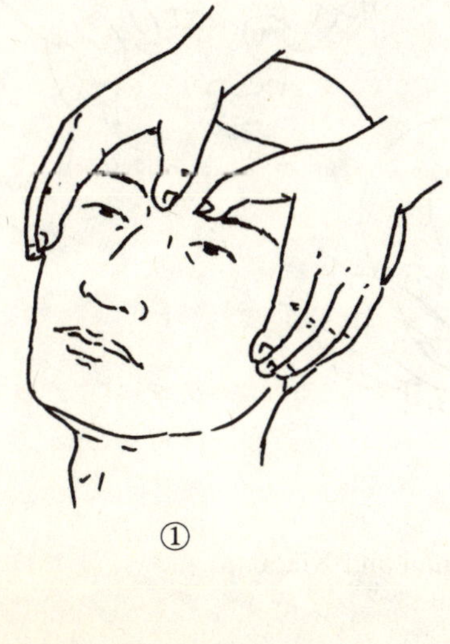

①

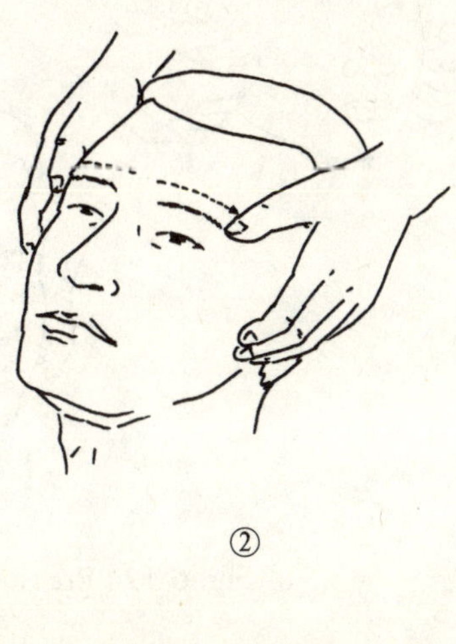

②

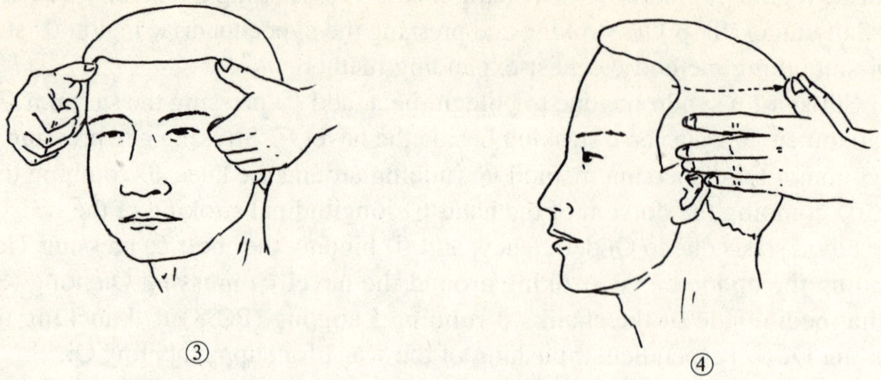

Fig. 6-123 Forked pushing before the forehead

2) Pressing Shangguan and Xiaguan (Fig. 6-124)

[Method] The doctor puts the tips of the thumbs and index fingers on Shangguan (GB 3) and Xiaguan (ST 7) of the patient to press and rub for 1-2 minutes. Then the thumbs are pushed upward to Touwei (ST 8) and the index fingers pushed downward to Jiache (ST 6) 5-10 times.

[Acupoints] Shangguan: Located at the upper border of the cheekbone and directly above Xiaguan. Xiaguan: Located in the depression between the cheekbone and mandible. Touwei: Located 0.5 *cun* directly above the forehead angle. Jiache: Located in a depression one transverse finger anterior and superior to the mandible angle.

[Pithy formula] The thumbs and index fingers are used to press Shangguan and Xiaguan and push to Touwei and Jiache. This manipulation is effective in treating tinnitus deafness and migraine, and stopping pain by dispersing wind.

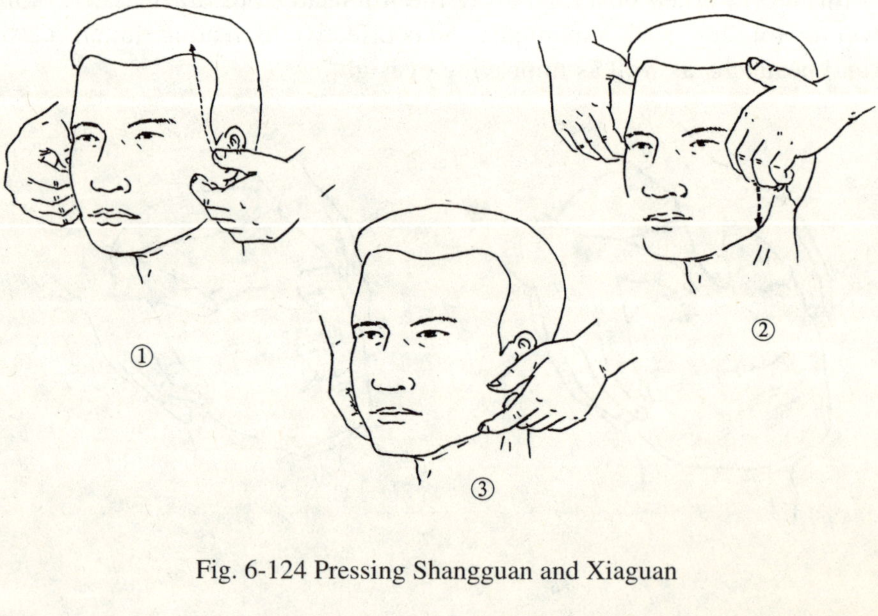

Fig. 6-124 Pressing Shangguan and Xiaguan

3) Pressing Wangu (Fig. 6-125)

[Method] The doctor puts the palmar side of a thumb on Wangu (GB 12) on the affected side and presses for 1-2 minutes. Then the thumb is pushed to Yifeng (TE 17). This manipulation is performed 2-3 times.

[Acupoints] Wangu: Located in the depression below the mastoid process. Yifeng: Located anterior and interior to the mastoid process and in the depression parallel to the lower border of the antilobium.

[Pithy formula] Pressing and pushing from Wangu to Yifeng relieves headache; cures ear disorder, a distorted face and shoulder and neck injuries; and disperses wind to stop pain.

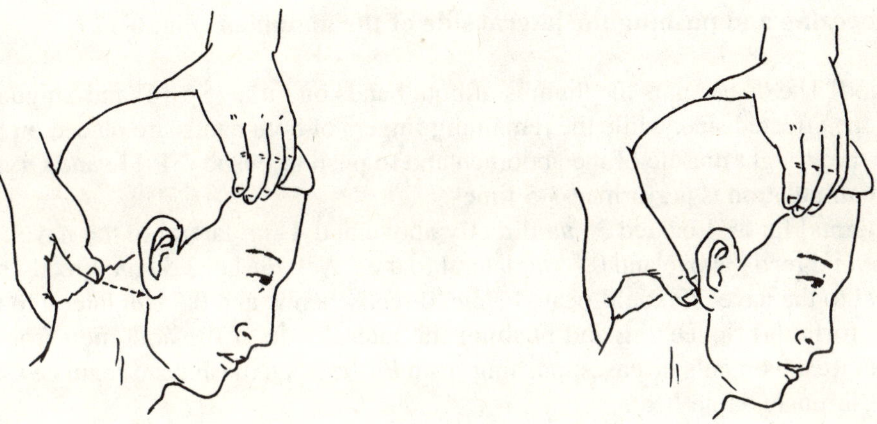

① ②

Fig. 6-125 Pressing Wangu

4) Point-pressing the lateral sides of the chest and abdomen (Fig. 6-126)

[Method] The doctor puts the four fingers of one hand on Qihu (ST 13) on the affected side and performs point-pressing along the costal spaces and from Yingchuang (ST 16), Qimen (LR14), Daheng (SP 15) and Fushe (SP 13) to Qichong (ST 30). This manipulation is performed 2-3 times.

[Acupoints] Qihu: Located on the lower border of the clavicle and 4 *cun* lateral to the front midline. Yingchuang: Located directly below Qihu and in the third costal space. Qimen: Located directly below the nipple and in the sixth costal space. Daheng: Located beside and 4 *cun* lateral to the navel. Fushe: Located 5 *cun* directly below Daheng. Qichong: Located 5 *cun* directly below the navel and 2 *cun* lateral to the navel.

[Pithy formula] Point-pressing the sides of the chest and abdomen from Qihu to Qichong relieves dull pain in the upper gastrium, regulating Qi, strengthening the spleen and eliminating dampness.

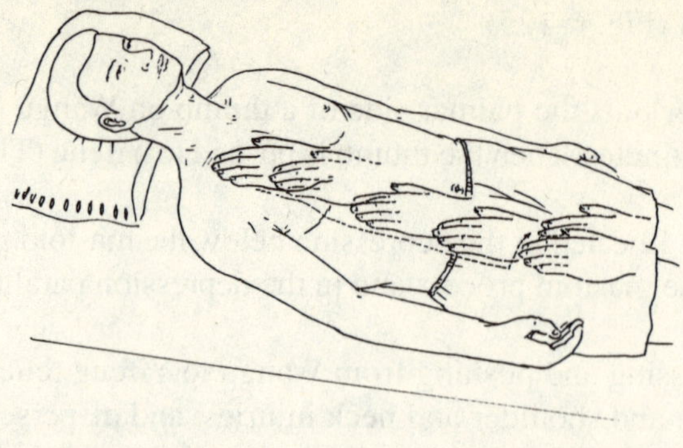

Fig. 6-126 Point-pressing the lateral sides of the chest and abdomen

5) Squeezing and pushing the lateral side of the abdomen (Fig. 6-127)

[Method] The doctor puts the thumbs of both hands on Fu'ai (Sp 16) and Shiguan (KI 18) located on the affected side, while the remaining fingers of both hands are placed on both sides to squeeze the straight muscle of the abdomen and to push to Fushe (SP 13) and Qixueshu (KI 13). This manipulation is performed 3-5 times.

[Acupoints] Fu'ai: Located 3 *cun* directly above and 4 *cun* lateral to the navel. Shiguan: Located 3 *cun* directly above and 0.5 *cun* lateral to the navel. Fushe: 3.5 *cun* directly below and 4 *cun* lateral to the navel. Qixue: Located 3 *cun* directly below and 0.5 *cun* lateral to the navel.

[Pithy formula] Squeezing and pushing the lateral side of the abdomen from Fu'ai to Shiguan can treat women's diseases; pushing from Fushe to Qixueshu can regulate Qi, activate blood and eliminate damp-heat.

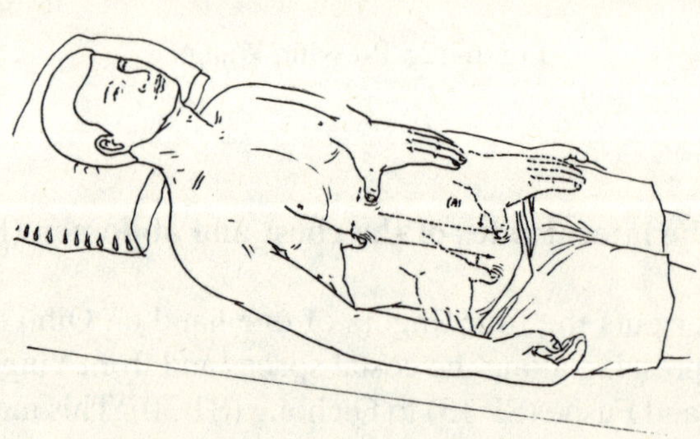

Fig. 6-127 Squeezing and pushing the lateral side of the abdomen

6) Rubbing and pinching the medial side of the thigh (Fig. 6-128)

[Method] The doctor puts the fingers on Yinlian (LR11) and Zuwuli (LR10) on the affected lower limb to rub and pinch the muscles on the medial side of the thigh from Yinbao (LR9) to Ququan (LR8). This manipulation is performed 3-5 times.

[Acupoints] Yinlian: Located 2 *cun* lateral to and 2 *cun* directly below the middle point of the upper border of the pubic symphysis. Zuwuli: Located 1 *cun* below Yinlian. Yinbao: Located 4 *cun* above the epicondyle of the femur and on the posterior border of the sartorius muscle. Ququan: Located in the depression above the medial crease of a bent knee.

[Pithy formula] Rubbing and pinching Yinlian, Yinbao and Ququan can relieve pain in the waist, leg and knee, remove coldness in the lower abdomen, and activate blood to resolve stasis and warm the meridians.

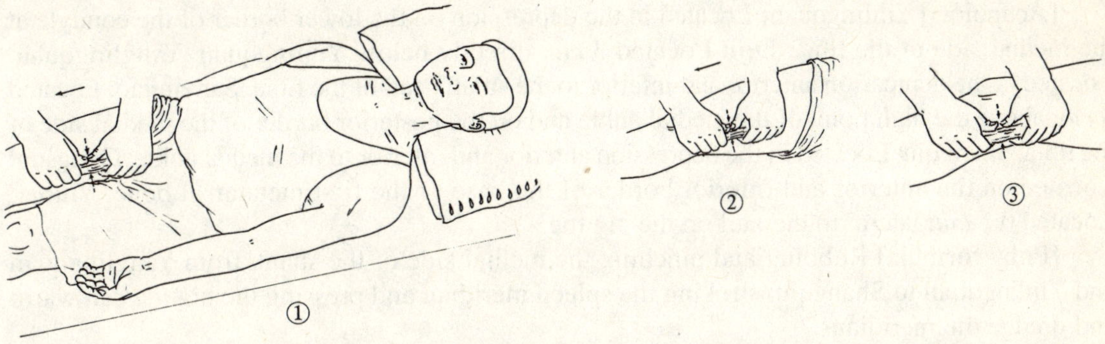

Fig. 6-128 Rubbing and pinching the medial side of the thigh

7) Rubbing Zusanli (Fig. 6-129)

[Method] The doctor puts the thumb of one hand on Zusanli (ST 36) on the affected side to press and rub and the remaining four fingers on Yanglingquan (GB 34), pushing downward to Xuanzhong (GB 39). This manipulation is performed for 1-2 minutes.

[Acupoints] Zusanli: Located one transverse finger lateral to the anterior crest of the femur. Yanglingquan: Located in the depression anterior to the small head of the fibia. Xuanzhong: Located 3 *cun* above the high point of the lateral malleolus and on the anterior border of the fibia.

[Pithy formula] Rubbing Zusanli from Yanglingquan to Xuanzhong can improve overstrain, strengthen the limbs and reinforce the spleen and tendons.

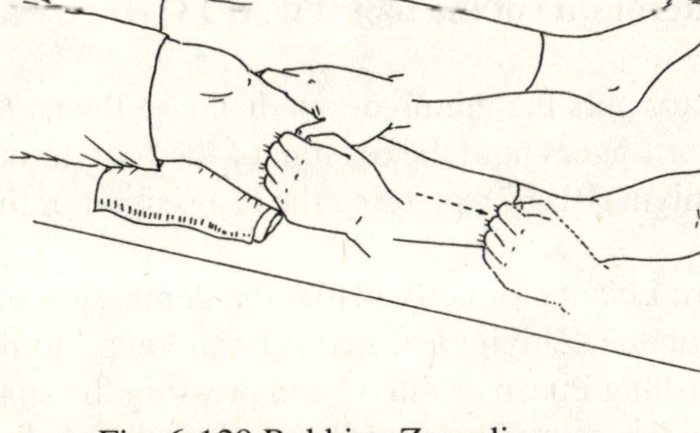

Fig. 6-129 Rubbing Zusanli

8) Rubbing and pinching the medial side of the shank (Fig. 6-130)

[Method] The doctor puts four fingers of both hands on Yinlingquan (SP 9) and Diji (SP 8) on the affected side and thumbs of both hands on Yanglingquan (GB 34) to press and rub. The other hand rubs and pinches downward along the medial side of the shank from Sanyinjiao (SP 6) to Shangqiu (SP 5) 3-5 times. The palms of both hands stroke downward along the medial side of the shank from Gongsun (SP 4) to Yinbai (SP 1), pressing the big toe at the same time, 5-10 times.

[Acupoints] Yinlingquan: Located in the depression on the lower border of the condyle at the medial side of the tibia. Diji: Located 3 *cun* directly below Yinlingquan. Yanglingquan: Located in the depression anterior and inferior to the small head of the fibia. Sanyinjiao: Located 3 *cun* above the high point of the medial ankle and on the posterior border of the medial side of the tibia. Shangqiu: Located in the depression anterior and inferior to the medial ankle. Gongsun: Located on the anterior and inferior border of the base of the first metatarsal bone. Yinbai: Located 0.1 *cun* lateral to the nail on the big toe.

[Pithy formula] Rubbing and pinching the medial side of the shank from Yanglingquan and Yinlingquan to Shangqiu, stroking the spleen meridian and pressing the big toe can warm and dredge the meridians.

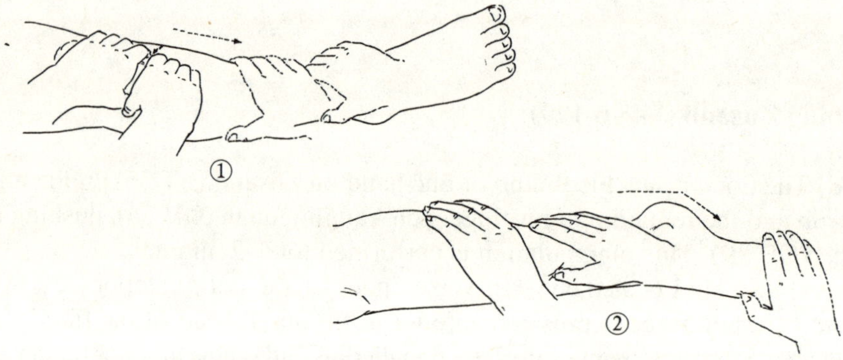

Fig. 6-130 Rubbing and pinching the medial side of the shank

9) Pushing the lateral side of the foot (Fig. 6-131)

[Method] The doctor puts the thumb of one hand on Pucan (BL 61) on the affected side, while the remaining four fingers hold the dorsum of the foot, to push from the lateral side (the bladder meridian) to Zhiyin (BL 67), pressing the last section of the small toe downward at the same time, 5-10 times.

[Acupoints] Pucan: Located directly below the depression between the high point of the lateral ankle and heel tendon. Zhiyin: Located 0.1 *cun* lateral to the nail on the small toe.

[Pithy formula] Pushing Pucan to Zhiyin and pressing the small toe can treat ankle injury, lumbago and foot flaccidity as well as dredge the meridians and activate the collaterals.

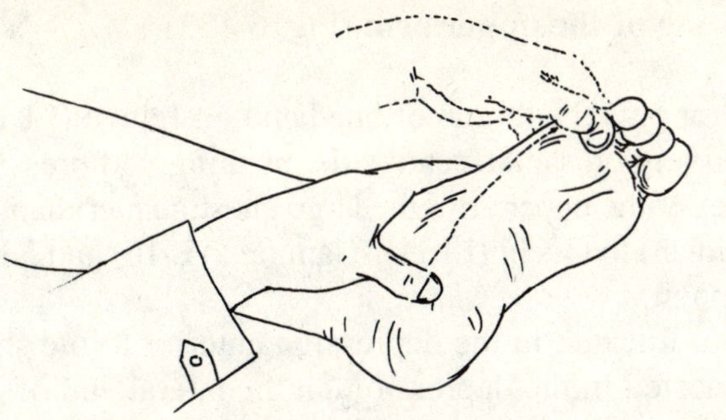

Fig. 6-131 Pushing the lateral side of the foot

10) Dorsal bending of the ankle (Fig. 6-132)

[Method] The doctor puts four fingers of one hand on the dorsum of the foot on the affected side and the thumb on Yongquan (KI 1), the thumb and four fingers of the other hand on Shuiquan (KI 5) and Pucan (BL 61), to sway, bend and extend the foot, pressing and rubbing the acupoints at the same time, for 30-60 seconds.

[Acupoints] Yongquan: Located 1/3 anterior to the sole. Shuiquan: Located 1 *cun* directly below the depression between the high point of the medial ankle and heel tendon. Pucan: Located directly below the depression between the high point of the lateral ankle and heel tendon.

[Pithy formula] Dorsal bending of the ankle can resolve prolonged stasis, treat dysuria and foot flaccidity, dredge the meridians, promote urination, subdue swelling and relieve pain.

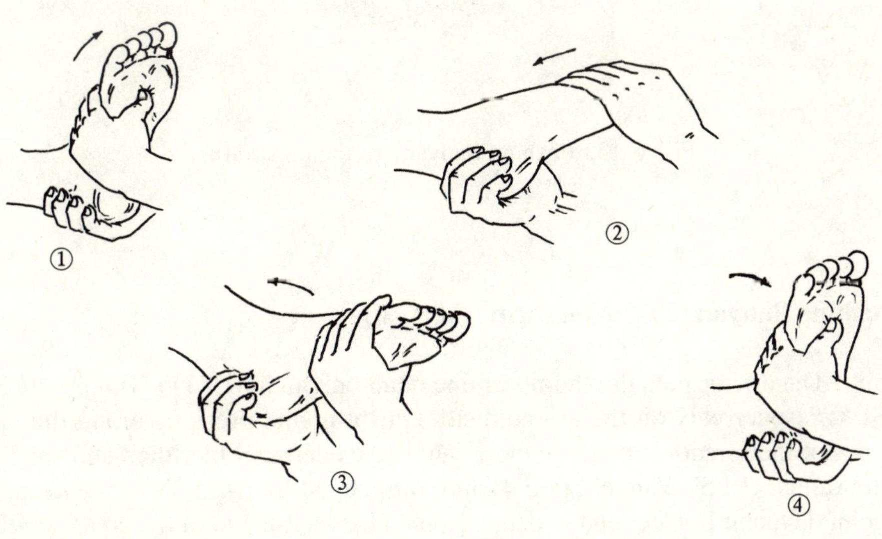

Fig. 6-132 Dorsal bending of the ankle

11) Pushing Sanyang of the upper arm (Fig. 6-133)

[Method] The doctor puts the thumb of one hand on Jianyu (LI 15), Jianliao (TE 14) and Jianzhen (SI 9) respectively on the affected side, pushing and pressing downward along the lateral and posterior sides of the upper arm (the large intestine meridian, triple energizer meridian and small intestine meridian) to Quchi (LI 11), Tianjing (TE 10) and Xiaohai (SI 8) respectively, 3-5 times for each acupoint.

[Acupoints] Jianyu: Located in the depression anterior to the shoulder when it is raised horizontally. Quchi: Located in the depression on the lateral end of the crease on the elbow. Jianliao: Located in the depression posterior to Jianyu. Tianjing: Located 1 *cun* above olecranon. Jianzhen: Located 1 *cun* above the folds in the armpit. Xiaohai: Located in the depression between olecranon and epicondle of the humerus.

[Pithy formula] Pushing three Yang acupoints on the upper arm can treat pain in the shoulder, arm and elbow, subdue cheek swelling, relieve pain and clear away heat by dredging collaterals.

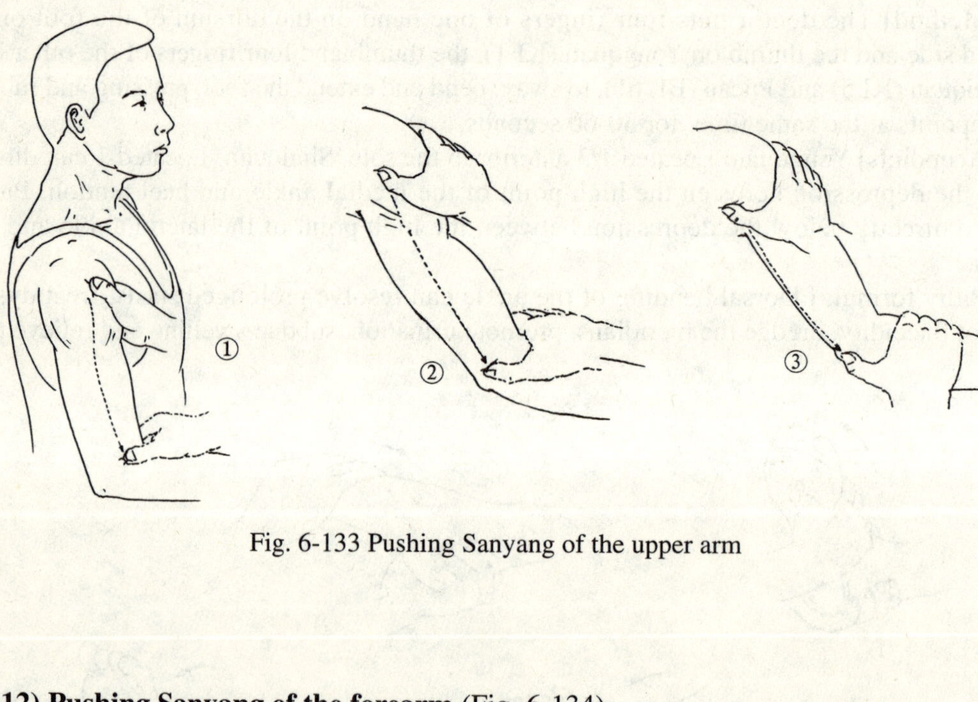

Fig. 6-133 Pushing Sanyang of the upper arm

12) Pushing Sanyang of the forearm (Fig. 6-134)

[Method] The doctor puts the thumb of one hand on Quchi (LI 11), Tianjing (TE 10) and Xiaohai (SI 8) respectively on the affected side, pushing and pressing along the lateral and posterior sides of the forearm (the large meridian, triple energizer meridian and small intestine meridian) to Yangxi (LI 5), Yangchi (TE 4) and Yanggu (SI 5), 3-5 times for each acupoint.

[Acupoints] Quchi: Located in the depression on the lateral end of the crease on the elbow. Yangxi: Located in the depression between the tendons of the long and short extensors of the thumb. Tianjing: Located 1 *cun* above the olecranon. Yangchi: Located in the depression at the ulnar border of the tendon of the general extensor. Xiaohai: Located in the depression between the olecranon of the ulna and the epicondyle of the humerus. Yanggu: Located in the depression anterior to the styloid process of the ulna.

[Pithy formula] Pushing the three Yang acupoints on the forearm can treat spasms of the elbow and arm, stop throat pain, activate the blood to relieve convulsions and eliminate stagnation and fire.

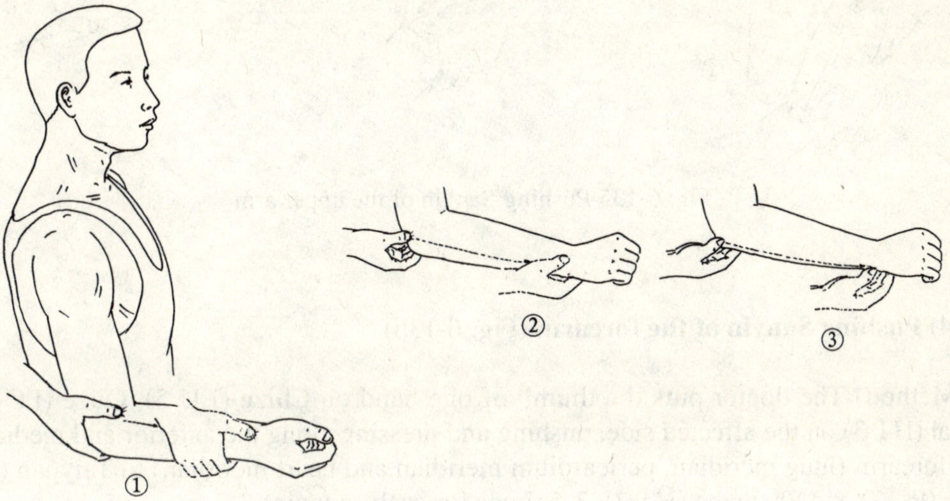

Fig. 6-134 Pushing Sanyang of the forearm

13) Pushing Sanyin of the upper arm (Fig. 6-135)

[Method] The doctor puts the thumb of one hand on Tianfu (LU 3), Tianquan (PC 2) and Jiquan (HT 1) on the affected side, pushing and pressing along the anterior and medial sides of the forearm (lung meridian, pericardium meridian and heart meridian) to Chize (LU 5), Quze (PC 3) and Shaohai (HT 3), 3-5 times for each acupoint.

[Acupoints] Tianfu: Located 3 *cun* below the horizontal line lateral to the upper side of the folds in the armpit and on the lateral border of the cubital biceps. Chize: Located on the radial border of the humeral biceps and in the cubital transverse folds. Tianquan: Located between the short and long ends of the humeral biceps and 2 *cun* below the horizontal line on the upper end of the folds anterior to the armpit. Quze: Located on the ulnar border of the tendon of humeral biceps. Jiquan: Located in the middle of the armpit. Shaohai: Located on the middle point of the line connecting the medial border of the cubital transverse crease and the epicondyle of the humerus.

[Pithy formula] Pushing the three Yin meridians on the forearm can relieve cold sensation in the chest, back and limbs, and attenuate finger numbness by means of warming and dredging the meridians.

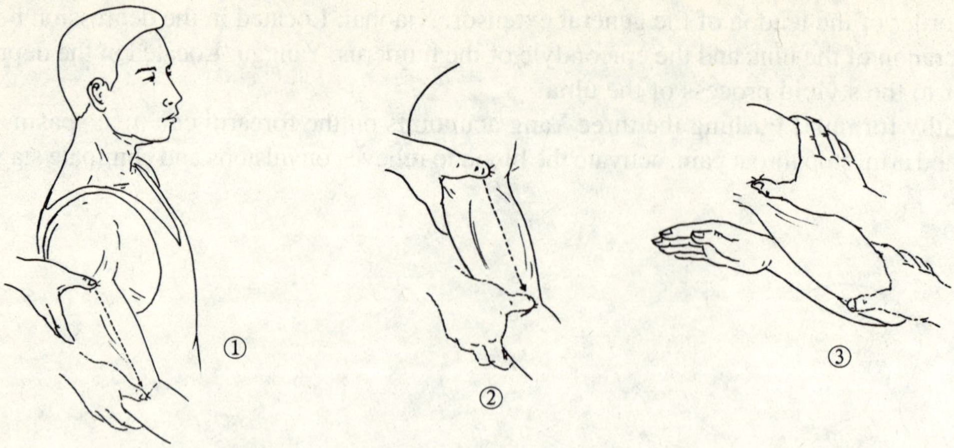

Fig. 6-135 Pushing Sanyin of the upper arm

14) Pushing Sanyin of the forearm (Fig. 6-136)

[Method] The doctor puts the thumb of one hand on Chize (LU 5), Quze (PC 3) and Shaohai (HT 3) on the affected side, pushing and pressing along the anterior and medial sides of the forearm (lung meridian, pericardium meridian and heart meridian) to Taiyuan (LU 9), Daling (PC 7) and Shenmen (HT 7), 3-5 times for each acupoint.

[Acupoints] Chize: Located on the radial border of the humeral biceps and in the cubital transverse folds. Taiyuan: Located on the ulnar side of the humeral biceps, Quze: Located on the ulnar border of the tendon of humeral biceps. Daling: Located between the long palmar tendon and radial flexor. Shaohai: Located on the middle point on the line connecting the medial border of the cubital transverse crease and epicondyle of the humerus. Shenmen: Located in the depression at the radial side of the tendon of the ulnar flexor muscle of the wrist.

[Pithy formula] Pushing the three Yin meridians of the forearm with fingers from He-sea to Shu-stream can treat cough, asthma, palpitation and pain in the elbow and wrist as well as promoting Qi flow and relieving convulsions.

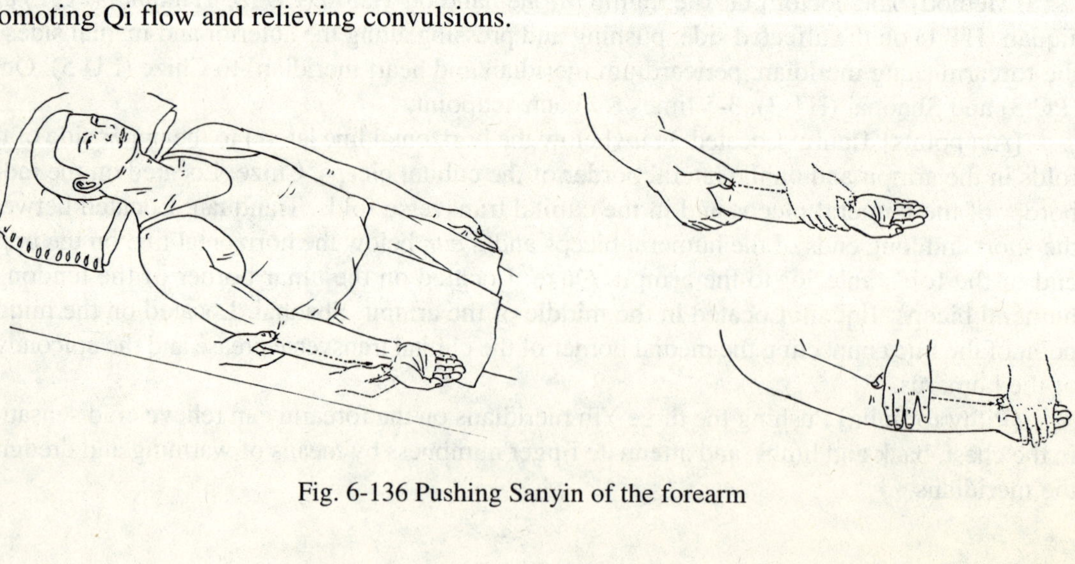

Fig. 6-136 Pushing Sanyin of the forearm

15) Pressing Neiguan and Waiguan (Fig. 6-137)

[Method] The doctor puts the thumb of one hand on Neiguan (PC 6) on the affected side, and the remaining four fingers on Waiguan (TE 15) to press against each other for 30-60 seconds. Then the thumb pushes and presses downward from Daling (PC 7) and Yangchi (TE 4) to Laogong (PC 8) and Zhongchong (PC 9), each acupoint being pressed and rubbed for 3-5 seconds. This manipulation is repeated 2-5 times.

[Acupoints] Neiguan: Located 2 *cun* above the crease on the wrist and between the long palmar muscle tendon and tendon of the radial flexor of the wrist. Waiguan: Located 2 *cun* above the crease on the back of the wrist and between the radius and ulna. Daling: Located in the middle of the wrist crease and between the long palmar tendon and flexor. Yangchi: Located in the middle of the crease on the back of the wrist and in the depression at the ulnar side of the tendon of the general extensor. Laogong: Located in the middle of the palmar crease and between the second and third metacarpal bones. Zhongchong: Located in the middle of the tip of the middle finger.

[Pithy formula] Rubbing and pressing Neiguan, Waiguan, Laogong and Zhongchong can stop fright at night, relieve stomachache and dysphoria, clear the heart and tranquilize the mind.

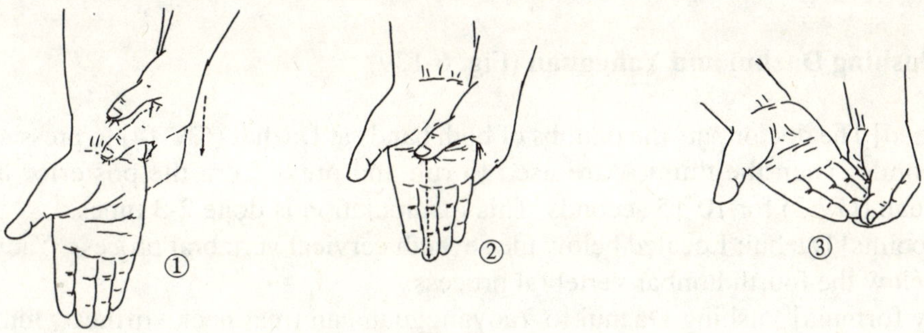

Fig. 6-137 Pressing Neiguan and Waiguan

16) Pinching neck muscles (Fig. 6-138)

[Method] The doctor puts the fingers of both hands at Fengchi (GB 20) on the affected side, the thumb at the lateral side of the neck muscles and the remaining fingers at the medial side, to lift up the neck muscles and hold from the upper to the lower, stopping at Jianzhongshu (SI 15). This manipulation is repeated 3-5 times.

[Acupoints] Fengchi: Located in the depression between the sternocleidomastoid muscle and the trapezius muscle and 1 *cun* directly above the point parallel to the posterior hairline. Jianzhongshu: 2 *cun* lateral to the seventh cervical vertebral process.

[Pithy formula] Pinching Fengchi to Jianzhongshu can treat pain in the shoulder and back. Rolling manipulation is used after pinching for the purpose of regulating Qi and blood as well as the meridians.

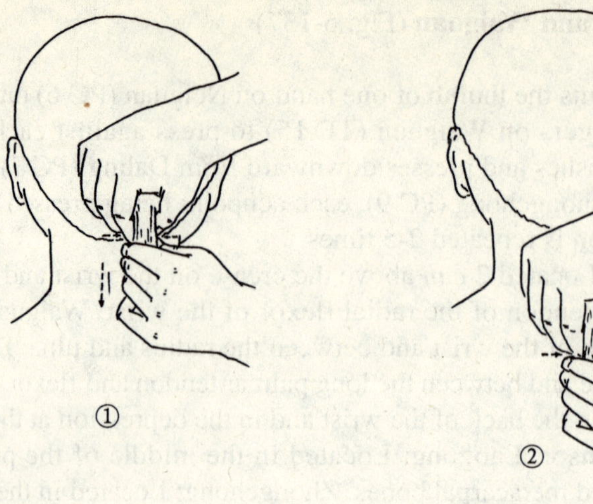

Fig. 6-138 Pinching neck muscles

17) Pushing Dazhui and Yangguan (Fig. 6-139)

[Method] The doctor puts the thumbs of both hands at Dazhui (GV 14) to press and rub for 10-15 seconds. Then the thumbs are used to rub and press from the posterior midline to Yaoyangguan (GV 3) for 10-15 seconds. This manipulation is done 2-3 times.

[Acupoints] Dazhui: Located below the seventh cervical vertebral process. Yaoyangguan: Located below the fourth lumbar vertebral process.

[Pithy formula] Pushing Dazhui to Yaoyangguan can treat neck stiffness, lumbago and febrile disease by means of dredging Yang and activating blood.

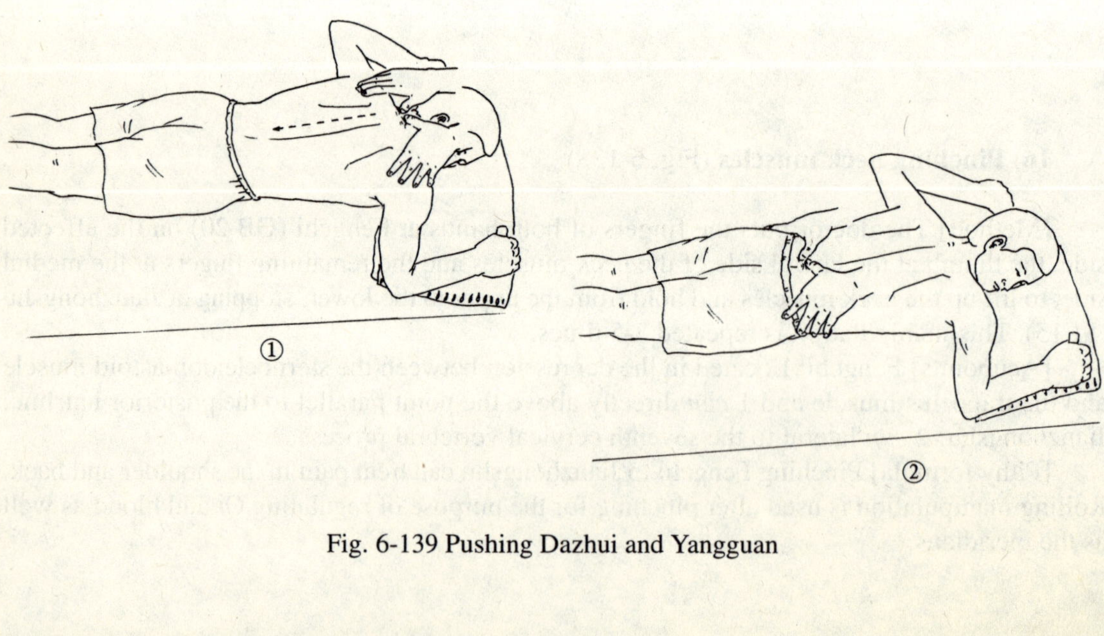

Fig. 6-139 Pushing Dazhui and Yangguan

18) Transverse stroking of the waist (Fig. 6-140)

[Method] The doctor puts one hand at Shenshu (BL 32), Qihaishu (CV 6) and Dachangshu (BL 25) on the healthy side to stroke to Daimai (GB 26) on the affected side, then to Daimai (GB 26) on the healthy side. This manipulation is repeated 15-20 times.

[Acupoints] Shenshu: Located 1.5 *cun* lateral to the lower point of the second lumbar vertebral process. Qihaishu: Located 1.5 *cun* lateral to the lower point of the third lumbar vertebral process. Dachangshu: Located 1.5 *cun* lateral to the lower point of the fourth lumbar vertebral process. Daimai: Located directly below the 11th rib and parallel to the navel.

[Pithy formula] Transverse rubbing and stroking of the waist can activate blood, dredge collaterals and strengthen tendons and bones.

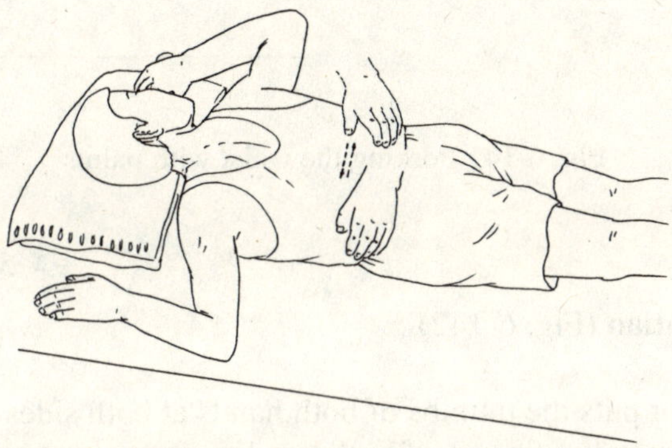

Fig. 6-140 Transverse stroking of the waist

19) Forking the waist with palms (Fig. 6-141)

[Method] The doctor puts the ends of both palms at Mingmen (GV 4) on the affected side and the fingers of both hands at the sides of the waist. The palms are used to push laterally in a forked way from Shenshu (BL 32) to Daimai (GB 26). This manipulation is repeated 5-10 times.

[Acupoints] Mingmen: Located below the second lumbar vertebral process. Shenshu: Located 1.5 *cun* lateral to Mingmen. Daimai: Located directly below the 11th rib and parallel to the navel.

[Pithy formula] Pushing Mingmen, Shenshu and Daimai can relieve spastic pain in the waist and spine, soothe the tendons, warm the kidney and quickly relieve pain.

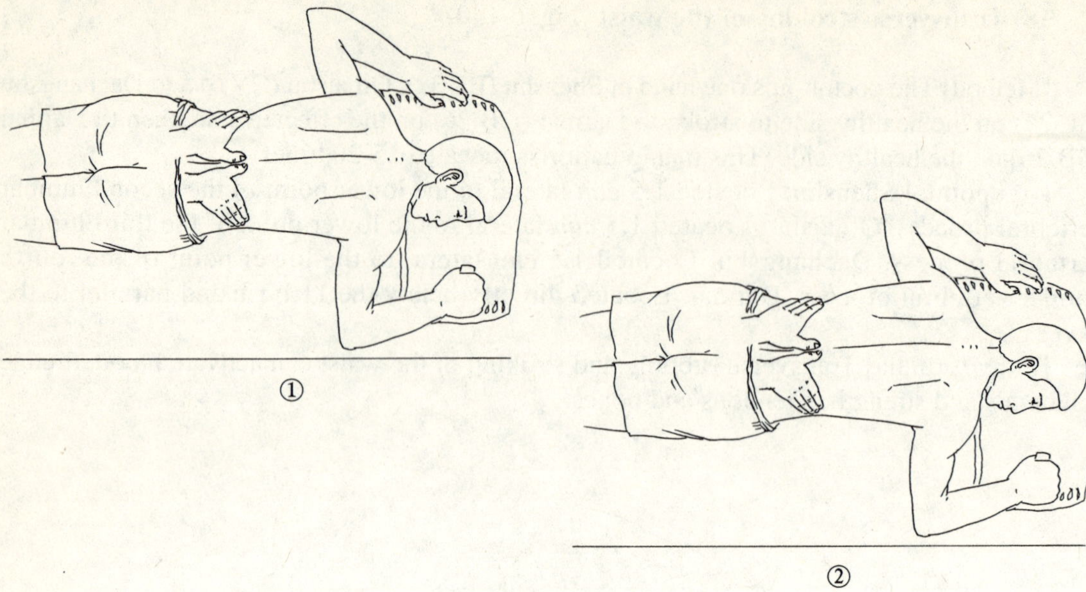

Fig. 6-141 Forking the waist with palms

20) Pressing Huantiao (Fig. 6-142)

[Method] The doctor puts the thumbs of both hands at both sides of Huantiao (GB 30) on the affected side. The remaining fingers of both hands are placed at both sides of the arms and the thumbs are used to press the acupoint from contrary directions for 15-30 seconds. This manipulation is repeated 3-5 times.

[Acupoint] Huantiao: Located at 1/3 of the lateral connecting line between the greater trochanter of the femur and sacral hiatus.

[Pithy formula] Pressing Huantiao with fingers, or with the elbow if necessary, can treat leg numbness by dredging the meridians, relieve convulsions and promote the flow of Qi and blood. Stroking manipulation must be used after pressing.

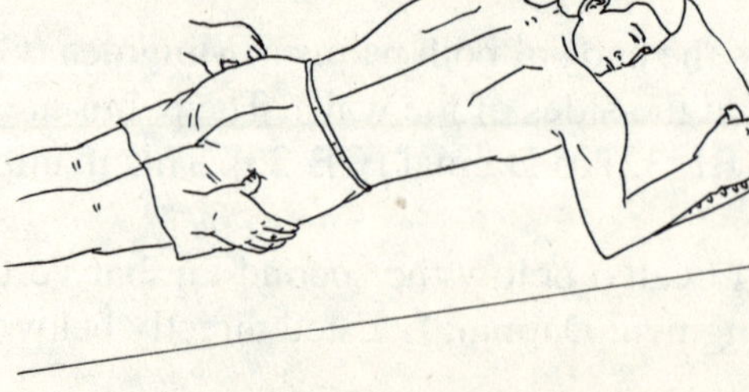

Fig. 6-142 Pressing Huantiao

21) Pushing the posterior side of the thigh (Fig. 6-143)

[Method] The doctor puts the thumbs of both hands at Chengfu (BL 36) on the affected limb and the remaining fingers of both hands at both sides of the thigh to push and press along the posterior midline of the leg (bladder meridian) from Yinmen (BL 37), Weizhong (BL 40) and Chengshan (BL 57) and the heel tendon. This manipulation is repeated 3-5 times.

[Acupoints] Chengfu: Located in the middle of the gluteal groove. Yinmen: Located 6 *cun* directly below Chengfu. Weizhong: Located on the middle of the popliteal crease. Chengshan: Located on the tip of the depression between the gastrocnemius muscle and abdominal muscle.

[Pithy formula] Pushing Chengfu, Yinmen and Weizhong can treat pain in the waist and leg. Pushing from Chengshan to the heel tendon can disperse cold, eliminate dampness and dredge the meridians and collaterals.

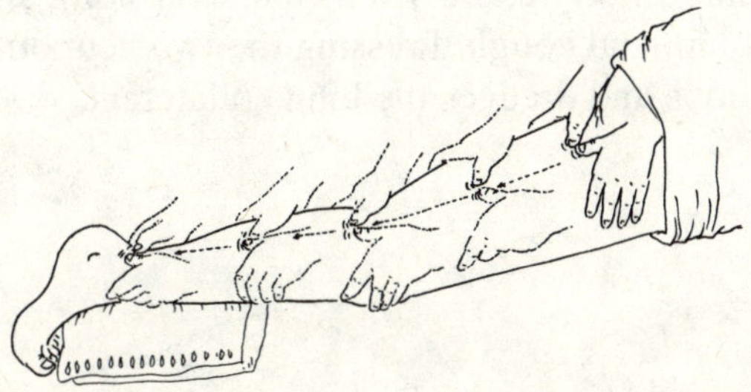

Fig. 6-143 Pushing the posterior side of the thigh

22) Holding Kunlun (Fig. 6-144)

[Method] The doctor puts the thumb and index finger of one hand at Sanyinjiao (SP 6) and Xuanzhong (GB 39) on the affected limb to push to Taixi (K13) and Kunlun (BL 60). The heel tendon is lifted 3-5 times with great strength.

[Acupoints] Sanyinjiao: Located 3 *cun* above the high point of the medial ankle and on the posterior border of the medial side of the tibia. Xuanzhong: Located 3 *cun* above the high point of the lateral ankle and on the anterior border of the fibia. Taixi: Located in the depression between the high point of the medial ankle and the heel tendon. Kunlun: Located in the depression between the high point of the lateral ankle and the heel tendon.

[Pithy formula] Holding Kunlun and Xuanzhong with fingers and pushing Sanyinjiao to Taixi can treat flaccidity, pain and distension of the waist and leg, as well as soothe tendons and activate the blood.

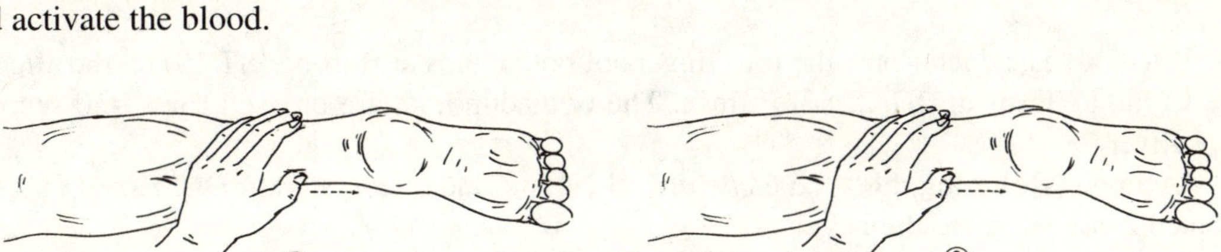

①　②

Fig. 6-144 Holding Kunlun

(2) Combination of the manipulations

1) Wind-phlegm blockage the collaterals

① Pressing Zhongfu and Yunmen (Fig. 6-145)

[Method] The doctor slightly forks the four fingers of one hand and puts them at the inner border of the greater pectoral muscle to stroke, like combing, from the inner to the outer along the costal spaces to Zhongfu (LU 1) and Yunmen (LU 2) 5-10 times. The two acupoints are pressed 2-3 times, 10-15 seconds each time.

[Acupoints] Zhongfu: Located 6 *cun* lateral to the anterior midline and parallel to the first costal space. Yunmen: Located 6 *cun* lateral to the anterior midline and at the lower border of the sternum.

[Pithy formula] Pressing Zhongfu and Yunmen and stroking along the costal spaces in a combing way treats chest pain and cough. Pressing the two acupoints relieves numbness and feverish sensation in the limbs and dredges the lung collaterals.

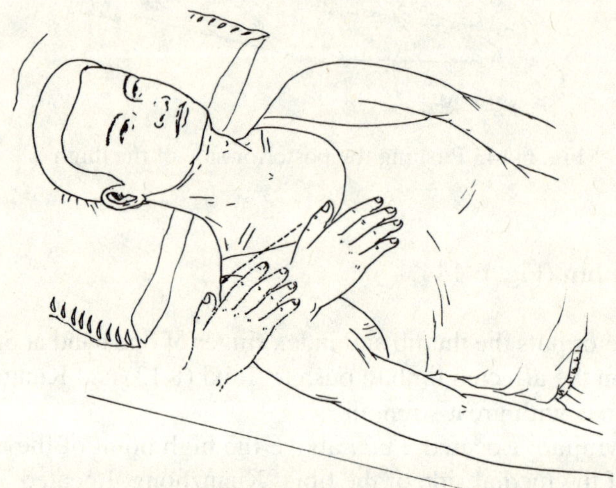

Fig. 6-145 Pressing Zhongfu and Yunmen

② Stroking and pressing the upper abdomen (Fig. 6-146)

[Method] The doctor puts the four fingers of both hands at Burong (ST 19) on the affected side to rub to Tianshu (ST 25) 3-5 times. The two acupoints are pressed for 15-30 seconds respectively.

[Acupoints] Burong: Located 6 *cun* directly above and 2 *cun* lateral to the navel. Tianshu: Located 2 *cun* lateral to the navel.

[Pithy formula] Pressing and rubbing the upper abdomen from Burong to Tianshu can relieve upper abdominal distension and stomachache as well as regulating Qi and strengthening the spleen.

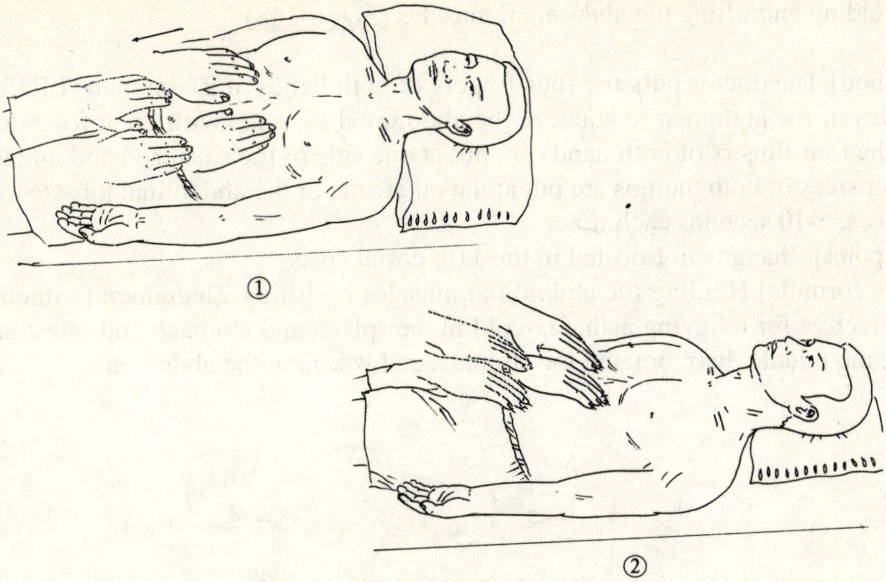

Fig. 6-146 Stroking and pressing the upper abdomen

③ Pressing the middle of the abdomen (Fig. 6-147)

[Method] The doctor puts the four fingers of one hand at Shangwan (CV 13) to press downward through Xiawan (CV 10) and Guanyuan (CV 4) to Qugu (CV 2). Each acupoint is pressed for 3-5 seconds. This manipulation is repeated 3-5 times.

[Acupoints] Shangwan: Located 5 *cun* directly above the navel. Xiawan: Located 2 *cun* directly above the navel. Guanyuan: Located 3 *cun* directly below the navel. Qugu: Located 5 *cun* directly below the navel.

[Pithy formula] Pressing the upper abdomen with the fingers to Qugu can treat diarrhea with undigested food, relieve stomach cold, warm the middle and harmonize the stomach.

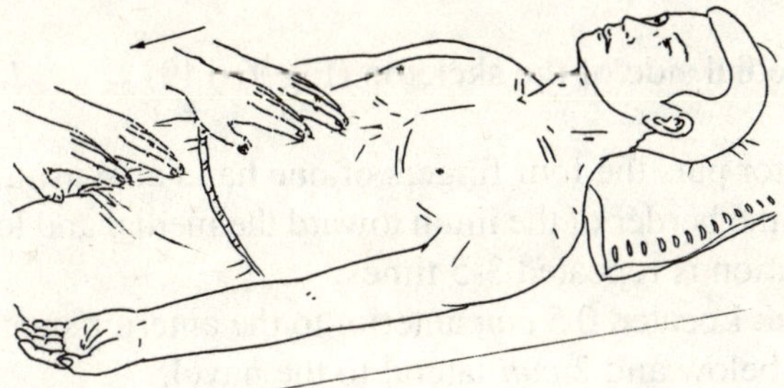

Fig. 6-147 Pressing the middle of the abdomen

④ Holding and lifting the abdominal muscles (Fig. 6-148)

[Method] The doctor puts the four fingers of both hands at Zhangmen (LR13) on both lateral sides of the abdomen to squeeze the abdominal muscles with great force toward the middle. The four fingers of both hands are put at one side of the squeezed abdominal muscle. The palmar sides of both thumbs are put at the other side of the abdominal muscle to hold and lift 3-5 times, 5-10 seconds each time.

[Acupoint] Zhangmen: Located in the 11th costal space.

[Pithy formula] Holding the abdominal muscles by lifting Zhangmen (without causing pain) is effective for relieving asthenia-cold in the spleen and stomach and intestinal spasm, regulating the middle, harmonizing the stomach and warming the abdomen.

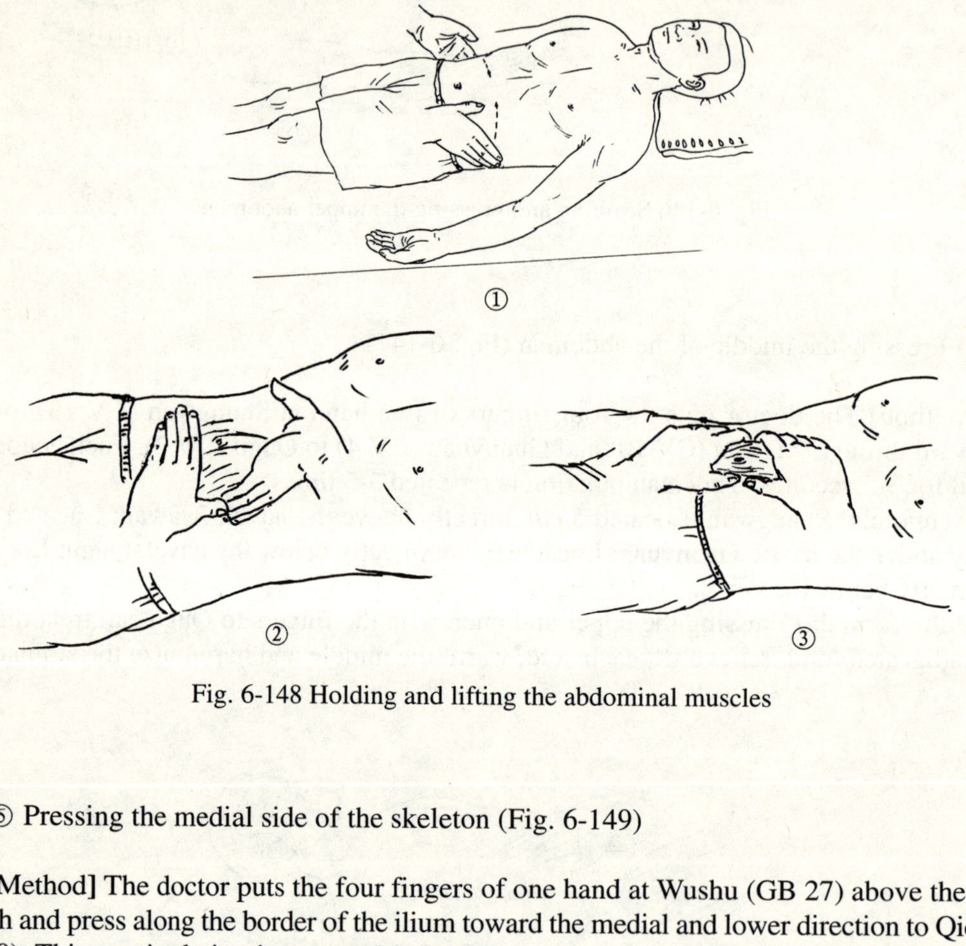

Fig. 6-148 Holding and lifting the abdominal muscles

⑤ Pressing the medial side of the skeleton (Fig. 6-149)

[Method] The doctor puts the four fingers of one hand at Wushu (GB 27) above the ilium to push and press along the border of the ilium toward the medial and lower direction to Qichong (ST 30). This manipulation is repeated 3-5 times.

[Acupoints] Wushu: Located 0.5 *cun* anterior to the anterior superior iliac spine. Qichong: Located 5 *cun* directly below and 2 *cun* lateral to the navel.

[Pithy formula] Pushing and pressing from the inner side of the ilium to Wushu and Qichong can relieve cold pain in the lower limb and cold sensation in the lower abdomen, warm Yang, dredge the meridians and promote the flow of Qi and blood.

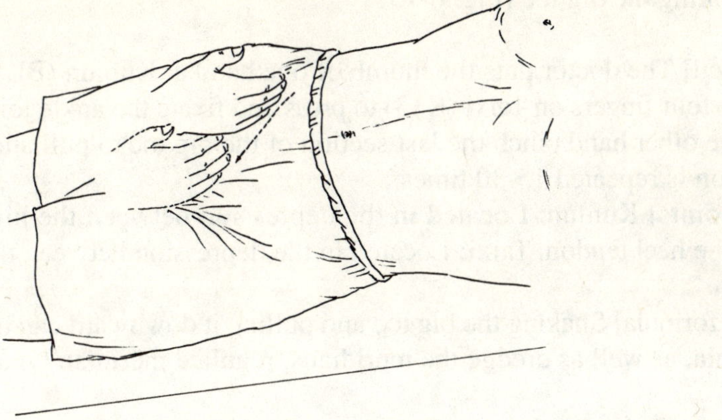

Fig. 6-149 Pressing the medial side of the skeleton

⑥ Rubbing Xuanzhong (Fig. 6-150)

[Method] The doctor puts the thumb of one hand at Xuanzhong (GB 39) on the affected limb, the thumb of the other hand at Tiaokou (ST 38) and the remaining four fingers at Chengshan (BL 57) to press and rub for 1-2 minutes with great strength.

[Acupoints] Xuanzhong: Located 3 *cun* above the high point of the lateral ankle and on the anterior border of the fibia. Tiaokou: Located 5 *cun* directly below and one transverse finger lateral to the anterior crest of the tibia. Chengshan: Located at the top of the depression between the two bellies of the gastrocnemius muscle.

[Pithy formula] Pressing and rubbing Xuanzhong, Tiaokou and Chengshan can subdue swelling, relieve numbness and spasms of the knee and shank, promote Qi flow and activate blood.

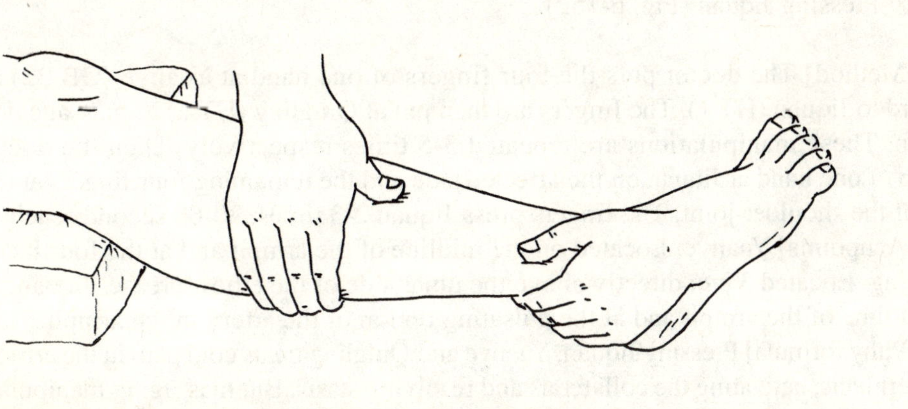

Fig. 6-150 Rubbing Xuanzhong

⑦ Shaking the big toe (Fig. 6-151)

[Method] The doctor puts the thumb of one hand at Kunlun (BL 60) on the affected limb and the rest four fingers on Taixi (K13) to press and fixate the ankle joint. The thumb and index finger of the other hand pinch the last section of the big toe to pull and shake downward. This manipulation is repeated 15-30 times.

[Acupoints] Kunlun: Located in the depression between the high point of the external ankle and the heel tendon. Taixi: Located in the depression between the internal ankle and the heel tendon.

[Pithy formula] Shaking the big toe and pulling it downward can treat dizziness, dysphoria and insomnia, as well as dredge the meridians, regulate meridian Qi and soothe the chest.

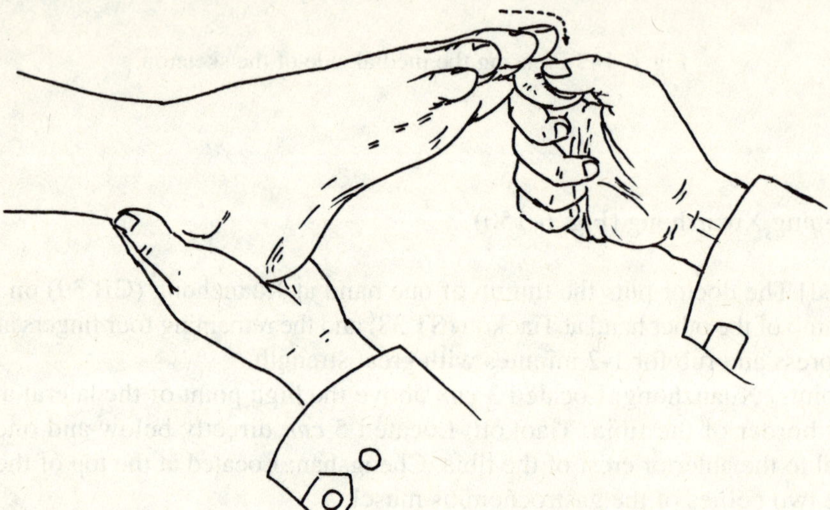

Fig. 6-151 Shaking the big toe

⑧ Pressing Jiquan (Fig. 6-152)

[Method] The doctor puts the four fingers of one hand at Yuanye (GB 22) to massage upward to Jiquan (HT 1). The fingers are then put at Qingling (HT 2) to massage downward to Jiquan. These manipulations are repeated 3-5 times respectively. Then the doctor puts the thumb of one hand at Jiquan on the affected side and the remaining four fingers at the posterior side of the shoulder joint. The fingers press Jiquan 2-3 times, 30-60 seconds each time.

[Acupoints] Yuanye: Located on the midline of the armpit and at the fourth costal space. Qingling: Located 3 *cun* directly above the ulnar side of the elbow crease. Jiquan: Located on the midline of the armpit and at the pulsating region of the artery in the armpit.

[Pithy formula] Pressing Jiquan, Yuanye and Qingling treats cold pain in the arm by warming the meridians, activating the collaterals and resolving stasis. But massaging manipulation cannot be performed for a long time.

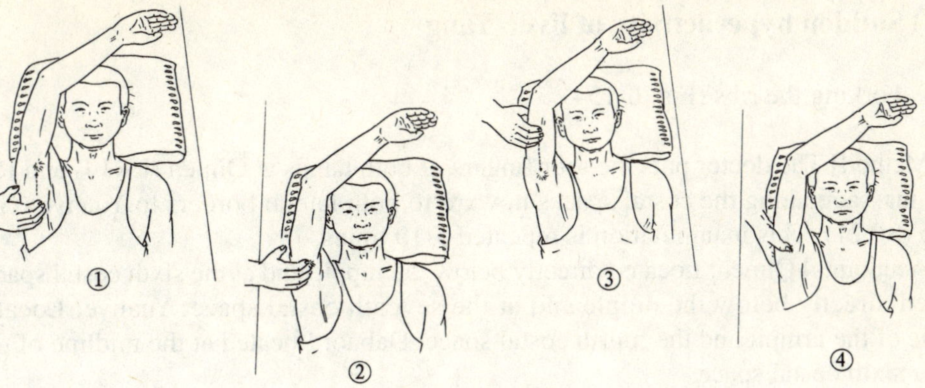

Fig. 6-152 Pressing Jiquan

⑨ Forked pushing of the occipital region (Fig. 6-153)

[Method] The doctor puts the palmar sides of the thumbs of both hands at Fengfu (GV 16) to push in a forked way downward and laterally along Fengchi (GB 20), Wangu (GB 12) and Yifeng (TE 17), then upward around the back of the ear (triple energizer meridian), by Chimai (TE 18), Luxi (TE 19), Jiaosun (TE 20) and Er'heliao (TE 22). These acupoints are pushed and rubbed 2-3 times.

[Acupoints] Fengfu: Located 1 *cun* directly above the posterior hairline. Fengchi: Located in the depression between the sternocleidomastoid muscle and trapezius muscle parallel to Fengfu. Wangu: Located in the depression posterior to the mastoid process. Yifeng: Located anterior and inferior to the mastoid process and in the depression parallel to the lower border of the earlobe. Chimai: Located in the middle of the mastoid process, at the lower 1/3 and upper 2/3 on the line connecting Yifeng and Jiaosun along the helix. Luxi: Located at the upper 1/3 on the line connecting Chimai. Jiaosun: Located on the hairline at the top of the ear. Er'heliao: Located at the posterior border of the temples, parallel to the auricle and on the posterior border of the superficial temporal artery.

[Pithy formula] Pushing Fengfu and Er'heliao in a forked way from the occipitus can treat ear disease. Pushing and rubbing the acupoints located on the triple energizer meridian behind the ear can tranquilize the mind, open the orifice and promote meridian Qi flow.

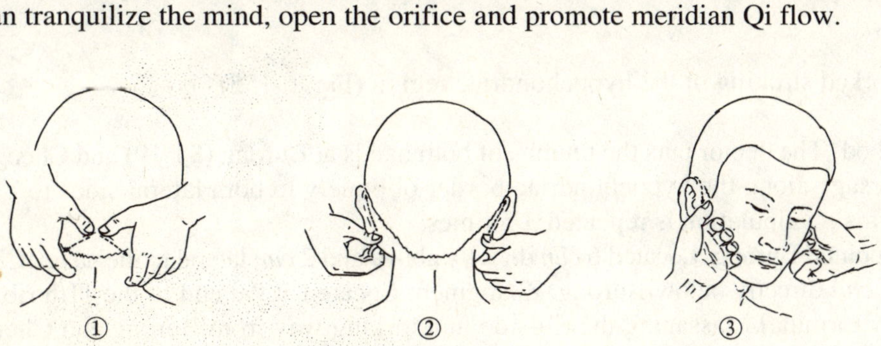

Fig. 6-153 Forked pushing of the occipital region

2) Sudden hyperactivity of liver-Yang

① Forking the ribs (Fig. 6-154)

[Method] The doctor puts the four fingers of both hands at Qimen (LR14) and Riyue (GB 24) to massage along the costal spaces upward to both lateral borders to Yuanye (GB 22)and Dabao (SP 21). This manipulation is repeated 5-10 times.

[Acupoints] Qimen: Located directly below the nipple and at the sixth costal space. Riyue: Located directly below the nipple and at the seventh costal space. Yuanye: Located at the midline of the armpit and the fourth costal space. Dabao: Located at the midline of the armpit and the sixth costal space.

[Pithy formula] Massaging Qimen and Riyue in a forked way treats thoracic and costal injury. Massaging Yuanye and Dabao in a forked way can regulate the liver meridian and resolve blood stasis.

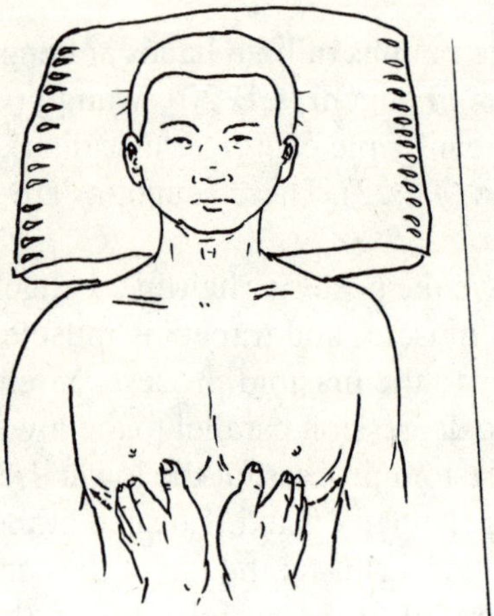

①

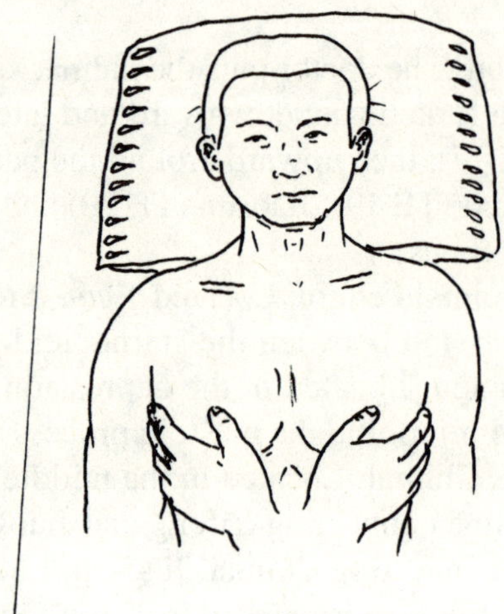

②

Fig. 6-154 Forking the ribs

② Forked stroking of the hypochondriac region (Fig. 6-155)

[Method] The doctor puts the thumbs of both hands at Burong (ST 19) and Chengman (ST 20) to massage along the hypochondriac border obliquely to both lateral sides to Zhangmen (LR13). This manipulation is repeated 3-5 times.

[Acupoints] Burong: Located 6 *cun* directly above and 2 *cun* lateral to the navel. Chengman: Located 1 *cun* directly below Burong. Zhangmen: Located at the end of the 11th rib.

[Pithy formula] Massaging the rib-side in a forking way from Burong and Chengman to Zhangmen can relieve chest oppression, cough and hypochondriac pain, regulate liver-Qi and stop pain.

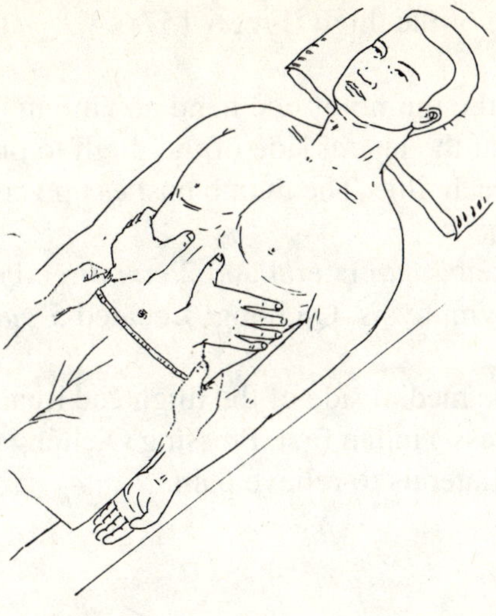

Fig. 6-155 Forked stroking of the hypochondriac region

③ Minor Qi-dispersing method (Fig. 6-156)

[Method] The doctor puts the four fingers of both hands at the upper border of Weidao (GB 28) on the affected side to massage along the medial and inferior direction to Qichong (ST 30). This manipulation is repeated 3-5 times.

[Acupoints] Weidao: Located 1 *cun* anterior and inferior to the anterior iliac spine and 3 *cun* directly below the point parallel to the navel. Qichong: Located 5 *cun* directly below and 2 *cun* lateral to the navel.

[Pithy formula] The minor Qi-dispersing method relieves abdominal distension. Massaging from Weidao to Qichong can treat oral ulceration, reduce heat and relieve borborygmus as well as clear away damp-heat.

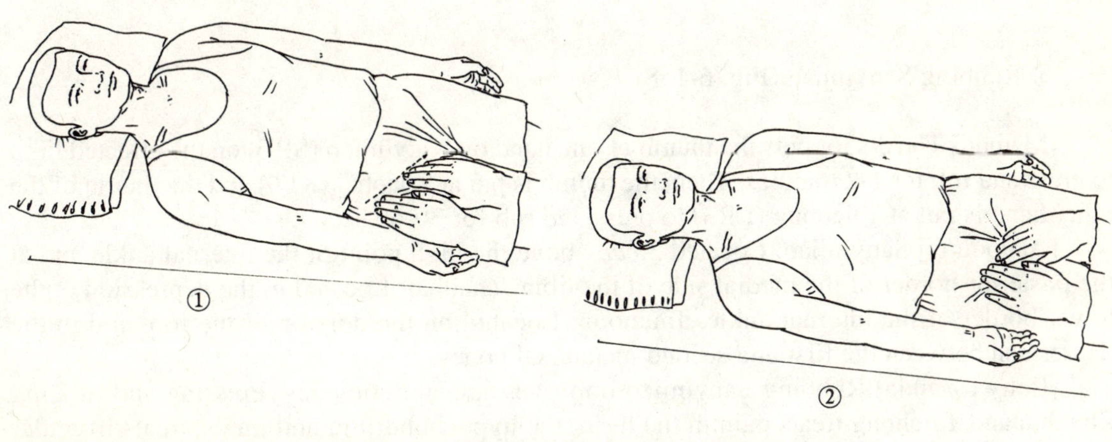

①

②

Fig. 6-156 Minor Qi-dispersing method

④ Pressing the medial side of the thigh (Fig. 6-157)

[Method] The doctor puts the thumb of one hand at Yinlian (LR11) on the affected side and the remaining four fingers at the lateral side of the thigh to press the acupoint with great force 3-5 times, 15-30 seconds each time. The thumb pushes upward to Qichong and presses 1-3 times, 30-60 seconds each time.

[Acupoints] Yinlian: Located 2 *cun* lateral and 2 *cun* directly below the middle point of the upper border of the pubic symphysis. Qichong: Located 5 *cun* directly below and 2 *cun* lateral to the navel.

[Pithy formula] Pressing the medial side of the thigh can treat cold obstruction syndrome by warming. It is advisable to press Yinlian first. Pressing Qichong is effective for dredging the meridians and activating the collaterals to relieve pain.

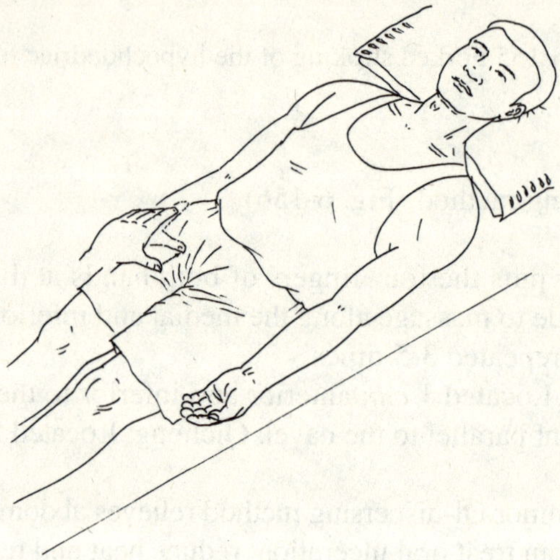

Fig. 6-157 Pressing the medial side of the thigh

⑤ Rubbing Sanyinjiao (Fig. 6-158)

[Method] The doctor puts the thumb of one hand on Sanyinjiao (SP 6) on the affected limb to press and rub for 1-2 minutes. Then, the thumb is put at Zhaohai (KI 6) and the thumb of the other hand is put at Taichong (LR3) to press and rub for 30-60 seconds.

[Acupoints] Sanyinjiao: Located 3 *cun* above the high point of the internal ankle and at the posterior border of the medial side of the tibia. Zhaohai: Located in the depression at the lower border of the internal ankle. Taichong: Located on the dorsum of the foot and in the depression between the first and second metatarsal bones.

[Pithy formula] Rubbing Sanyinjiao improves spleen deficiency. Pressing and rubbing Zhaohai and Taichong treats pain in the head, the hypochondrium and limbs, treats irregular menstruation, regulates Yin meridians and resolves stasis.

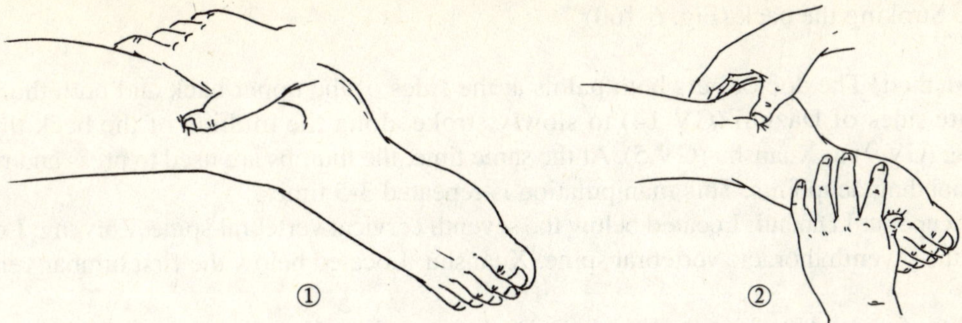

Fig. 6-158 Rubbing Sanyinjiao

⑥ Stroking and pressing the hypochondriac region (Fig. 6-159)

[Method] The doctor puts the four fingers of one hand at Burong (ST 19) and Chengman (ST 20) located on the hypochondrium and the four fingers of the other hand at Hunmen (BL 47) and Yanggang (BL 48) located on the back to press toward the midline of the armpit for 3-5 seconds. This manipulation is repeated 5-10 times.

[Acupoints] Burong: Located 6 *cun* directly above and 2 *cun* lateral to the navel. Chengman: Located 1 *cun* directly below Burong. Hunmen: Located below and 3 *cun* lateral to the ninth thoracic vertebral spine. Yanggang: Located below and 3 *cun* lateral to the 10th thoracic vertebral spine.

[Pithy formula] Stroking and pressing from Burong on the hypochondrium to the armpit, pressing first and then stroking can dredge liver Qi and relieve the backache.

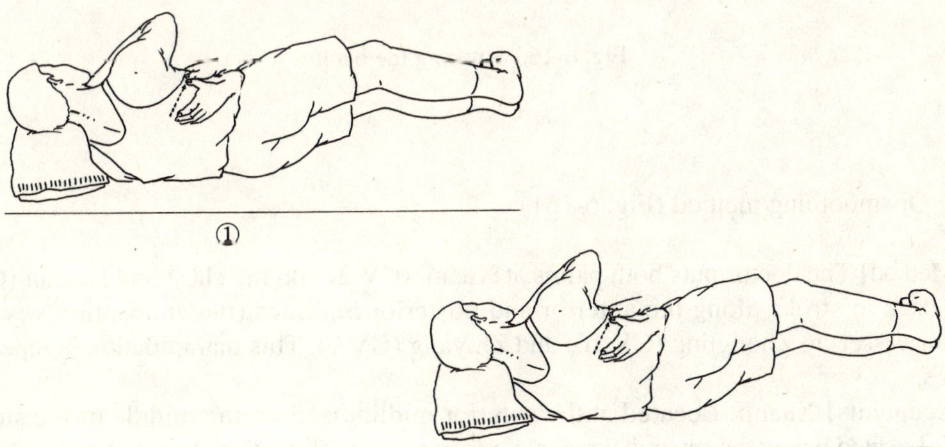

Fig. 6-159 Stroking and pressing the hypochondriac region

⑦ Stroking the back (Fig. 6-160)

[Method] The doctor puts both palms at the sides of the upper back and both thumbs at opposite sides of Dazhui (GV 14) to slowly stroke along the midline of the back through Zhiyang (GV 9) to Xuanshu (GV 5). At the same time, the thumbs are used to press and rub the corresponding acupoints. This manipulation is repeated 3-5 times.

[Acupoints] Dazhui: Located below the seventh cervical vertebral spine. Zhiyang: Located below the seventh thoracic vertebral spine. Xuanshu: Located below the first lumbar vertebral spine.

[Pithy formula] Stroking the back from Dazhui directly to Xuanshu can treat liver stagnation, spleen deficiency and diarrhea through relieving stagnation, strengthening the spleen and regulating the intestines and stomach.

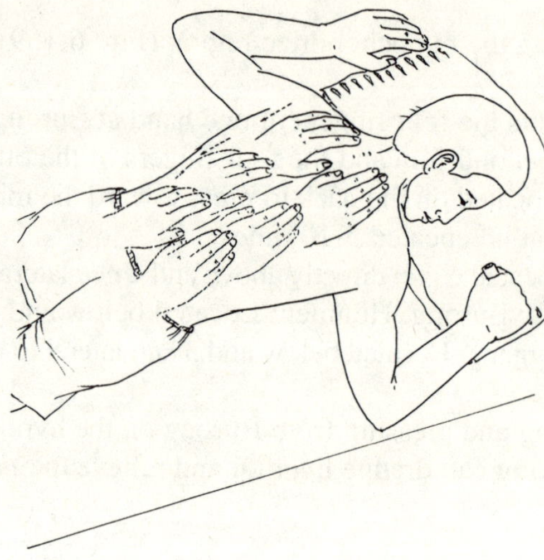

Fig. 6-160 Stroking the back

⑧ Qi-smoothing method (Fig. 6-161)

[Method] The doctor puts both palms at Xuanji (CV 21) on the chest and Dazhui (GV 14) on the back to stroke along the anterior and posterior midlines (the conception vessel and governor vessel) to Zhongting (CV 16) and Zhiyang (GV 9). This manipulation is repeated 5-10 times.

[Acupoints] Xuanji: Located at the anterior midline and on the middle of the sternum. Dazhui: Located below the seventh cervical vertebral spine. Zhongting: Located on the midpoint of the xiphosternal synchondrosis. Zhiyang: Located below the seventh thoracic vertebral spine.

[Pithy formula] Smoothing Qi by stroking Xuanji and Dazhui can treat pain in the chest and back. Stroking from Zhongting to Zhiyang can descend Qi and soothe the chest.

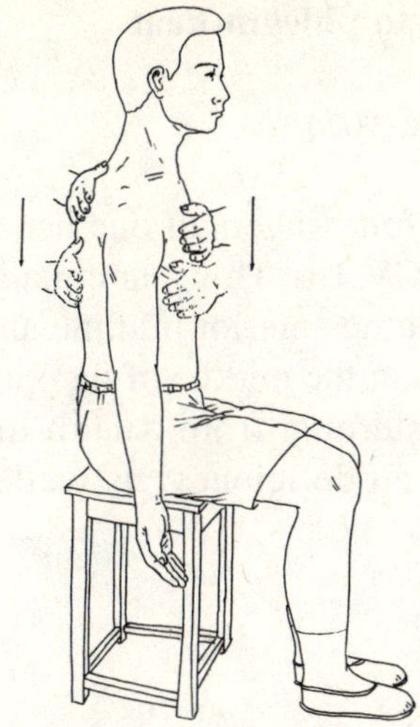

Fig. 6-161 Qi-smoothing method

⑨ Chest-expanding method (Fig. 6-162)

[Method] The doctor embraces the elbows of the patient with both hands and puts the knee on Zhiyang (GV 9) on the back. Then the doctor asks the patient to straighten the chest and breathe deep. At the same time, the doctor pulls the elbows of the patient backward, pushing and pressing the back with the knee until the patient inhales. This manipulation is repeated 3-5 times.

[Acupoint] Zhiyang: Located below the seventh thoracic vertebral spine.

[Pithy formula] Embracing the head with both hands of the patient can dilate the chest and relieve thoracic distension. Pulling the patient's elbows and pushing the patient's back when the patient breathes deep can regulate Qi activity and soothe the chest.

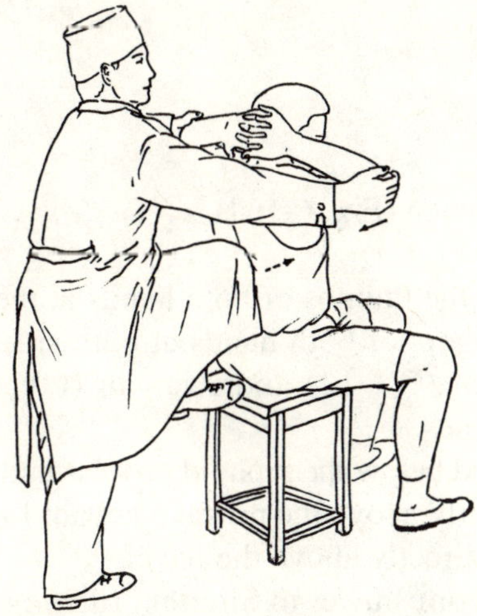

Fig. 6-162 Chest-expanding method

3) Sthenia-Fu syndrome due to phlegm-heat

① Pressing the sternum (Fig. 6-163)

[Method] The doctor puts the four fingers of one hand at Xuanji (CV 21) to press along the anterior midline to Zhongting (CV 16). This manipulation is repeated 3-5 times.

[Acupoints] Xuanji: Located at the anterior midline and on the middle of the manubrium of the sternum. Zhongting: Located at the middle of the xiphosternal synchondrosis.

[Pithy formula] Pressing the sternum from Xuanji to Zhongting can treat vomiting of phlegm, and insomnia due to spleen deficiency, as well as nourish Qi and strengthen the spleen.

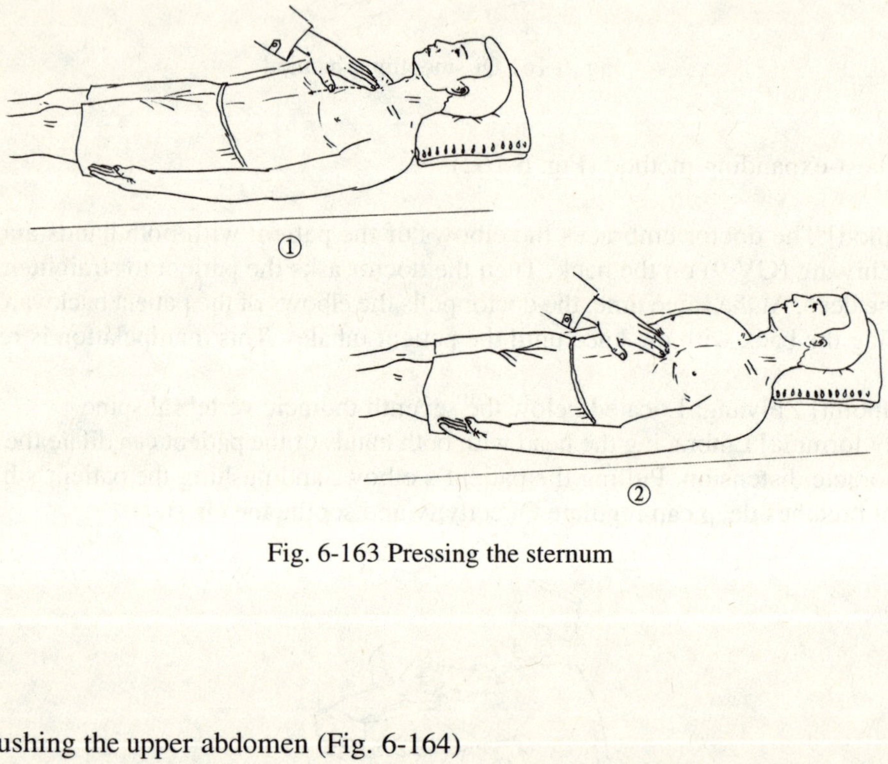

Fig. 6-163 Pressing the sternum

② Pushing the upper abdomen (Fig. 6-164)

[Method] The doctor puts the thumbs of both hands at the opposite sides of Jiuwei (CV 15) and the remaining four fingers of both hands at both sides of the chest to push and rub downward through Zhongwan (CV 12) and Xiawan (CV 10) to Shuifen (CV 9). This manipulation is repeated 3-5 times.

[Acupoints] Jiuwei: Located below the xiphoid process and 7 *cun* directly above the navel. Zhongwan: Located 4 *cun* directly above the navel. Xiawan: Located 2 *cun* directly above the navel. Shuifen: Located 1 *cun* directly above the navel.

[Pithy formula] Pushing from Jiuwei to Shuifen, rubbing and pressing lightly first and then heavily, can relieve epigastrium distension and regulate Qi activity.

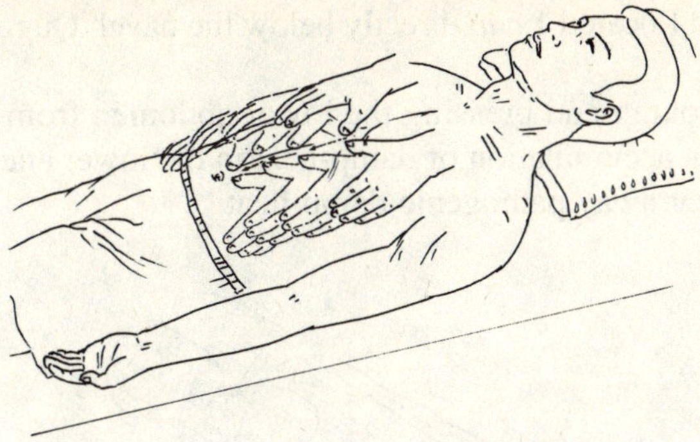

Fig. 6-164 Pushing the upper abdomen

③ Transverse stroking beside the navel (Fig. 6-165)

[Method] The doctor puts the four fingers of one hand at Daheng (SP 15) and Fujie (SP 14) to stroke transversely through Tianshu (ST 25) and Wailing (ST 26) to Daheng and Fujie on the affected side. This manipulation is repeated 5-10 times.

[Acupoints] Daheng: Located 4 *cun* lateral to the navel. Fujie: Located 1.3 *cun* below Daheng. Tianshu: Located 2 *cun* lateral to the navel. Wailing: Located 1 *cun* below Tianshu.

[Pithy formula] Stroking transversely beside the navel can treat constipation and hiccup. Unidirectionally stroking Daheng can regulate Qi activity and relax the body.

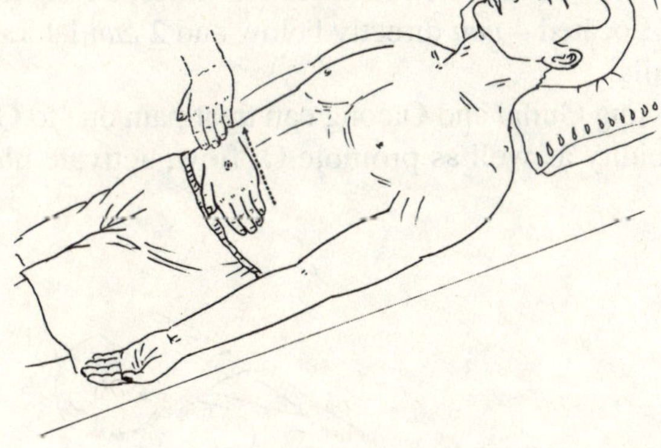

Fig. 6-165 Transverse stroking beside the navel

④ stroking and pressing the lower abdomen (Fig. 6-166)

[Method] The doctor puts the four fingers of one hand at Yinjiao (CV 7) to stroke downward along the midline on the abdomen (conception vessel) to Qugu (CV 2). This manipulation is repeated 5-10 times.

[Acupoints] Yinjiao: Located 1 *cun* directly below the navel. Qugu: Located 5 *cun* directly below the navel.

[Pithy formula] Stroking and pressing the lower abdomen from Yinjiao to Qugu (to be pressed heavily) can treat accumulation of damp-heat in the lower energizer and constipation, promote Qi flow and clear away pathogenic damp-heat.

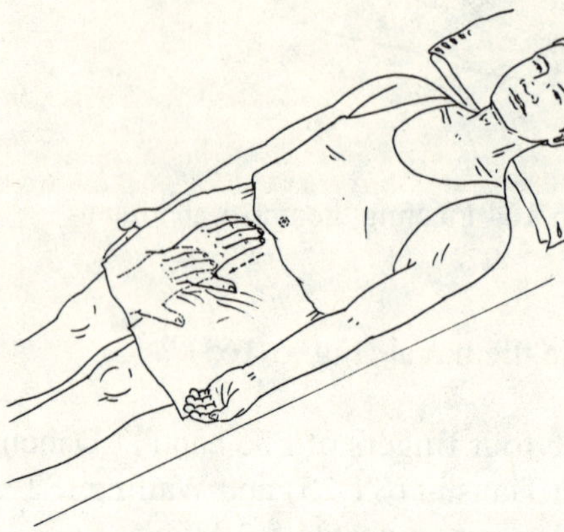

Fig. 6-166 Stroking and pressing the lower abdomen

⑤ Major Qi-dispersing method (Fig. 6-167)

[Method] The doctor puts the four fingers of both hands at Guilai (ST 29) and Qichong (ST 30) at the sides of the lower abdomen to press 1-3 times, 30-60 seconds each time.

[Acupoints] Guilai: Located 4 *cun* directly below and 2 *cun* lateral to the navel. Qichong: Located 1 *cun* below Guilai.

[Pithy formula] Pressing Guilai and Qicong can treat pain due to Qi stagnation, abdominal distension and foot flaccidity as well as promote Qi flow, activate blood and dredge vessels and meridians.

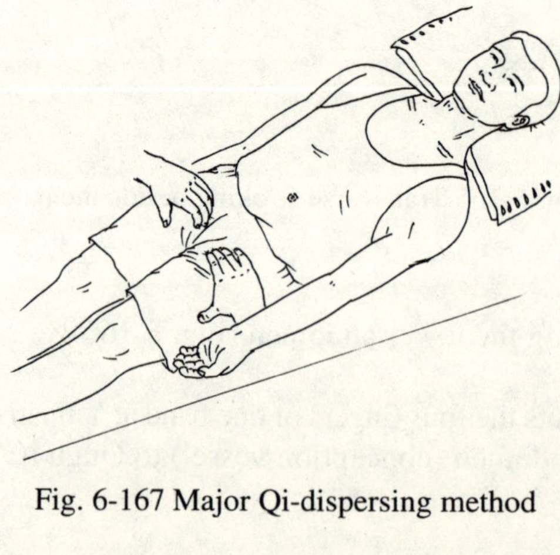

Fig. 6-167 Major Qi-dispersing method

⑥ Rubbing around the knee (Fig. 6-168)

[Method] The doctor puts the thumb of one hand at Xuehai (SP 10) on the affected limb and the thumb and index finger of the other hand at Xiyan (EX-LE 5) at the medial and lateral sides respectively to rub and press for 1-2 minutes. Then the thumb and index finger are put at Yinlingquan (SP 9) and Yanglingquan (GB 34) to press and rub for 30-60 seconds. Finally the palm is put on the knee and the fingers are put around the knee to rub and pinch for 1-2 minutes.

[Acupoints] Xuehai: Located 2 *cun* above the upper border of the patella. Medial Xiyan: Located in the depression medial to the tip of the patella. Lateral Xiyan: Located in the depression lateral to the tip of the patella. Yinlingquan: Located in the depression below the lower border of the medial condyle of the femur. Yanglingquan: Located in the depression below the small head of the fibia.

[Pithy formula] Rubbing around the knee, Xuehai and medial and lateral Xiyan is effective in relieving convulsion and pain. Rubbing Yinlingquan and Yanglingquan is effective in clearing away damp-heat and subdue swelling.

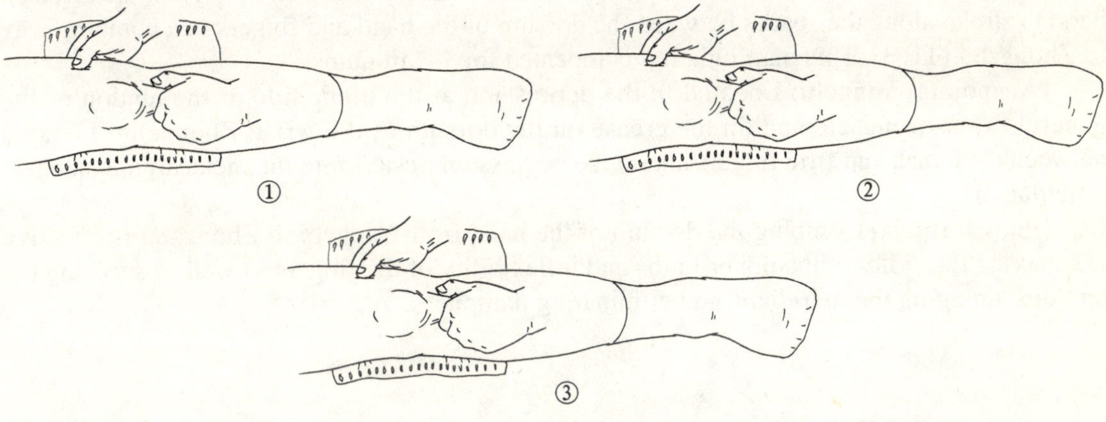

Fig. 6-168 Rubbing around the knee

⑦ Combing the dorsum of the foot (Fig. 6-169)

[Method] The doctor puts the four fingers of one hand at Jiexi (ST 41) on the affected foot to stroke in a combing way along the dorsum of the foot to the toes. At the same time, the thumb of the other hand is used to press and rub Jiexi. This manipulation is repeated for 1-2 minutes.

[Acupoints] Jiexi: Located at the middle of the crease on the dorsum-ankle joint and between the tendons of extensor muscles of the big toe and the other toes.

[Pithy formula] Combing the dorsum of the foot, pressing Jiexi and stroking the spaces between the toes can activate Qi and blood, relieve foot swelling, headache and pain in the waist and leg as well as relax the tendons, activate the collaterals and tranquilize the mind.

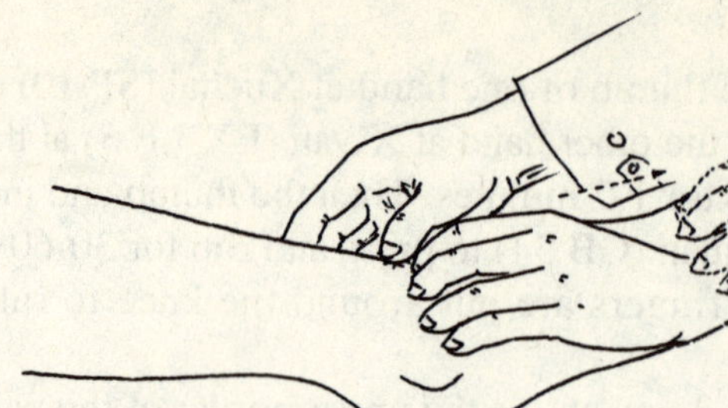

Fig. 6-169 Combing the dorsum of the foot

⑧ Combing the dorsum of hand (Fig. 6-170)

[Method] The doctor puts the four fingers of one hand at Yangchi (TE 4) on the affected hand to stroke along the spaces between the dorsum of the hand and fingers in a combing way to Zhongzhu (TE 3). This manipulation is repeated for 1-2 minutes.

[Acupoints] Yangchi: Located in the depression at the ulnar side of the tendon of the general extensor muscle and on the crease on the dorsum of the wrist. Zhongzhu: Located between the fourth and fifth fingers and in the depression posterior to the metacarpophalangeal articulation.

[Pithy formula] Combing the dorsum of the hand from Yangchi to Zhongzhu is effective in relieving flaccidity of the upper limbs and inflexibility of the fingers as well as soothing the tendons, dredging the meridians and eliminating dampness.

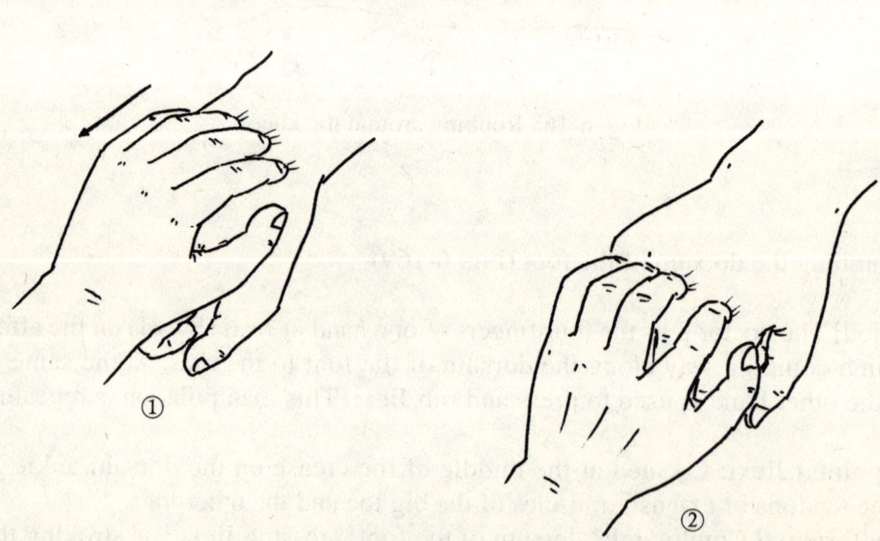

① ②

Fig. 6-170 Combing the dorsum of the hand

⑨ Longitudinal stroking of the waist (Fig. 6-171)

[Method] The doctor puts the four fingers of both hands at Weishu (BL 21) and Weicang (BL 50) to stroke directly downward through Shenshu (BL 23), Zhishi (BL 52) and Xiaochangshu (BL 27). This manipulation is repeated for 1-3 minutes.

[Acupoints] Weishu: Located below and 1.5 *cun* lateral to the 12th thoracic vertebral spine. Weicang: Located 1.5 *cun* lateral to Weishu. Shenshu: Located below and 1.5 *cun* lateral to the second lumbar vertebral spine. Zhishi: Located 1.5 *cun* lateral to Shenshu. Xiaochangshu: Located below and 1.5 *cun* lateral to the sacral vertebral spine.

[Pithy formula] Stroking the waist from Weishu to Xiaochangshu is effective in relieving pain in the waist and sacrum, soothing distension of the foot and knee, and strengthening the kidney and spleen.

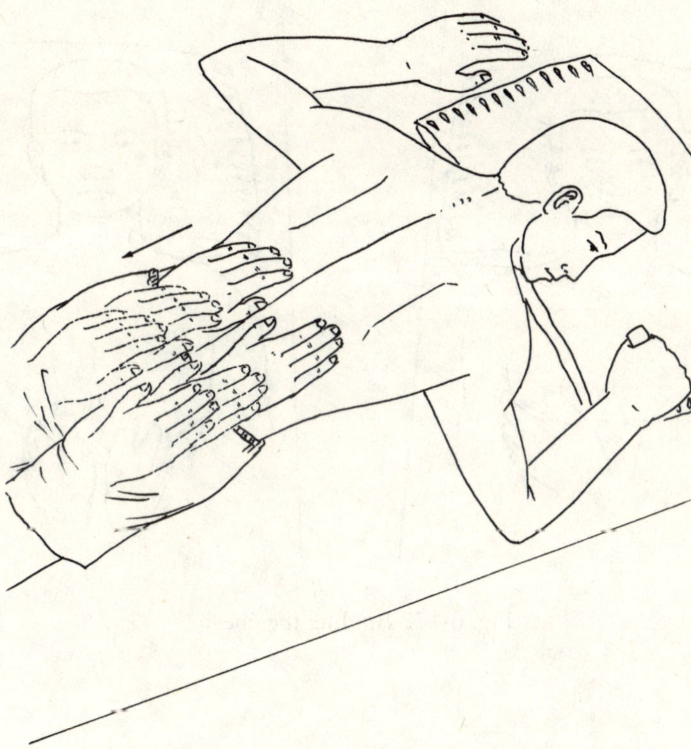

Fig. 6-171 Longitudinal stroking of the waist

4) Blood stasis due to Qi deficiency

① Binding the chest (Fig. 6-172)

[Method] The doctor puts both palms at Yuanye (GB 22) and Dabao (SP 21) on both sides of the patient and the remaining fingers at the intercostal spaces to embrace the thorax and obliquely stroke toward the anterior part of the chest and Qimen (LR14). This manipulation is repeated 5-10 times.

[Acupoints] Yuanye: Located at the midline of the armpit and in the fourth intercostal space. Dabao: Located at the midline of the armpit and in the sixth intercostal space. Qimen: Located directly below the nipple and in the sixth intercostal space.

[Pithy formula] Binding the chest by embracing the thorax and stroking from Yuanye to Qimen is effective in eliminating dysphoria, consolidating Qi and nourishing the heart.

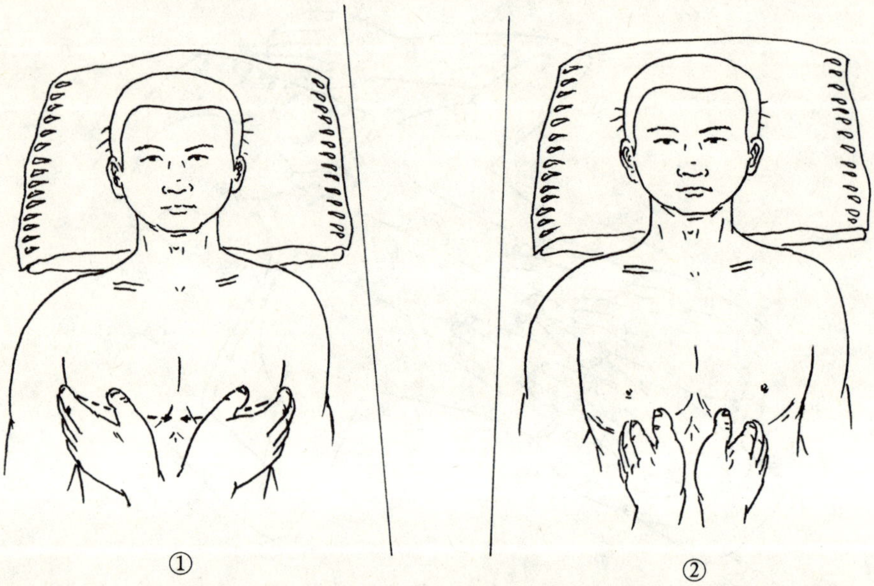

① ②

Fig. 6-172 Binding the chest

② Pressing Tianshu (Fig. 6-173)

[Method] The doctor puts the thumb and index finger of one hand at Tianshu (ST 25) to press and rub with great strength 3-5 times, 30-60 seconds each time.

[Acupoint] Tianshu: Located 2 *cun* lateral to the navel.

[Pithy formula] Pressing Tianshu is very effective in treating intestinal disorder, anorexia and diarrhea as well as strengthening the spleen, astringing the intestines and regulating Qi activity. Slight rubbing after pressing will improve the efficacy.

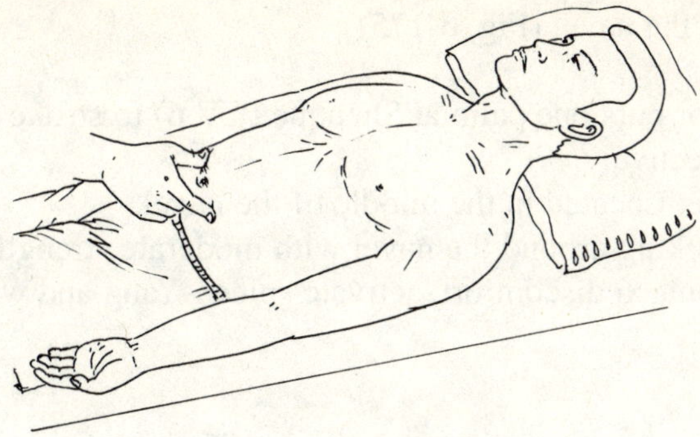

Fig. 6-173 Pressing Tianshu

③ Binding the abdomen (Fig. 6-174)

[Method] The doctor puts the four fingers of both hands at Zhangmen (LR13) and Jingmen (BL 63) to stroke the abdomen 3-5 times.

[Acupoints] Zhangmen: Located at the end of the 11th rib. Jingmen: Located at the end of the 11th rib.

[Pithy formula] Binding the abdomen with the fingers and stroking Zhangmen and Jingmen can relieve constipation, diarrhea, lumbago and hypochondriac pain due to deficiency, as well as regulate Qi and blood in the spleen and stomach.

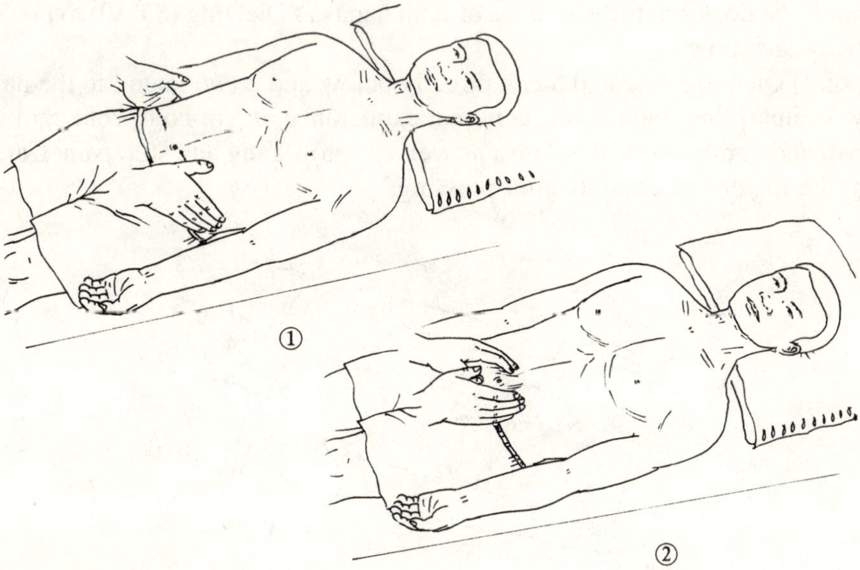

①

②

Fig. 6-174 Binding the abdomen

④ Stroking around the navel (Fig. 6-175)

[Method] The doctor puts one palm at Shenque (CV 6) to stroke clockwise and counter-clockwise 36 times respectively.

[Acupoint] Shenque: Located in the middle of the navel.

[Pithy formula] Stroking around the navel with moderate strength can treat diarrhea due to wind-cold, relieve stomach discomfort, activate spleen-Yang and warm the middle.

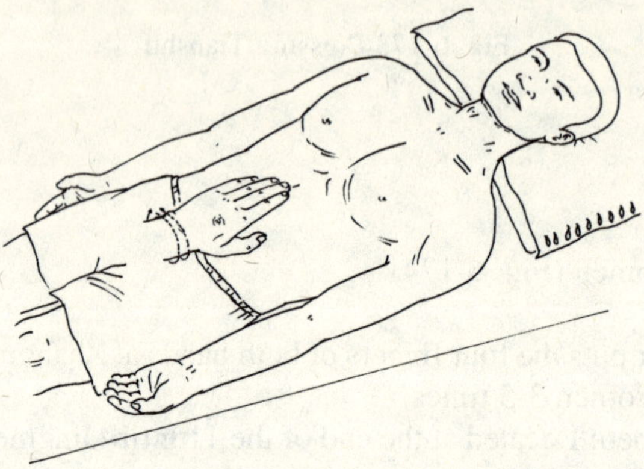

Fig. 6-175 Stroking around the navel

⑤ Pressing Qichong (Fig. 6-176)

[Method] The doctor puts the thumbs of both hands at Qichong (ST 30) to press 1-3 times, 15-30 seconds each time.

[Acupoint] Qichong: Located 5 *cun* directly below and 2 *cun* lateral to the navel.

[Pithy formula] Pressing Qicong can treat exuberance of Yin-cold, cold pain in the waist and abdomen and numbness of the limbs, as well as warm Yang and stop pain. Care should be taken to lift the finger immediately after pressing.

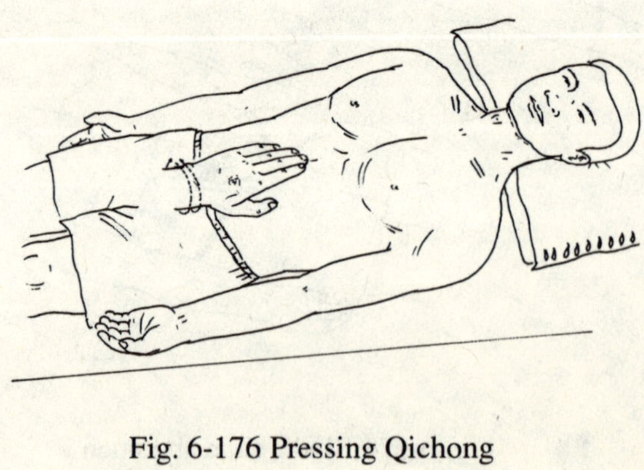

Fig. 6-176 Pressing Qichong

⑥ Pressing the medial side of the shank (Fig. 6-177)

[Method] The doctor puts the four fingers of one hand at Yinlingquan (SP 9) on the affected side to press and rub along the medial border of the tibia to Sanyinjiao (SP 6). At the same time, the four fingers of the other hand are put at Taixi (K13) to press and rub. This manipulation is repeated 3-5 times.

[Acupoints] Yinlingquan: Located in the depression on the lower border of the condyle at the medial side of the tibia. Sanyinjiao: Located 3 *cun* above the high point of the medial ankle and at the posterior border of the lateral side of the tibia. Taixi: Located in the depression between the high point of the medial ankle and the heel tendon.

[Pithy formula] Pressing Yinlingquan on the medial side of the shank to Sanyinjiao and Taixi can treat swelling of the lower limbs and flaccidity of the foot, strengthen the spleen, promote urination and smooth the flow of Qi and blood.

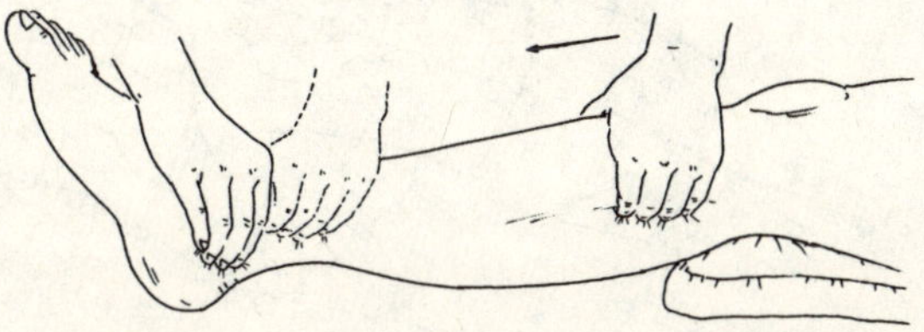

Fig. 6-177 Pressing the medial side of the shank

⑦ Rubbing Laogong (Fig. 6-178)

[Method] The doctor puts the thumb of one hand at Daling (PC 7) on the affected limb and the remaining four fingers at the back of the wrist to push obliquely downward to Laogong (PC 8). The thumb is used to press and rub the acupoints for 30-60 seconds and then pushed to the second metacarpophalangeal crease. This manipulation is repeated 3-5 times.

[Acupoints] Daling: Located at the middle of the wrist crease and between the tendons of the long palmar extensor muscle and radial flexor muscle of the wrist. Laogong: Located on the middle of the palmar crease and between the second and third metacarpal bones.

[Pithy formula] Rubbing Laogong and pushing Daling to the finger crease can treat severe palpitation, insomnia due to fright and numbness of the fingers, stop fear, tranquilize the mind and promote the flow of Qi and blood.

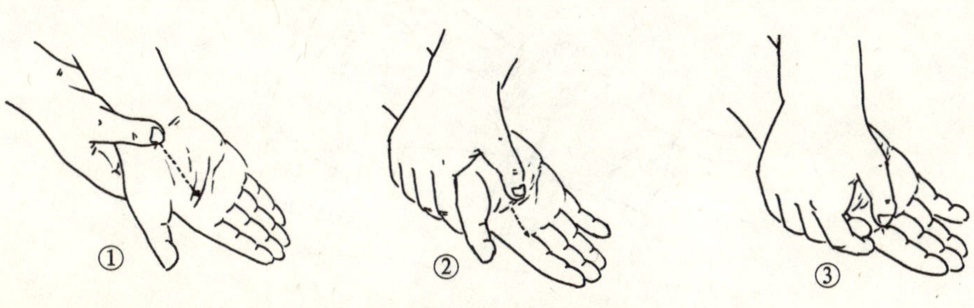

Fig. 6-178 Rubbing Laogong

⑧ Knocking the rib for supplementing Qi (Fig. 6-179)

[Method] The doctor dorsally bends the index fingers of both hands and puts them at Dazhu (BL 11) to press along the costal spaces through Xinshu (BL 15) to Geshu (BL 17). This manipulation is repeated 3-5 times.

[Acupoints] Dazhu: Located below and 1.5 *cun* lateral to the first thoracic vertebral spine. Xinshu: Located below and 1.5 *cun* lateral to the fifth thoracic vertebral spine. Geshu: Located below and 1.5 *cun* lateral to the seventh thoracic vertebral spine.

[Pithy formula] Bending the index fingers at Dazhu to press the rib-side can supplement Qi to treat palpitation. Pressing costal spaces, Xinshu and Geshu can supplement Qi and strengthen the heart.

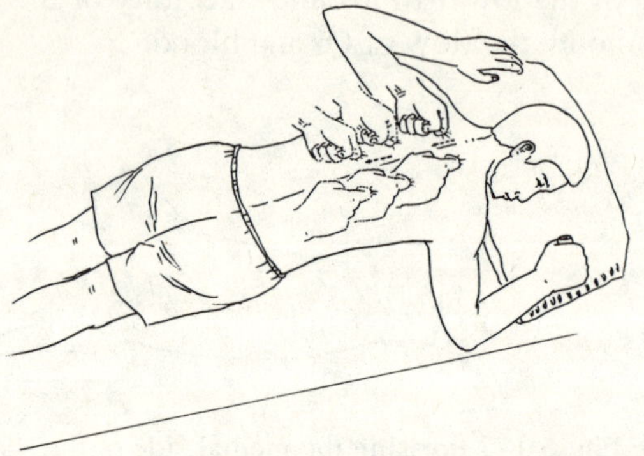

Fig. 6-179 Knocking the rib for supplementing Qi

⑨ Perpendicular pushing of the waist for supplementing Qi (Fig. 6-180)

[Method] The doctor puts the four fingers of both hands at Shenshu (BL 23), Qihai (CV 6) and Dachangshu (BL 25) to push and press for 30-60 seconds respectively.

[Acupoints] Shenshu: Located below and 1.5 *cun* lateral to the second lumbar vertebral spine. Qihai: Located below and 1.5 *cun* lateral to the third lumbar vertebral spine. Dachangshu: Located below and 1.5 *cun* lateral to the fourth lumbar vertebral spine.

[Pithy formula] Perpendicular pushing of the waist from Shenshu to Qihai and Dachangshu can treat insufficiency of kidney-Qi and frequent urination at night, supplement the kidney and nourish Qi.

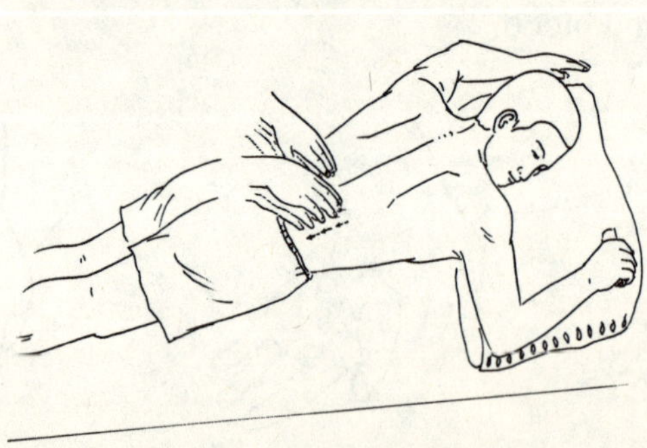

Fig. 6-180 Perpendicular pushing of the waist for supplementing Qi

5) Disturbance of wind due to Yin deficiency

① Pressing the head from both sides (Fig. 6-181)

[Method] The doctor puts the four fingers of both hands at Touwei (ST 8) located at both forehead angles to stroke in a posterior direction to Houding (GV 19) 5-10 times. Then the doctor puts both palms at the temple and ear of the patient to press from both sides for 15-30 seconds.

[Acupoints] Touwei: Located 0.5 *cun* directly above the temple hair. Houding: Located 5.5 *cun* directly above the midpoint of the posterior hairline.

[Pithy formula] Pressing the temples with both palms and stroking from Touwei to Houding can treat dizziness, strengthen the brain, tranquilize the mind and regulate Qi.

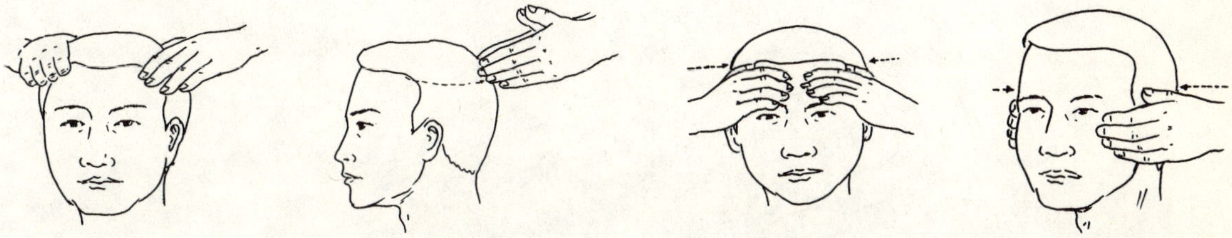

① ② ③ ④

Fig. 6-181 Pressing the head from both sides

② Pinching Sishencong (Fig. 6-182)

[Method] The doctor puts the thumbs of both hands at Luoque (BL 8), Qianding (GV 21), Houding (GV 19) and Baihui (GV 20) on both sides of the vertex to pinch first and then rub. This manipulation is repeated for 20-30 seconds.

[Acupoints] Luoque: Located 5.5 *cun* directly above and 1.5 *cun* lateral to the midpoint of the anterior hairline. Qianding: Located 3.5 *cun* directly above the midpoint of the anterior hairline. Houding: Located 6.5 *cun* directly above the midpoint of the anterior hairline. Baihui: Located 5 *cun* directly above the midpoint of the anterior hairline.

[Pithy formula] Pinching Sishencong, Luoque, Qianding, Houding and Baihui can treat palpitation due to fright, resuscitate the brain and improve eyesight.

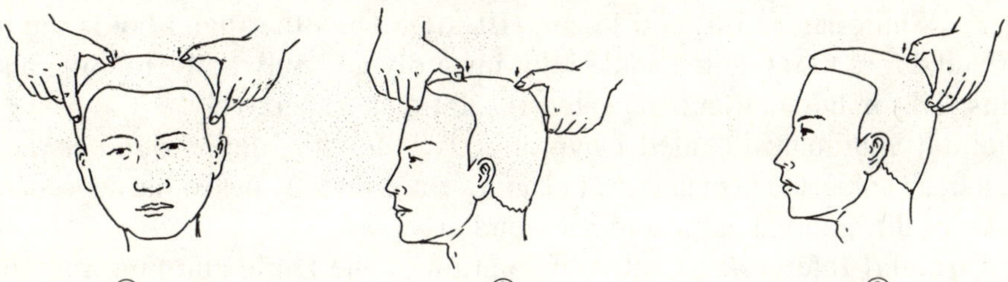

① ② ③

Fig. 6-182 Pinching Sishencong

③ Expanding the chest (Fig. 6-183)

[Method] The doctor puts both palms at Yuanye (GB 22) and Dabao (SP 21) and the thumbs of both hands at Tianchi (PC 1) and Shidou (SP 17) to shake and press for 30-60 seconds.

[Acupoints] Yuanye: Located on the midline of the armpit and in the fourth costal space. Dabao: Located on the midline of the armpit and in the sixth costal space. Tianchi: Located 1 *cun* lateral to the nipple and in the middle of the fourth costal space. Shidou: Located 6 *cun* lateral to the anterior midline and in the middle of the fifth costal space.

[Pithy formula] Shaking and pressing in line with the rhythm of respiration to expand the chest can eliminate chest fullness and dysphoria, regulate Qi, expand the chest, relieve stagnation and disperse heat.

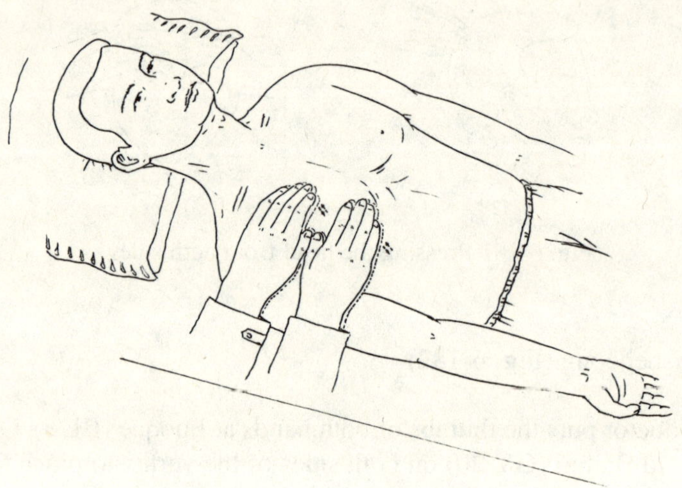

Fig. 6-183 Expanding the chest

④ Internal and external rotation of the ankle (Fig. 6-184)

[Method] The doctor holds the heel of the patient's affected foot and puts the thumb and index finger at Shuiquan (KI 5) and Pucan (BL 61). The other hand holds the toes of the patient's affected foot to rotate the ankle joint inwardly and outwardly, rubbing and pressing the acupoints. This manipulation is repeated 10-20 times respectively.

[Acupoints] Shuiquan: Located 1 *cun* directly below the depression between the high point of the medial ankle and heel tendon. Pucan: Located directly below the depression between the high point of the external ankle and heel tendon.

[Pithy formula] Internal and external rotation of the ankle and pressing and rubbing Shuiquan and Pucan can treat foot droop and strephenopodia, dredge the meridian Qi and relieve spasms.

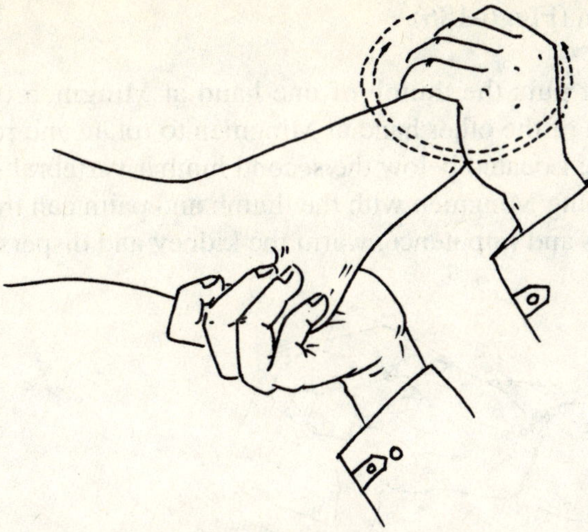

Fig. 6-184 Internal and external rotation of the ankle

⑤ Rubbing Yongquan (Fig. 6-185)

[Method] The doctor holds the heel tendon of the patient's affected foot and pulls downward with one hand and puts the thumb of the other hand at Yongquan (KI 1) to push upward, rotate and rub clockwise and counter-clockwise 50 times respectively.

[Acupoint] Yongquan: Located 1/3 anterior to the sole and in the depression when the toes are bent.

[Pithy formula] Pushing Yongquan and pulling the heel can treat throat disorder, dysuria, dysphoria and insomnia, as well as nourish Yin and relieve stagnation.

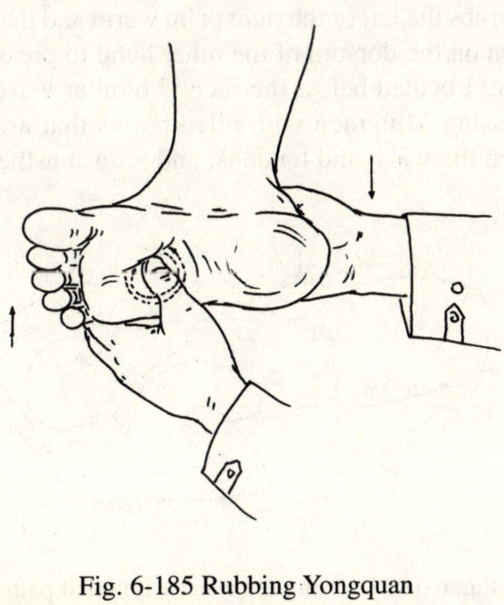

Fig. 6-185 Rubbing Yongquan

⑥ Rubbing Mingmen (Fig. 6-186)

[Method] The doctor puts the thumb of one hand at Mingmen (GV 4) to rub for 1-2 minutes and puts the palm of the other hand at Mingmen to rotate and rub for 1-2 minutes.

[Acupoint] Mingmen: Located below the second lumbar vertebral spine.

[Pithy formula] Rubbing Mingmen with the thumb and palm can treat deficiency-cold of the kidney, spinal stiffness and impotence, warm the kidney and disperse cold.

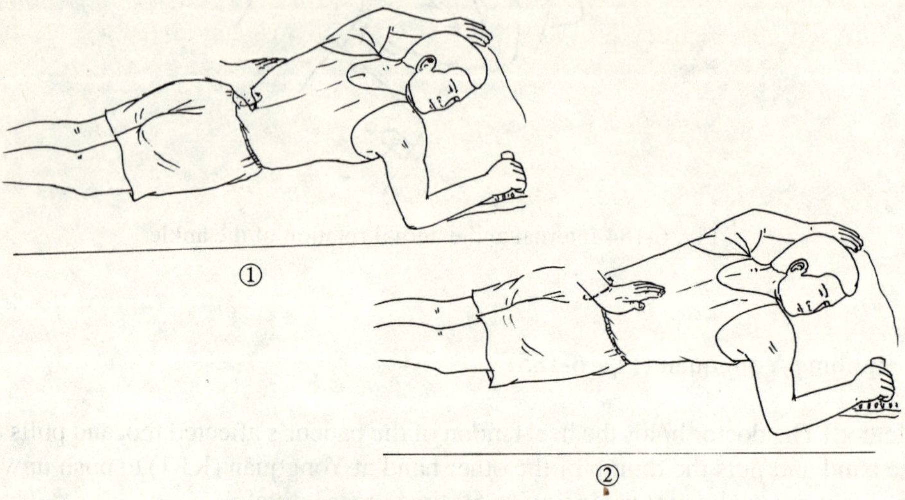

Fig. 6-186 Rubbing Mingmen

⑦ Pressing the waist with piled palms (Fig. 6-187)

[Method] The doctor rubs the left or the right palm warm and then puts the palm at Mingmen (GV 4) and the other palm on the dorsum of the other hand to press rhythmically 10-15 times.

[Acupoint] Mingmen: Located below the second lumbar vertebral spine.

[Pithy formula] Pressing Mingmen with piled palms that are rubbed warm can relieve spinal stiffness, strengthen the waist and tendons, and reduce asthenia-fire.

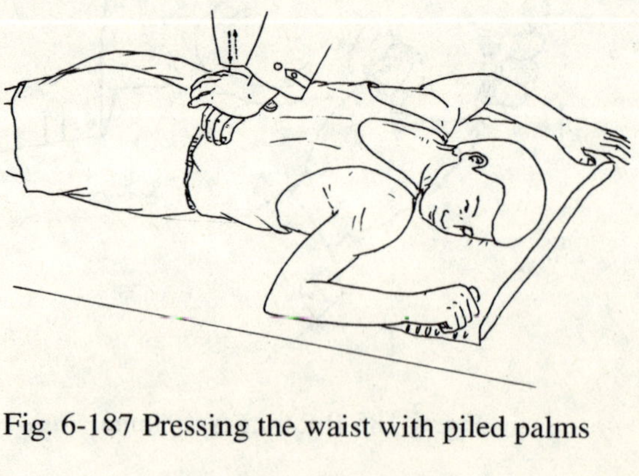

Fig. 6-187 Pressing the waist with piled palms

⑧ Forking the waist with fingers (Fig. 6-188)

[Method] The doctor puts the thumbs of both hands at Shenshu (BL 23) and the remaining four fingers at the waist to push medially and laterally to Daimai (GB 26). This manipulation is repeated 5-10 times.

[Acupoints] Shenshu: Located below and 1.5 *cun* lateral to the second lumbar vertebral spine. Daimai: Located directly below and parallel to the end of the 11th rib.

[Pithy formula] Pushing the waist with the thumbs in a forking way to Daimai can treat spasms and pain of the lumbar muscles and relieve convulsions.

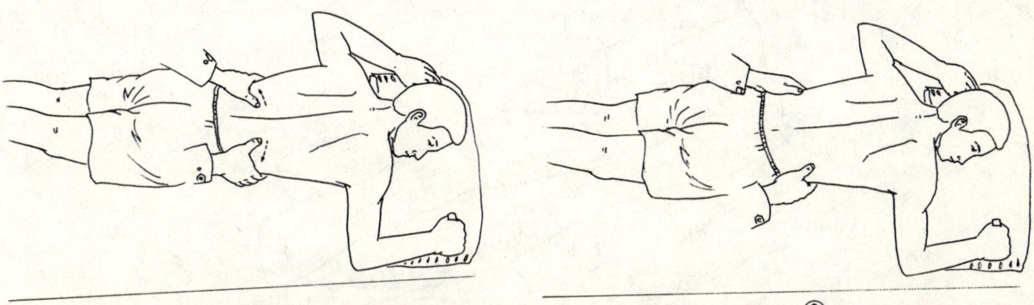

①　②

Fig. 6-188 Forking the waist with fingers

⑨ Rubbing the sides of the waist (Fig. 6-189)

[Method] The doctor forms one hand into a soft fist and puts it below Jingmen (GB 25) to rub for 1-3 minutes.

[Acupoint] Jingmen: Located at the end of the 11th rib.

[Pithy formula] Rubbing the sides of the waist below Jingmen can treat weakness of the waist and knee and constipation, regulate Qi and promote blood circulation.

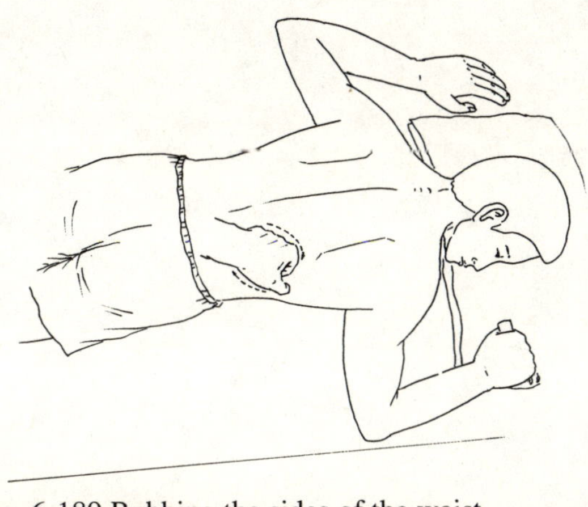

Fig. 6-189 Rubbing the sides of the waist

⑩ Rubbing Weizhong (Fig. 6-190)

[Method] The doctor puts the thumb of one hand at Weizhong (BL 40) to press and rub forcefully for 1-3 minutes.

[Acupoint] Weizhong: Located on the middle of the popliteal crease.

[Pithy formula] Rubbing Weizhong with the thumb can treat lumbago, flaccidity of the lower limbs and difficulty in extending the tendons, as well as reduce stagnant heat and dredge meridian Qi.

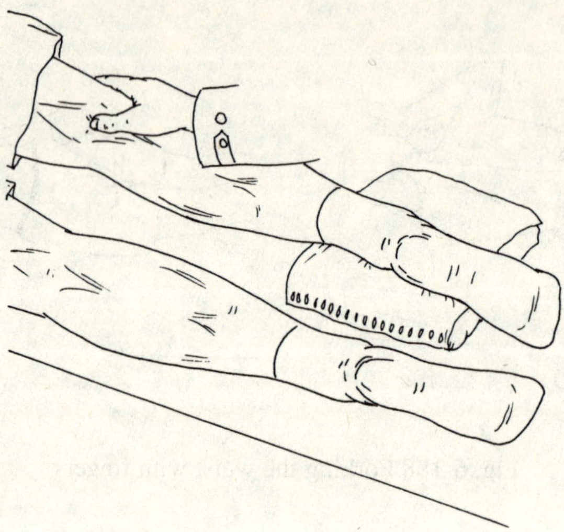

Fig. 6-190 Rubbing Weizhong

Chapter 7

ILLUSTRATED TECHNIQUES FOR CORRECTING DEFORMITY AT THE SEQUELAE STAGE

The sequelae stage refers to the period half a year after treatment and rehabilitation. Various sequelae, especially dysfunction of the affected limbs, may appear due to individual pathological condition, nature of the disease and constitution as well as functional training. Since paralysis after wind stroke is central paralysis due to injury of the cerebral neural cells, muscular tension of some muscles on the affected limb may be intensified and cause abnormal contraction, leading to spasms or stiffness of the joints, such as adhesion of the shoulder joint due to adduction and intorsion muscles on the shoulder; or hyper function of the muscles responsible for bending the elbow joint, leading to spasms of the elbow joint; or hyper function of the muscles responsible for pronation, leading to posterior turning of the palm; or hyper function of the muscles responsible for bending the wrist joint and finger joints, making the fingers appearing like "monkey talons"; or hyper function of the muscles responsible for abduction and eversion of the hip joint, leading to lifting of the hip joint and oblique walking; or hyper function of the muscles responsible for extending the knee joint, leading to stiff walking and a swaying leg in walking; or hyper function of the muscles responsible for bending the metatarsal bones, leading to foot droop and strephenopodia. Besides, in syndromes of the shoulder and hand, the disorder of the sympathetic nerve system may lead to pain of the shoulder, elbow and finger joints on the affected upper limb, swelling and stiffness of the fingers and wrist, profuse sweating, change of skin color and temperature, restricted movement of the joints, or even spasm of the tendons, muscular atrophy and deformity of the shoulder and hand joints. Semiluxation of the shoulder joint is caused by flaccid paralysis of the affected upper limb, loosening of the articular capsule and paralysis and hypo function of the muscles around the shoulder joint.

It is generally believed that half a year after onset of the disease it is difficult to restore the functions of the nerve, but it is possible to restore the functions of the limbs and other compensatory functions of the cerebral tissues. Sometimes, it is due to the fact that some patients fail to make full use of the rehabilitated neural functions because they do not actively do functional exercise after onset of the disease. So, it is very important to take measures to correct deformity with selected and focal therapy.

1. LIFTING THE HIP FOR OBLIQUE ORTHOPEDIC TREATMENT

(1) Bending the hip and knee joints for intorsion of the hip (Fig. 7-1)

[Method] The patient lies in a supine position in a functional posture with both lower limbs naturally extended. The doctor (or nurse) holds the knee and foot on the affected limb of the patient, and slowly and forcefully bends the hip and knee to the patient's tolerance. Then the doctor slowly rotates the hip inward and after 30-60 seconds, returns to the normal position slowly. This manipulation is repeated 3-5 times. After performance of this manipulation, the doctor rubs and strokes the medial side of the thigh and the lateral side of the buttocks on the affected side for 1-2 minutes respectively.

[Effect] To contract the muscles responsible for bending the hip and knee joints as well as intorsion of the hip joint; and to restrain hyper function of the muscles responsible for extension and eversion of the hip joint to reduce spasms.

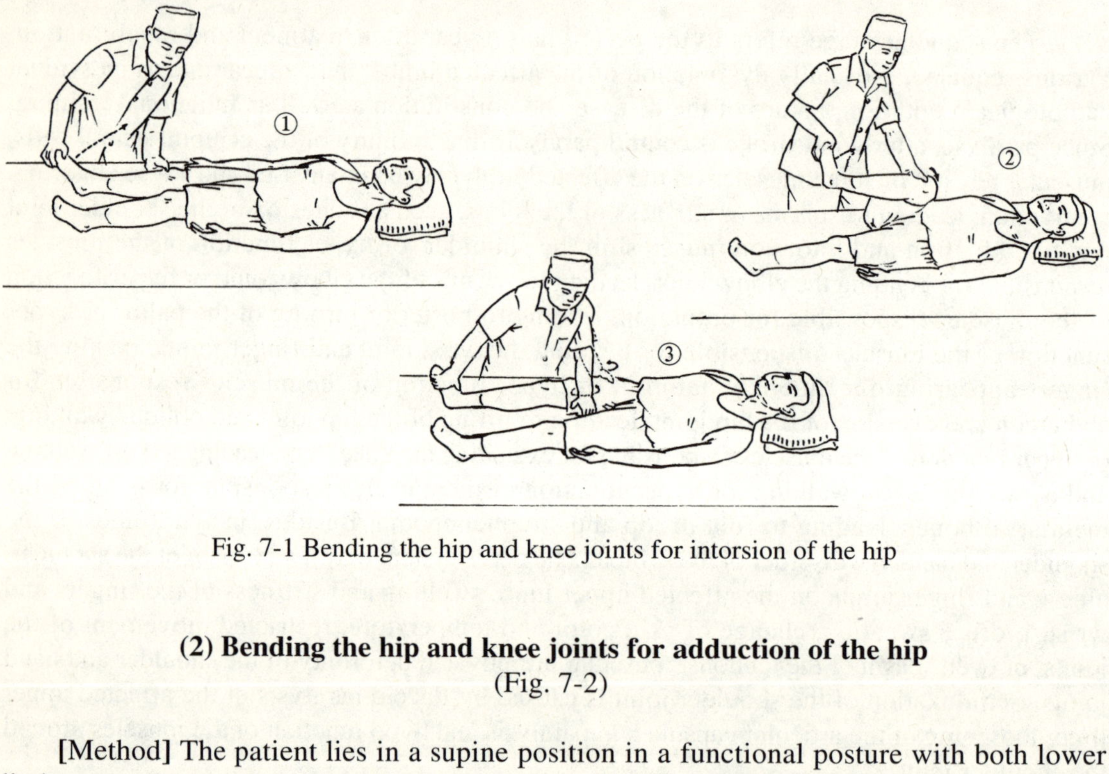

Fig. 7-1 Bending the hip and knee joints for intorsion of the hip

(2) Bending the hip and knee joints for adduction of the hip (Fig. 7-2)

[Method] The patient lies in a supine position in a functional posture with both lower limbs naturally extended. The patient inhales and slowly bends the hip and knee on the affected side as much as possible. Then the patient exhales and slowly adducts the hip, extends the knee with the affected foot put at the rear of the healthy knee in a cross position, then returning to the normal position. This manipulation is repeated 5-10 times.

[Effect] To train the muscles responsible for bending and extending the hip and knee joints, as well as to adduct the hip joint; to restrain hyper function of the muscles responsible for extending and abducting the hip joint; and to reinforce the tension of the abdominal muscles and improve the functions of the heart and lungs.

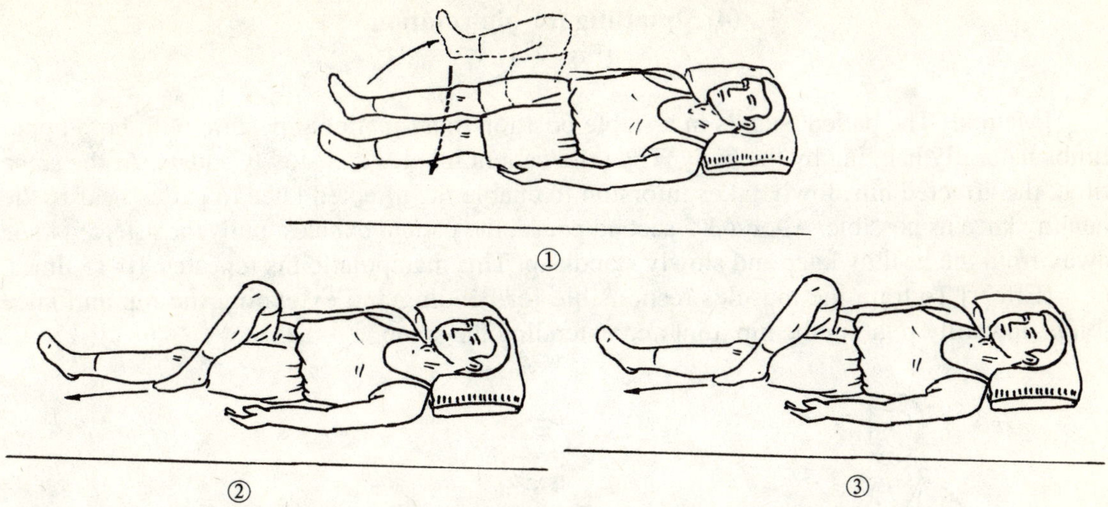

Fig. 7-2 Bending the hip and knee joints for adduction of the hip

(3) Rubbing and pinching the medial side of the thigh
(Fig. 7-3)

[Method] The doctor (or nurse) puts the fingers of both hands at Yinlian (LR11) and Zuwuli (LR10) to rub and pinch the medial muscles downward through Yinbao (LR9) to Ququan (LR8). This manipulation is repeated 3-5 times.

[Acupoints] Yinlian: Located 2 *cun* lateral to and 2 *cun* directly below the midpoint on the lower border of the pubic symphysis. Zuwuli: Located 1 *cun* below Yinlian. Yinbao: Located 4 *cun* above the medial epicondyle of the femur and on the posterior border of the sartorius muscle. Ququan: Located in the depression above the end of the medial crease on the knee.

[Pithy formula] Rubbing and pinching Yinlian, Yinbao and Ququan can relieve cold pain in the waist, leg and knee as well as activate blood, resolve stasis and warm the meridians.

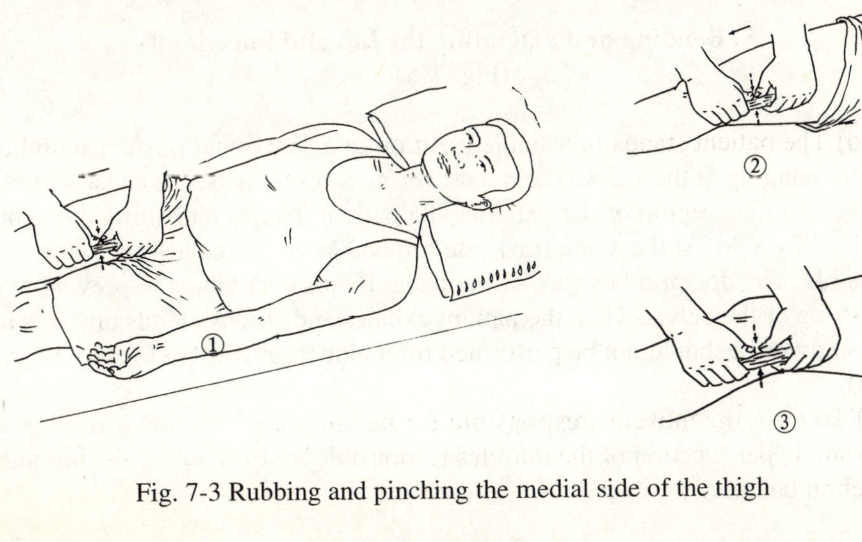

Fig. 7-3 Rubbing and pinching the medial side of the thigh

(4) Squatting for hip rotation

(Fig. 7-4)

[Method] The patient stands in a stable position in a functional posture with both upper limbs naturally hanging by the body. Then the patient inhales and slowly squats. At the same time, the affected hip slowly takes intorsion to enable the affected knee to get as near to the healthy knee as possible. After a 3-5 second pause, the patient exhales, pulls the affected knee away from the healthy knee and slowly stands up. This manipulation is repeated 10-15 times.

[Effect] To train the muscles responsible for bending and extending the hip and knee joints, inwardly rotating the hip joint and extending the spine.

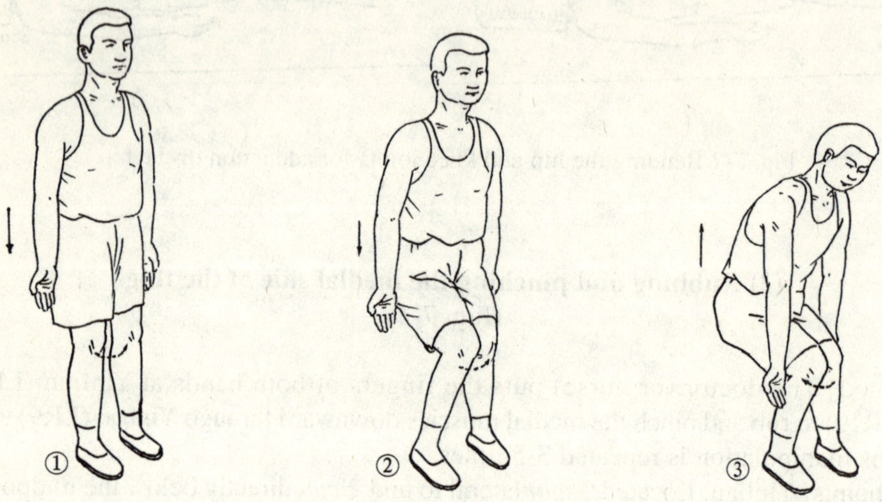

Fig. 7-4 Squatting for hip rotation

(5) Bending and extending the hip and knee joints

(Fig. 7-5)

[Method] The patient stands in a stable position in a functional posture with both upper limbs naturally hanging at the sides. The doctor (or nurse) stands beside the affected side and holds the knee and iliac region of the patient. The patient inhales and shifts the center of the body to the healthy side. At the same time, the hip and knee on the affected side are bent as much as possible. The doctor takes care of the patient with both hands to prevent eversion of the hip and lifting of the pelvis. Then the patient exhales and slowly stands up. This activity is repeated 10-30 times (it should not be performed for a longer time lest deformity be caused due to overstrain).

[Effect] To train the muscles responsible for bending and extending the hip and knee joints; to restrain hyper function of the muscles responsible for eversion of the hip joint; and to improve cerebral balance.

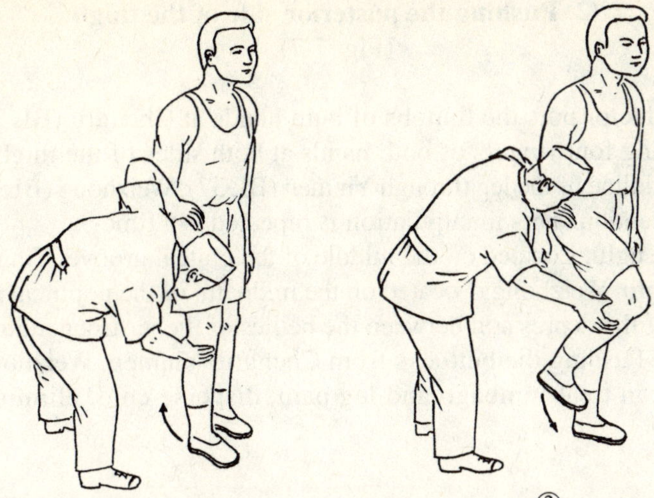

Fig. 7-5 Bending and extending the hip and knee joints

2. ORTHOPEDIC TREATMENT FOR SWINGING THE LEG AND WALKING SIDEWAYS

(1) Bending and extending the knee joint (lying position) (Fig. 7-6)

[Method] The patient lies in pronation in a functional posture with both lower limbs naturally extended. The patient inhales and slowly bends the knee on the affected limb and pauses for 3-5 seconds. Then the patient exhales and slowly extends the knee. This activity is performed 10-20 times (the hip should not be bent).

[Effect] To train the muscles responsible for bending and extending the knee joint; and to separate the common movement of the hip and knee joints to reduce spasms.

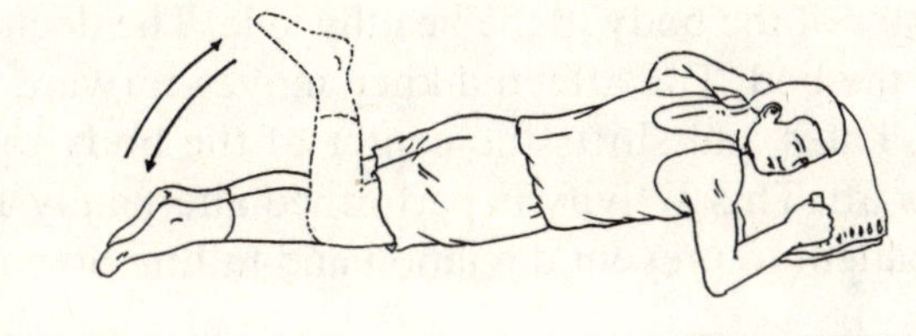

Fig. 7-6 Bending and extending the knee joint (lying position)

(2) Pushing the posterior side of the thigh
(Fig. 7-7)

[Method] The doctor puts the thumbs of both hands at Chengfu (BL 36) on the affected side and the remaining four fingers of both hands at both sides of the thigh to push and press along the posterior midline of the leg through Yinmen (BL 37), Weizhong (BL 40) and Chengshan (BL 57) to the heel tendon. This manipulation is repeated 3-5 times.

[Acupoints] Chengfu: Located on the middle of the gluteal groove. Yinmen: Located 6 *cun* directly below Chengfu. Weizhong: Located on the midpoint of the popliteal crease. Chengshan: Located on the top of the depression between the bellies of the gastrocnemius muscle.

[Pithy formula] Pushing the buttocks from Chengfu, Yinmen, Weizhong and Chengshan to the heel tendon can treat lumbago and leg pain, disperse cold, eliminate dampness and dredge the meridians.

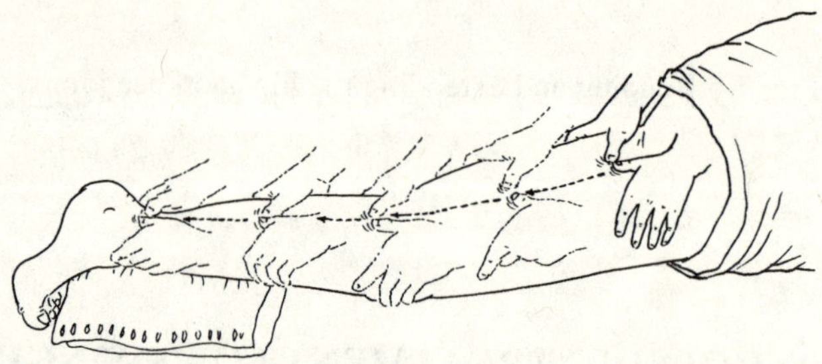

Fig. 7-7 Pushing the posterior side of the thigh

(3) Walking with both knees
(Fig. 7-8)

[Method] The patient kneels down with both knees on a thickly cushioned bed with the neck, back and waist extended as much as possible. The doctor (or nurse) stands by the affected side of the patient and holds the iliac region and the sole of the patient. The patient inhales and shifts the center of the body to the healthy side. The doctor helps the patient raise the affected shank from the bed. The affected knee moves forward and slowly touches the bed. The patient then exhales and shifts the center of the body to the affected side. The healthy knee moves forward. This activity is performed alternately 10-50 times. The doctor should take care of the patient to prevent deviation and falling down (a weak patient should not undertake this activity).

[Effect] To train the muscles responsible for bending the knee joint; to restrain hyper function of the muscles responsible for extending the knee; and to separate the common movement of the hip and knee joints to reduce spasms.

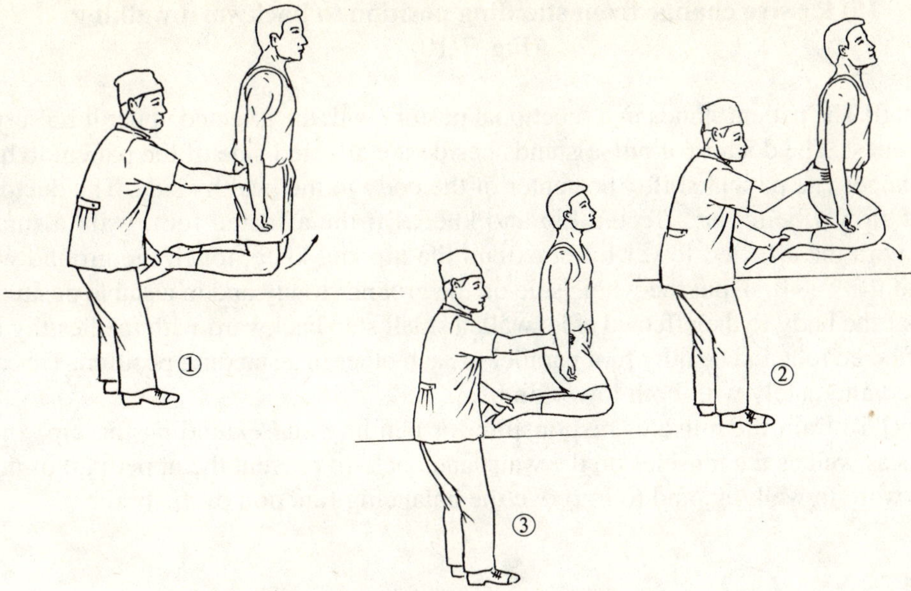

Fig. 7-8 Walking with both knees

(4) Bending and extending the knee joint (sitting position) (Fig. 7-9)

[Method] Sitting straight in a functional posture, the patient inhales and slowly bends the knee on the affected limb as much as possible, extending and lifting the affected foot, pausing for 3-5 seconds. Then the patient exhales and slowly extends the knee and bends the affected foot. This activity is performed 10-20 times.

[Effect] To train the muscles responsible for bending and extending the knee joint as well as dorsal bending and metatarsal bending of the ankle joint; to separate common movement of the knee and ankle joints to reduce spasms; and to prevent spasms of the knee joint.

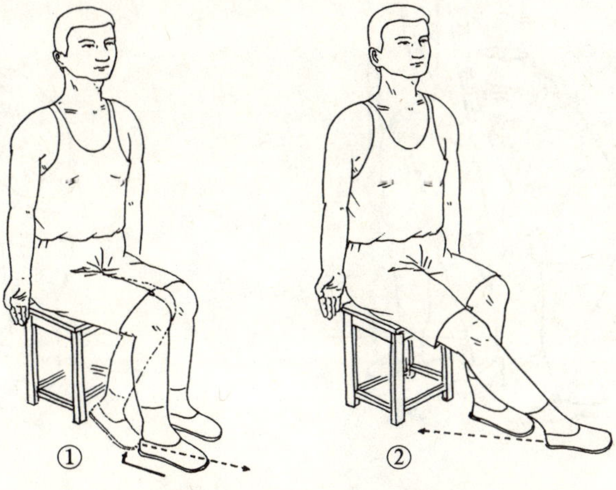

Fig. 7-9 Bending and extending the knee joint

(5) Passive change from standing position to backward walking (Fig. 7-10)

[Method] The patient stands in a functional posture with the affected upper limb suspended before the chest. The doctor (or nurse)stands beside the affected side of the patient to hold the waist and knee. The patient shifts the center of the body to the healthy side. The doctor helps the patient slowly bend the affected hip and knee, lift the affected foot, walk a small step backward with the affected lower limb, extend the hip and knee, touch the ground with the front part of the sole first, put the whole sole on the ground slowly and in a stable position, shift the center of the body to the affected side, walk a small step backward with the healthy limb to keep the affected foot and healthy foot parallel to each other in a standing position. This activity is performed alternately with both lower limbs.

[Effect] To train the muscles responsible for bending and extending the hip, knee and ankle joints as well as the muscles on the waist and back; to prevent the upper part of the body leaning forward in walking; and to improve the balancing function of the brain.

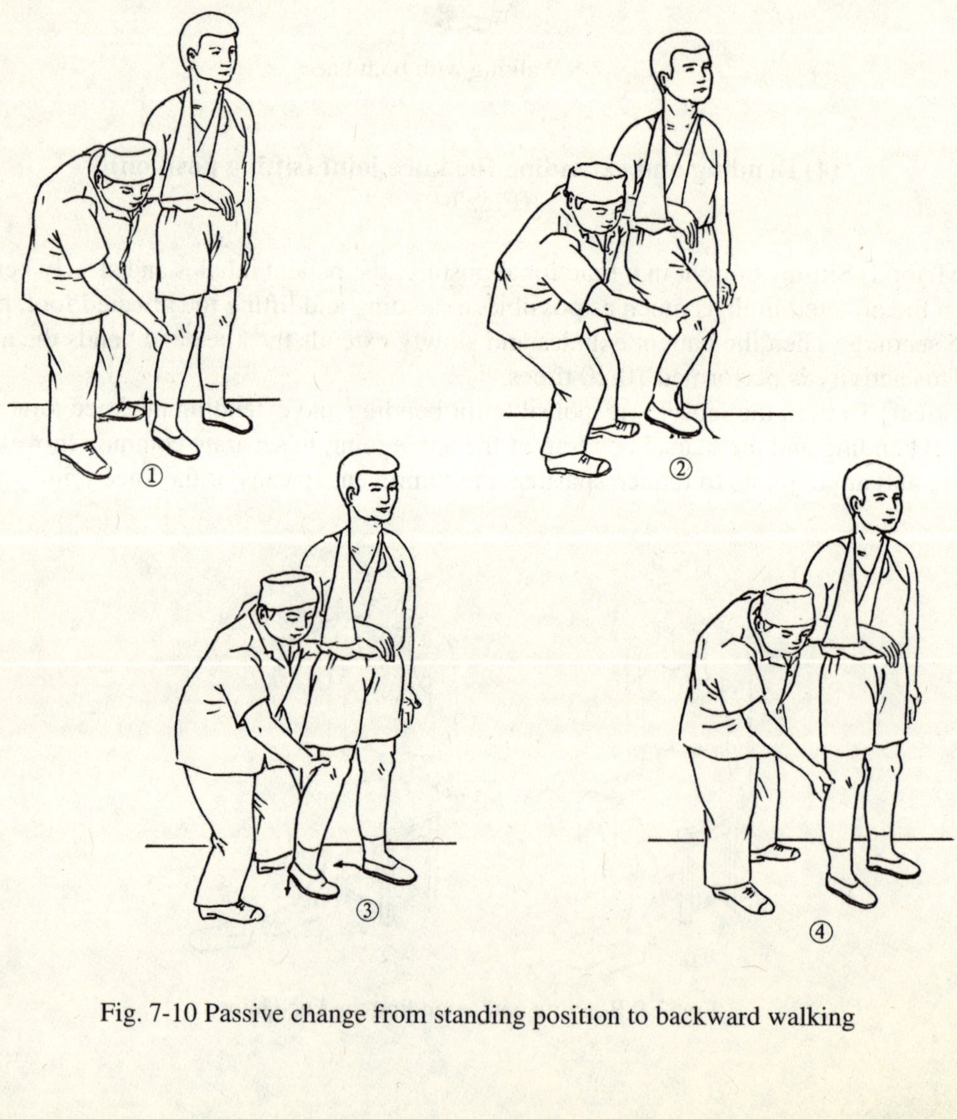

Fig. 7-10 Passive change from standing position to backward walking

3. ORTHOPEDIC TREATMENT FOR SWINGING THE SHANK IN WALKING

(1) Bending the knee and rotating the hip
(Fig. 7-11)

[Method] Lying in a supine position in a functional posture with the lower limbs naturally extended, the patient inhales, bends the affected knee slowly, touching the bed in a stable position with the sole, fixing such a position with the healthy foot at the beginning, rotating inwardly the affected hip as much as possible and pausing for 3-5 seconds. Then the patient exhales and slowly relaxes. This activity is performed 20-50 times.

[Effect] To train the muscles responsible for bending the knee joint and inwardly rotating the hip joint.

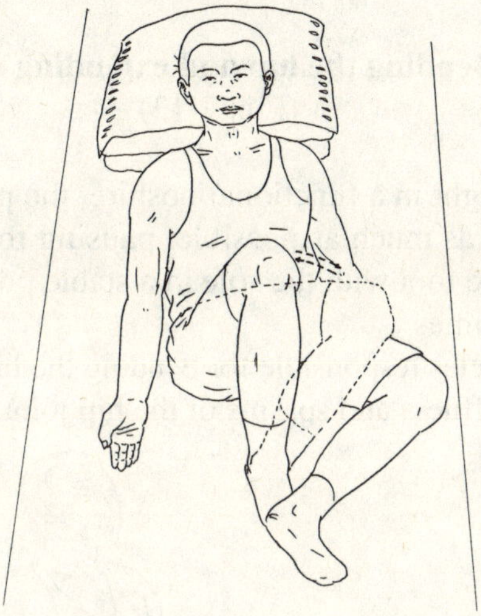

Fig. 7-11 Bending the knee and rotating the hip

(2) Rubbing around the knee
(Fig. 7-12)

[Method] The doctor puts the thumb of one hand at Xuehai (SP 10) on the affected limb and the thumb and index finger of the other hand at Neixiyan (EX-LE 4) and Waixiyan to rub with fingers of both hands for 1-2 minutes. Then the doctor puts the thumb and index finger at Yinlingquan (SP 9) and Yanglingquan (GB 34) to press and rub for 30-60 seconds. Finally the doctor puts one palm over the knee to rub and pinch around with the fingers for 1-2 minutes.

[Acupoints] Xuehai: Located 2 *cun* above the upper border of the patella at the medial side. Neixiyan: Located in the depression medial to the tip of the patella. Waixiyan: Located in the depression lateral to the tip of the patella. Yinlingquan: Located in the depression below the lower border of the tibia at the medial side. Yanglingquan: Located in the depression below and anterior to the small head of the fibia.

[Pithy formula] Rubbing the knee from Xuehai, Neixiyan, Waixiyan, Yinlingquan and Yanglingquan with great strength can relieve spastic pain, clear away damp-heat and subdue swelling.

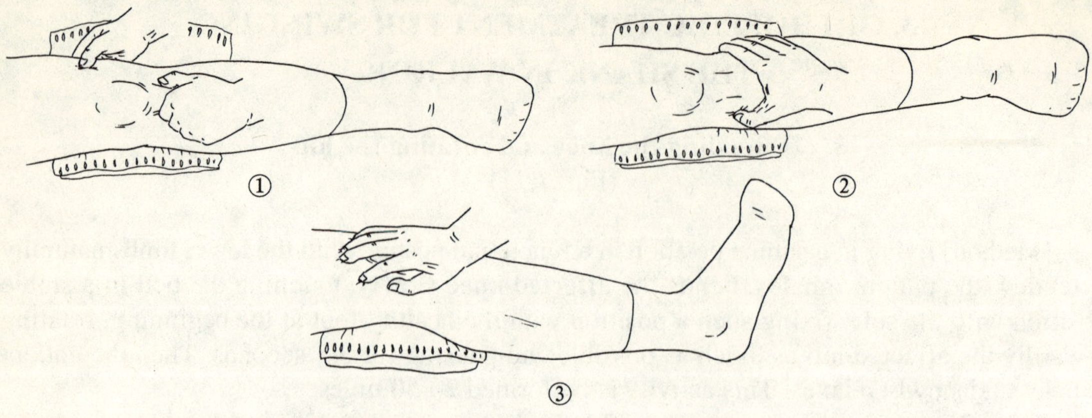

Fig. 7-12 Rubbing around the knee

(3) Bending the hip and extending the foot
(Fig. 7-13)

[Method] Standing straight in a functional posture, the patient inhales and slowly bends the hip and extends the foot as much as possible, pausing for 3-5 seconds. Then the patient exhales and slowly lowers the foot with the sole in a stable position touching the ground. This activity is performed 10-15 times.

[Effect] To train the muscles responsible for bending the hip joint and dorsal bending of the ankle joint; and to prevent stiffness and spasms of the hip joint, foot droop and strephenopodia.

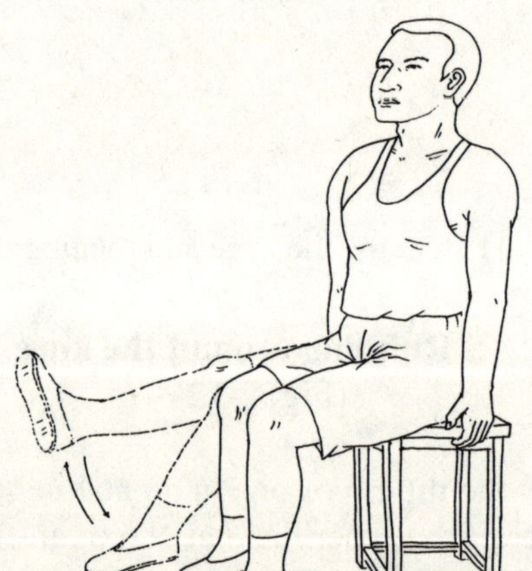

Fig. 7-13 Bending the hip and extending the foot

(4) Squatting with forward lunge
(Fig. 7-14)

[Method] Standing in a stable position in a functional posture with the upper limbs naturally hanging at the sides, the patient inhales and bends the hip and knee slowly as much as possible with the lower limbs in a forward lunge, pausing for 3-5 seconds. Then the patient exhales and slowly extends with the lower limbs in a half-squatting posture. This activity is performed 10-50 times.

[Effect] To train the muscles responsible for bending and extending the hip and knee joints; and to reinforce the stability of the knee joint.

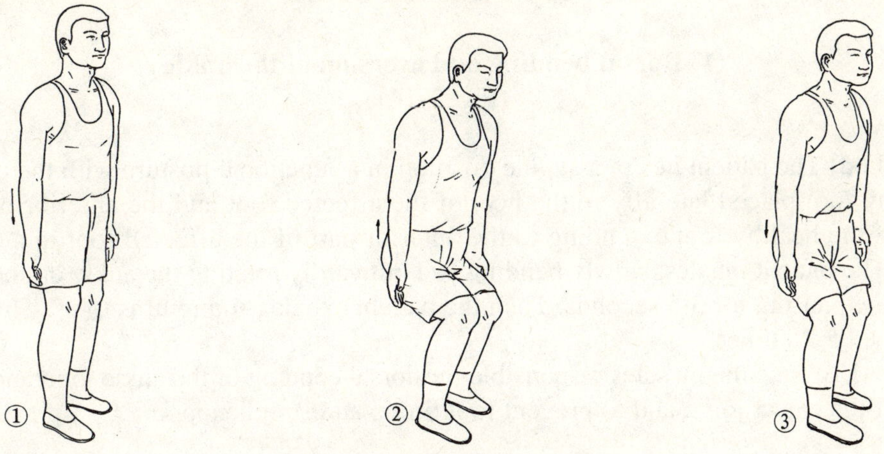

Fig. 7-14 Squatting with forward lunge

(5) Percussing the popliteal fossa
(Fig. 7-15)

[Method] The patient stands in a stable position in a functional posture and holds a pole for support with the healthy hand. The patient shifts the center to the affected side as much as possible and percusses the popliteal fossa on the affected limb with the dorsum of the healthy foot with moderate strength, light at first and then heavy, until a numb sensation is felt without bending the knee joint. Such a percussion is done 10-30 times.

[Effect] To reinforce the stability of the joints of the affected lower limb; and to achieve a certain effect on patients with lumbago or back pain by dredging the meridians and activating the vessels.

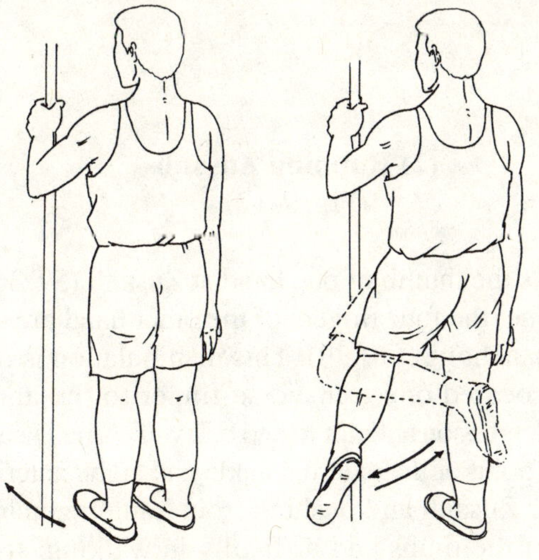

Fig. 7-15 Percussing the popliteal fossa

4.ORTHOPEDIC TREATMENT FOR FOOT DROOP AND STREPHENOPODIA

(1) Dorsal bending and eversion of the ankle
(Fig. 7-16)

[Method] The patient lies in a supine position in a functional posture with the dorsum of the healthy foot placed laterally to the heel of the affected foot and the anterior part of the dorsum of the healthy foot extending to the anterior part of the affected foot in a crossover position. The patient inhales, slowly bending and outwardly rotating the ankle on the affected limb, before pausing for 3-5 seconds. Then the patient exhales and returns to 0°. This activity is performed 5-20 times.

[Effect] To train the muscles responsible for dorsal bending of the ankle joint and external rotation of the calcar joint; and to prevent foot droop and strephenopodia.

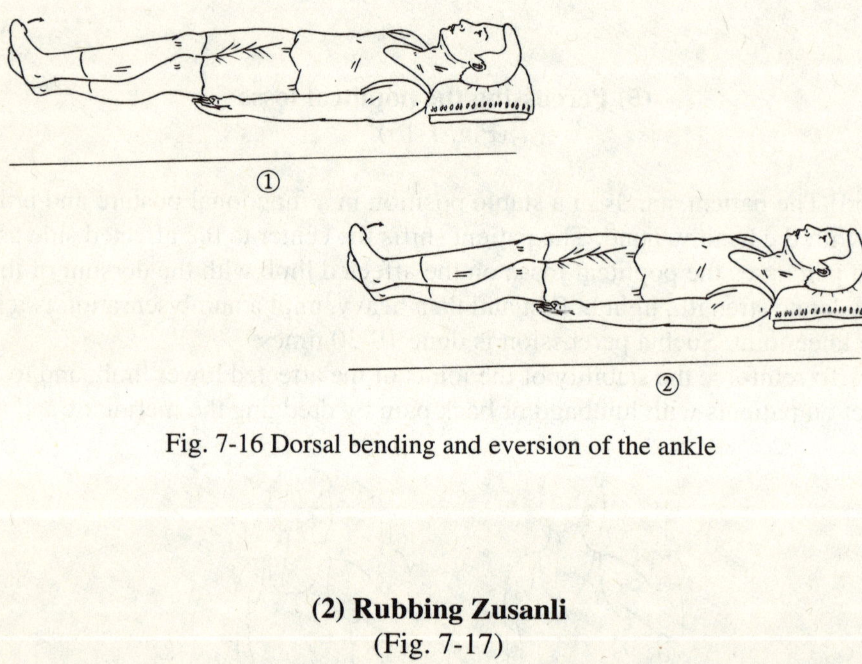

Fig. 7-16 Dorsal bending and eversion of the ankle

(2) Rubbing Zusanli
(Fig. 7-17)

[Method] The doctor puts the thumb of one hand at Zusanli (ST 36) on the affected limb to press and rub. At the same time, the four fingers of the other hand are put at Yanglingquan (GB 34) to push downward to Xuanzhong (GB 39). This manipulation is repeated for 1-2 minutes.

[Acupoints] Zusanli: Located one transverse finger to the anterior crest of the tibia. Yanglingquan: Located in the depression anterior to and below the small head of the fibia. Xuanzhong: Located 3 *cun* above the high point of the external ankle and at the anterior border of the fibia.

[Pithy formula] Rubbing Zusanli and pushing from Yanglingquan to Xuanzhong with the fingers can treat flaccidity of the limbs and difficulty in walking, strengthen the spleen and reinforce the tendons.

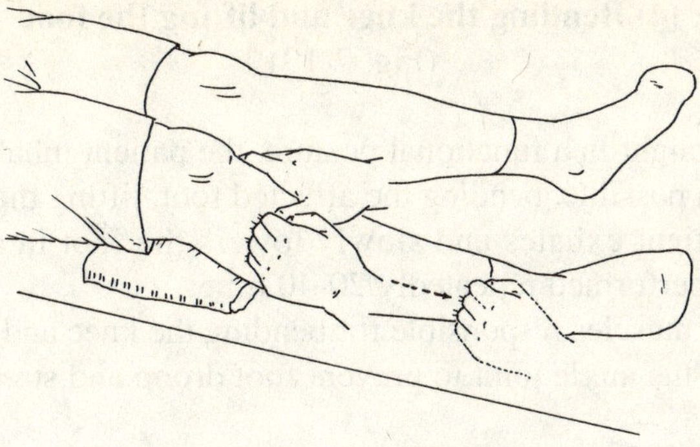

Fig. 7-17 Rubbing Zusanli

(3) Dorsal bending of the ankle
(Fig. 7-17)

[Method] The doctor puts four fingers of one hand at the dorsum of the affected foot and the thumb at Yongquan (KI 1). The thumb and the remaining four fingers of the other hand are put at Shuiquan (KI 5) and Pucan (BL 61). Then the doctor shakes, bends and extends the foot of the patient, pressing and rubbing the acupoints at the same time. This manipulation is done for 30-60 seconds.

[Acupoints] Yongquan: Located 1/3 anterior to the sole and in the depression when the toes and metatarsal bones are bent. Shuiquan: Located 1 *cun* directly below the depression between the high point of the medial ankle and heel tendon. Pucan: Located directly below the depression between the high point of the external ankle and heel tendon.

[Pithy formula] Dorsal bending, intorsion and eversion of the ankle can treat dysuria and foot flaccidity, promote menstruation and urination, subdue swelling and relieve pain.

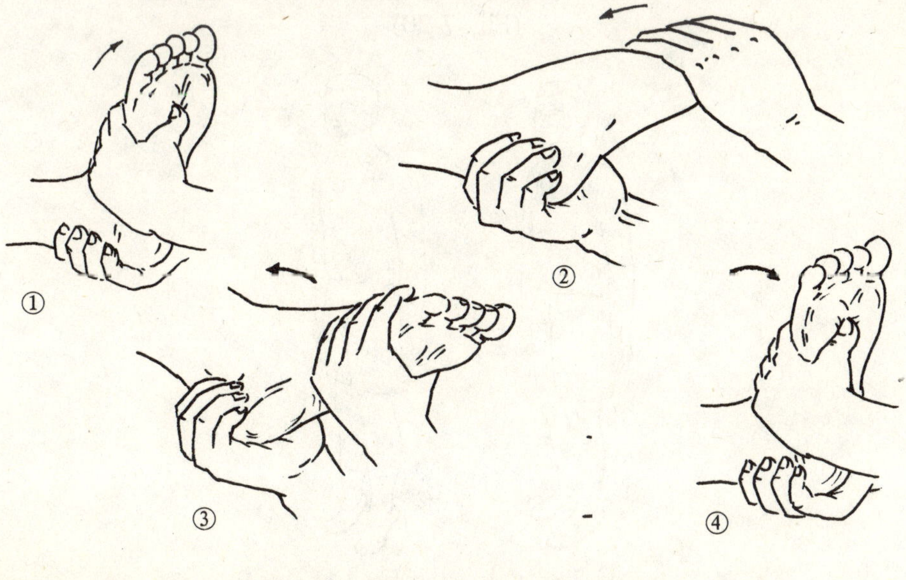

Fig. 7-18 Dorsal bending of the ankle

(4) Bending the knee and lifting the foot
(Fig. 7-19)

[Method] Sitting straight in a functional posture, the patient inhales and slowly bends the affected limb as much as possible, bending the affected foot, lifting the heel and pausing for 3-5 seconds. Then the patient exhales and slowly lowers the foot in a stable position on the ground. This activity is performed repeatedly 20-40 times.

[Effect] To train the muscles responsible for bending the knee and metatarsal joints; and to reinforce the stability of the ankle joint to prevent foot droop and strephenopodia.

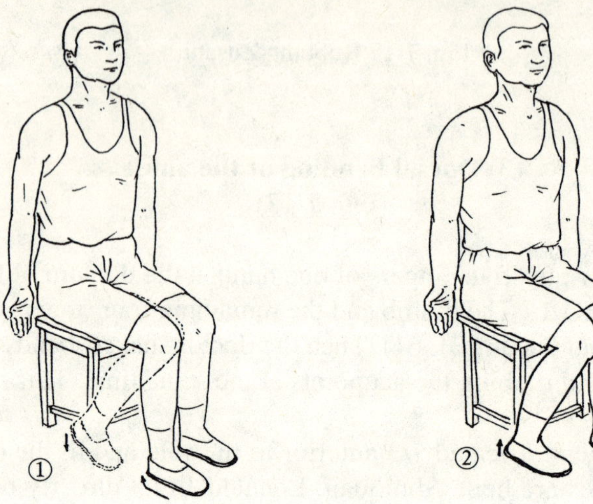

Fig. 7-19 Bending the knee and lifting the foot

(5) Metatarsal and dorsal bending of the ankle joint
(Fig. 7-20)

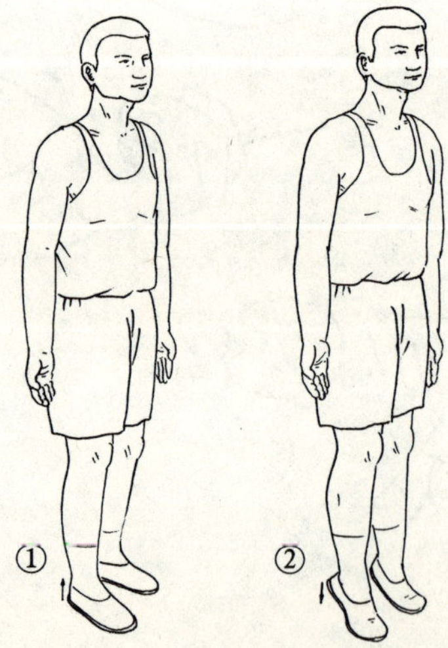

Fig. 7-20 Metatarsal and dorsal bending of the ankle

[Method] The patient stands in a stable position in a functional posture with the upper limbs hanging naturally at the side. The patient inhales and slowly lifts the heels as much as possible, bending the ankle joint, touching the ground with the anterior part of the sole, shifting the center of the body gradually to the affected side, and pausing for 3-10 seconds. Then the patient exhales and slowly lowers the heels, extending to 0°. This activity is repeated 10-20 times.

[Effect] To train the muscles responsible for metatarsal and dorsal bending of the ankle joint; and to reinforce the stability of the ankle joint to prevent foot droop and strephenopodia.

(6) Kneeling down with forward lunge
(Fig. 7-21)

[Method] Standing in a stable position in a functional posture (the doctor or nurse standing on the affected side), the patient shifts the center of the body to the healthy side and slowly stretches the affected foot in "forward lunge." The doctor helps the patient slowly kneel down with the healthy knee on the ground, shift the center of the body to the affected side, touch the ground in a stable position with the affected sole, straighten the chest and absorb the abdomen in a squatting position for 1-2 minutes. Then the patient stands up slowly with the help of the doctor. This activity is performed 5-10 times (patients with weak constitution should not undertake such an activity).

[Effect] To train the muscles responsible for bending the hip, knee and ankle joints; to restrain hyper function of the muscles responsible for extending the hip, knee and ankle joints; and to prevent stiffness of the hip and knee joints as well as foot droop and strephenopodia.

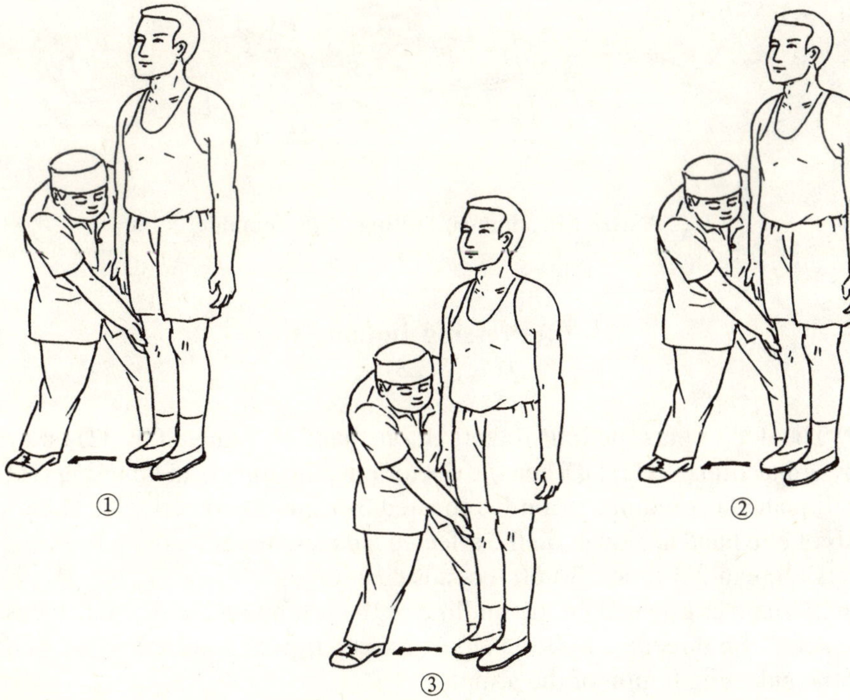

Fig. 7-21 Kneeling down with forward lunge

5. ORTHOPEDIC TREATMENT FOR SHOULDER AND HAND SYNDROME

(1) Anterior bending and lifting of the shoulder joint

(Fig. 7-22)

[Method] Lying in a supine position in a functional posture with the fingers on the healthy hand forking between the fingers on the affected hand in an extended position, the affected elbow extended and the palms facing each other, the patient inhales, slowly bending in an anterior way and lifting the affected shoulder and pausing for 5-10 seconds. Then the patient exhales and slowly lowers the shoulder. This activity is performed 10-50 times.

[Effect] To strengthen the function of bending and extending the shoulder joint; to restrain hyper function of the muscles responsible for bending the elbow, wrist and fingers as well as the pronator muscle; and to prevent adhesion of the shoulder joint and spasms and deformity of the joints on the affected upper limb.

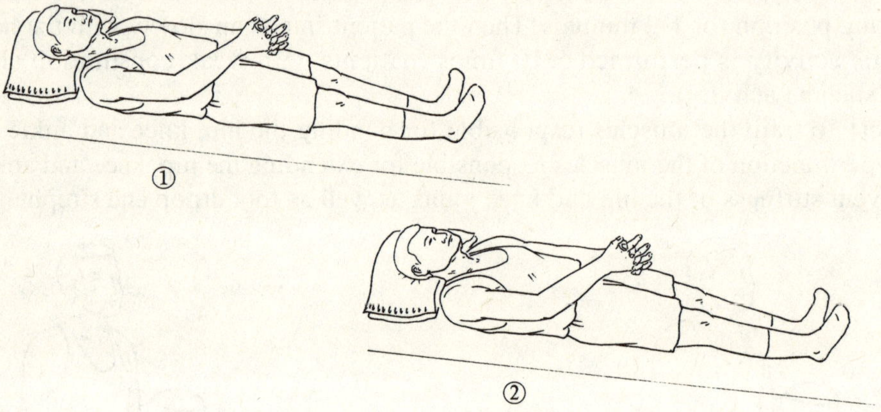

Fig. 7-22 Anterior bending and lifting of the shoulder joint

(2) Pressing Jiquan

(Fig. 7-23)

[Method] The doctor puts the four fingers of one hand at Yuanye GB 32) on the affected side to rub upward to Jiquan (HT 1). Then the doctor puts the fingers at Qingling (HT 2) to rub downward to Jiquan. This manipulation is repeated 3-5 times respectively. Then the doctor puts the thumb of one hand at Jiquan on the affected side and the remaining four fingers at the shoulder to press Jiquan 2-3 times, 30-60 seconds each time.

[Acupoints] Yuanye: Located on the midline of the armpit and at the fourth costal space. Qingling: Located 3 *cun* directly above the elbow crease. Jiquan: Located on the middle of the armpit and at the pulsating region of the armpit.

[Pithy formula] Pressing Jiquan, Yuanye and Qingling can treat cold pain of the arm, warm the meridians, activate the collaterals and resolve stasis.

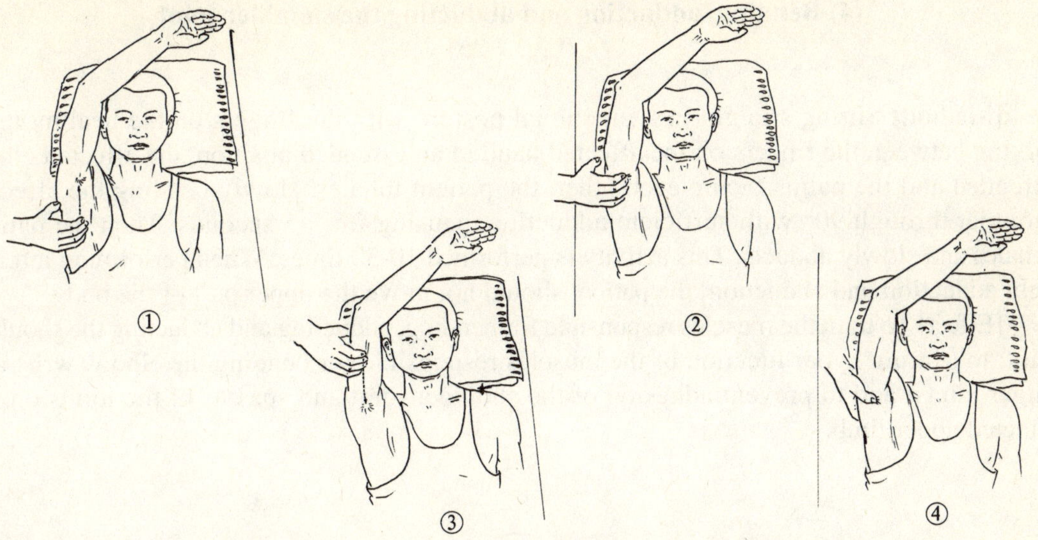

Fig. 7-23 Pressing Jiquan

(3) Pressing around the shoulder
(Fig. 7-24)

[Method] The doctor puts the thumbs of both hands at both sides of Naoshu (SI 10) on the affected side, then at Binao (LI 14) and Jianzhen (SI 9). Finally, the doctor puts the thumb of one hand at Jiquan (HT 1) and the remaining four fingers at Zhongfu (LU 1) and Yunmen (LU 2) to press and rub, 30-60 seconds each time for each acupoint. This manipulation is repeated 2-3 times.

[Acupoints] Naoshu: Located directly above the posterior folds of the armpit and in the depression at the lower border of the spine of the scapula. Binao: Located 7 *cun* directly above the lateral side of the elbow crease and below the deltoid muscle. Jianzhen: Located 1 *cun* above the posterior folds of the armpit. Jiquan: Located at the middle point of the armpit and at the pulsating region of the armpit. Zhongfu: Located 6 *cun* lateral to the anterior midline and parallel to the first costal space. Yunmen: Located 6 *cun* lateral to the anterior midline and at the lower border of the clavicle.

[Pithy formula] Pressing around the shoulder from Naoshu, Binao, Jianzhen, Jiquan, Zhongfu and Yunmen can activate blood, stop pain and dredge the meridians.

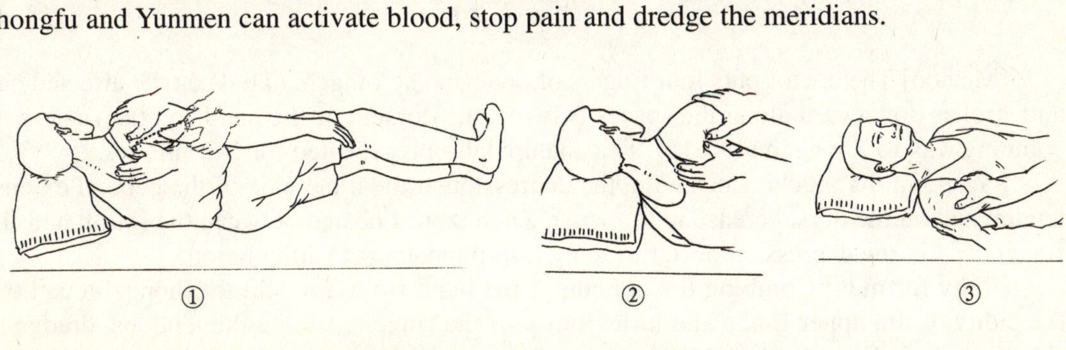

Fig. 7-24 Pressing around the shoulder

(4) Bending, adducting and abducting the shoulder joint
(Fig. 7-25)

[Method] Sitting straight in a functional posture with the fingers on the healthy hand forking between the fingers on the affected hand in an extended position, the affected elbow extended and the palms facing each other, the patient inhales, slowly bending the affected shoulder through 90° with sufficient adduction, pausing for 3-5 seconds. Then the patient exhales and slowly abducts. This activity is performed 10-30 times. When performing left and right adduction and abduction, the patient should not move the upper part of the body.

[Effect] To train the muscles responsible for bending, adducting and abducting the shoulder joint; to restrain hyper function of the muscles responsible for bending the elbow, wrist and finger joints; and to prevent adhesion of the shoulder joint and spasms of the joints on the affected upper limb.

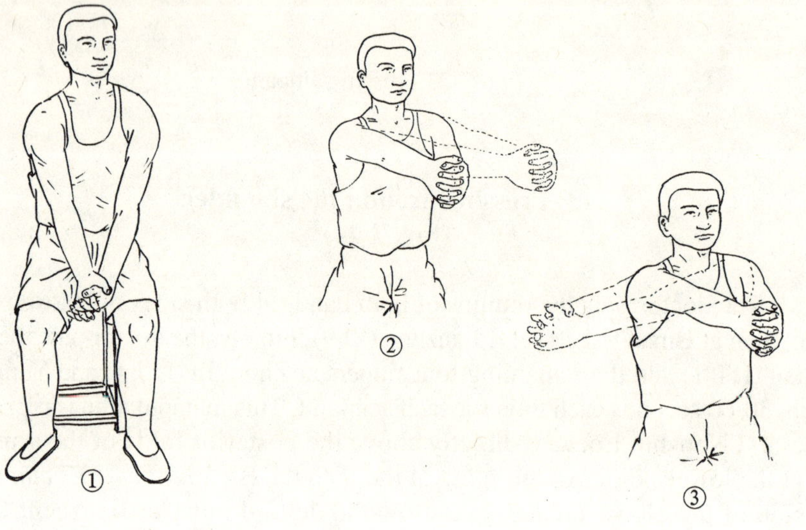

Fig. 7-25 Bending, adducting and abducting

(5) Combing the dorsum of the hand
(Fig. 7-26)

[Method] The doctor puts four fingers of one hand at Yangchi (TE 4) on the affected hand and strokes downward along the spaces between the dorsum of the hand and the fingers in a combing way to Zhongzhu (KI 15). This manipulation is repeated for 1-2 minutes.

[Acupoints] Yangchi: Located in the depression at the ulnar side of the general extensor tendon and on the dorsal crease of the wrist. Zhongzhu: Located between the fourth and fifth fingers and in the depression posterior to metacarpophalangeal articulation.

[Pithy formula] Combing the dorsum of the hand from Yangchi to Zhongzhu can treat flaccidity of the upper limbs and inflexibility of the fingers, soothe the tendons, dredge the meridians and eliminate dampness.

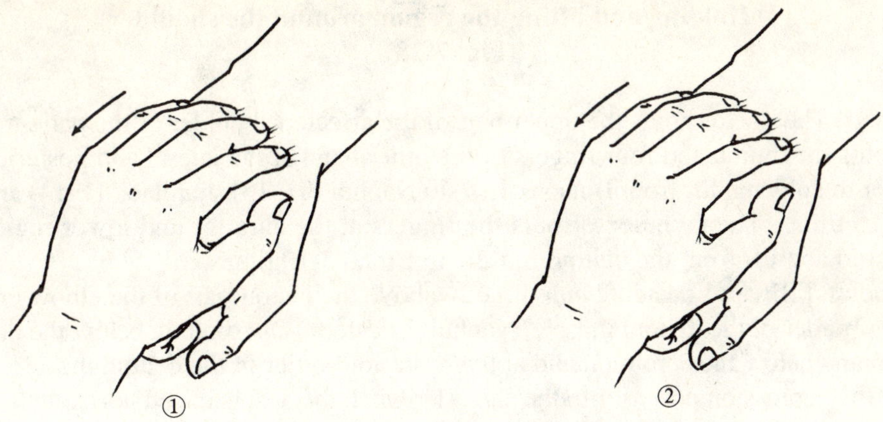

Fig. 7-26 Combing the dorsum of the hand

6. ORTHOPEDIC TREATMENT FOR SEMI-DISLOCATION OF THE SHOULDER JOINT

(1) Pressing and stroking around the shoulder (Fig. 7-27)

[Method] The doctor puts both palms at the neck on the affected side to rub from the acromion and the scapula 5-10 times, then rubbing and pressing from the acromion and the deltoid muscle to the elbow and wrist 5-10 times.

[Pithy formula] Rubbing around the shoulder from the acromion to the scapula can relieve spastic pain of the wrist and spasms of the shoulder and arm.

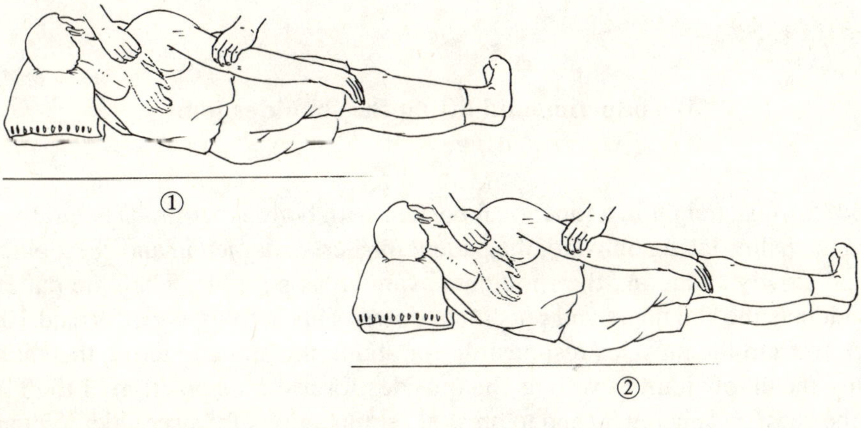

Fig. 7-27 Pressing and stroking around the shoulder

(2) Holding and lifting the region around the shoulder
(Fig. 7-28)

[Method] The doctor holds the upper part of the affected shoulder of the patient with one hand and puts the thumb and four fingers of the other hand at the lateral and posterior part of the shoulder to hold and lift from Binao (LI 14) to Naohui (TE 13), Jianliao (TE 14) and Jianyu (LI 15) 5-10 times. Then the doctor puts the fingers at the anterior and lower region of the armpit to hold and lift from the deltoid muscle to Binao 5-10 times.

[Acupoints] Binao: Located 7 *cun* directly above the lateral part of the elbow crease and at the lower border of the deltoid muscle. Naohui: Located 3 *cun* directly below the depression posterior to and below the acromion and at the posterior border of the deltoid muscle. Jianliao: Located in the depression posterior to the shoulder when the arm is raised horizontally. Jianyu: Located in the depression anterior to the shoulder when the arm is raised horizontally.

[Pithy formula] Holding and lifting the muscles around the shoulder can treat shoulder disorder, soothe the tendons and stop pain.

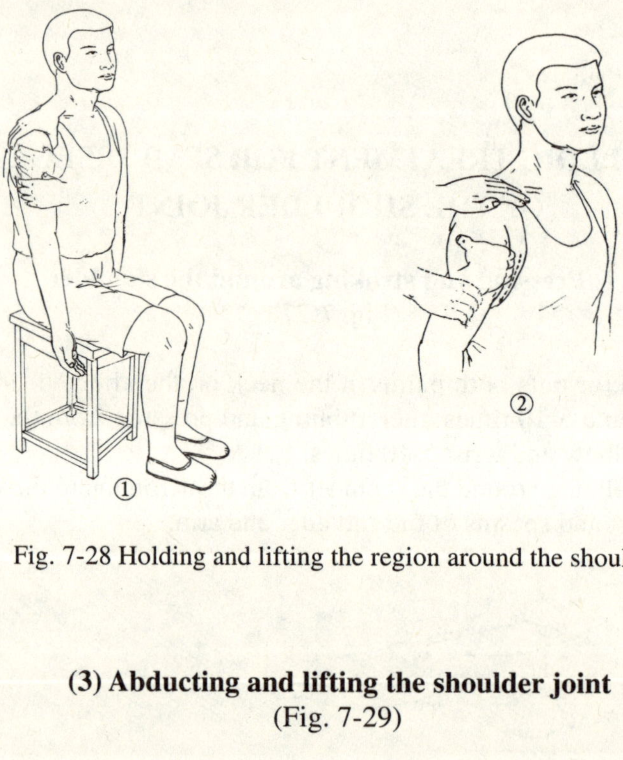

Fig. 7-28 Holding and lifting the region around the shoulder

(3) Abducting and lifting the shoulder joint
(Fig. 7-29)

[Method] Sitting straight in a functional posture with both upper limbs naturally put beside the body and the palms facing outward, the patient inhales, abdomen in and chest out, extending the elbow and slowly abducting the shoulders as much as possible. Then the patient exhales and slowly adducts the shoulders and puts them down. This activity is performed 10-30 times.

[Effect] To train the muscles responsible for abducting and adducting the shoulder joint and extending the elbow joint as well as the muscles for a supine position of the forearm and muscles on the chest and abdomen; and to prevent semiluxation of the shoulder joint and spasms of the elbow joint.

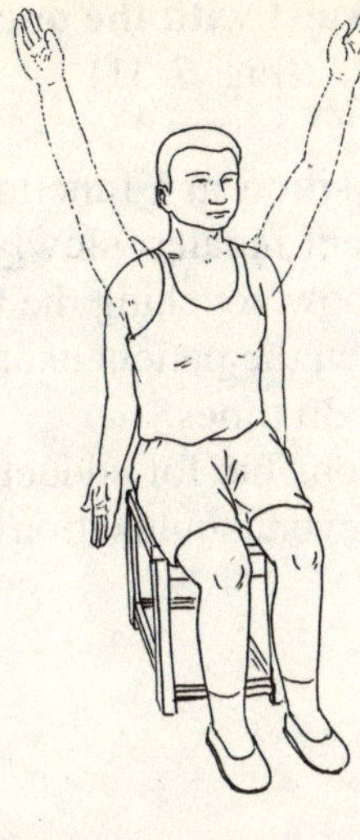

Fig. 7-29 Abducting and lifting the shoulder joint

(4) Pushing and pressing the three Yangming acupoints
(Fig. 7-30)

[Method] The doctor puts the thumb of one hand at Jianyu (LI 15) on the affected side to push and press along the lateral side of the arm (large intestine meridian) through Quchi (LI 11) to Hegu (LI 4). This manipulation is repeated 3-5 times.

[Acupoints] Jianyu: Located in the depression anterior to the shoulder when the arm is lifted horizontally. Quchi: Located in the depression at the lateral side of the elbow crease. Hegu: Located at the dorsum of the hand, between the first and second metatarsal bones and at about the midpoint of the second metatarsal bone.

[Pithy formula] Pushing and pressing the three Yangming acupoints from Jianyu and Quchi to Hegu can treat shoulder inflexibility, distorted face and sore throat, clear away heat, eliminate dampness and promote flow of Qi and blood.

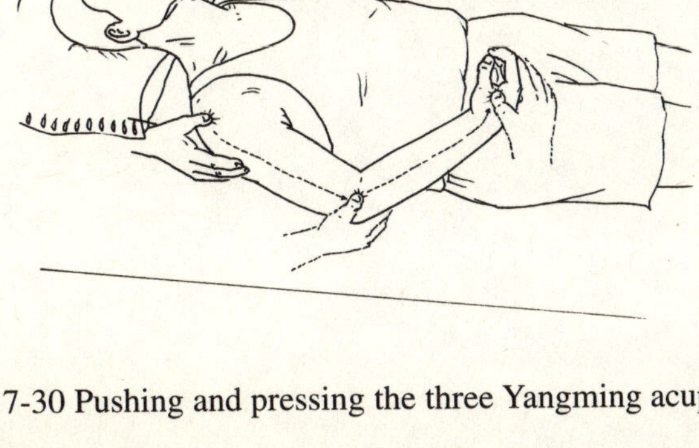

Fig. 7-30 Pushing and pressing the three Yangming acupoints

(5) Touching the waist with the dorsum of the hand
(Fig. 7-31)

[Method] Standing in a stable position in a functional posture with both upper limbs hanging naturally at the side, the patient inhales, slowly adducting the affected upper limb, extending the shoulder, bending the elbow, touching the waist with the dorsum of the affected hand, and pausing for 3-5 seconds. Then the patient exhales and slowly returns to the normal position. This activity is performed 20-30 times.

[Effect] To train the muscles responsible for adducting and extending the shoulder joint and bending the elbow joint; and to prevent subluxation of the shoulder joint and stiffness of the elbow joint.

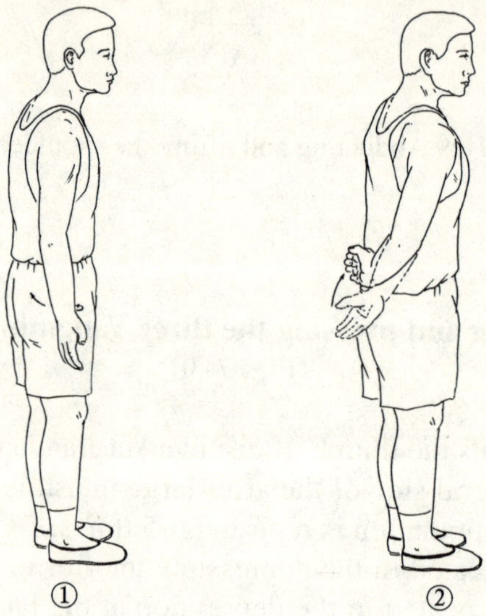

Fig. 7-31 Touching the waist with the dorsum of the hand

Chapter 8

TWENTY QUESTIONS CONCERNING APOPLECTIC PATIENTS

During the course of rehabilitation, apoplectic patients will ask various questions related to health-care and remedy, dining and living, washing and toileting as well as psychological changes and the pathological condition. In order to address such issues, we have selected 20 questions frequently confusing patients in order to enable them, their friends and relatives to cooperate with doctors. Under the guidance of doctors, patients can actively participate in exercises to recover as soon as possible and regain confidence in their future life.

1. HOW SHOULD THE PATIENTS TREAT THEMSELVES WITH CHINESE MEDICINAL BATHING?

Bathing treatment with Chinese medicinal herbs refers to the therapeutic method for the treatment of diseases with the composition of a special formula. The process is like this: First decoct the prescribed herbs; pour the liquid into a basin or a bathtub with hot water and fumigate and wash the patent's affected limbs or body. This treatment can help the patient dredge the meridians and activate the blood, ease swelling to relieve pain and lubricate the joints.

(1) Prescription for the remedy of apoplectic dyskinesia:

30 g of Danggui (Radix Angelicae Sinensis), 30 g of Chishao (Radix Paeoniae Rubra), 20 g of peach seed (Semen Persicae), 30 g of Sangjisheng (Herba Taxilli), 30 g of Ruxiang (Olibanum), 30 g of Moyao (Myrrha), 30 g of Dilong (Pheretima), 30 g of Honghua (Flos Carthami), 30 g of Zelan (Herba Lycopi), 20 g of Sumu (Lignum Sappan), 20 g of Muxiang (Radix Aucklandiae), 50 g of Haitongpi (Cortex Ergthrinae Orientalis), 50g of Shenjincao (Herba Lycopodii), 30 g of Jixueteng (Laulis Spatholobi), 30 g of Wushaoshe (Zaocys).

1) For patients with cold upper limbs, 20 g of Guizhi (Ramulus Cinnamomi) and 20 g of Jianghuang (Rhizoma Curcumae Longae) are added.

2) For patients with feverish upper limbs, 40 g of Sangzhi (Ramulus mori) and 30 g of Jiujun are added.

3) For patients with cold lower limbs, 30 g of Wuyao (Radix Linderae) and 40 g of Huainiuxi (Radix Cyathukae) are added.

4) For patients with feverish lower limbs, 30 g of Yemugua (Caulis et Folium Stauntoniae) and 30 g of Chuanniuxi (Radix Cyathulae) are added.

(2) Fumigation and washing method:

Decoct the medicinal herbs twice, mix the liquid, add 10 to 20 ml of liquor and pour the mixture into a basin for fumigation and washing.

Fumigate and wash the affected limbs once a day with the mixture. Fumigate the affected limbs with the vapor of the mixture first, and then wash them half an hour later when the temperature of the mixture has dropped to 50°C.

If possible, the patient can fumigate and wash the whole body once every three days for half an hour. Keep the water at 50°C to 60°C and the room temperature at 23°C to 30°C respectively. Keep the door and windows slightly open. The patient can drink about 200 ml of light salty water before washing.

(3)Caution: Change the medicinal herbs every two days; quit bathing in case of bruising or ulceration of the affected limbs.

2. HOW SHOULD THE PATIENTS TRAIN THEMSELVES IN USING THE BRAIN?

A patient with apoplexy suffers more or less from malfunction in terms of feeling, sensation, memory, association, thinking and even loss of memory. If the patient cannot rehabilitate his memory, he is likely to have cerebrovascular dementia. So, brain training is very important.

(1) Change both the ways and contents of thinking: After the patient with apoplexy finishes doing exercises for rehabilitation, he can read or study in moderation. The constant change of ways and contents of study can enable part of the cerebral neural cells to change from excitation to inhibition and another part from inhibition into excitation.

(2) Strengthening the ability to maintain attention: The patient with apoplexy usually focuses his attention only on one thing or one aspect of study, often stimulating the cerebral neural cells in charge of "attention," frequently exciting these cells and inhibiting the cells responsible for other activities.

(3) Stimulating interest: Keen interest propels the patient to read books related to his disease, providing him with a good opportunity to use the brain.

Doing the aforementioned exercises is extremely beneficial to rehabilitating the function of the patient's cerebral neural cells and preventing cerebrovascular dementia.

3. HOW SHOULD THE PATIENTS TRAIN THEMSELVES IN USING LANGUAGE?

It is not rare for the patient of apoplexy to suffer from aphasia. Cerebral edema leads to aphasia, which results from hemorrhage of the brain. It can be treated by dehydration therapy. With the improvement of the pathological condition, the ability to speak is restored quickly.

Aphasia caused by cerebral infarction results from ischemia that impairs the language center, which is difficult to improve.

In the treatment of this problem, the use of Chinese medicinal herbs or acupuncture is usually combined with language training.

(1) Language training: 1) vocalize numbers like "one, two, three—." 2) Pronounce letters: read letters such as "a, i, u, b, p, m..." aloud after the doctor or nurse. 3) Read words: ask the patient to read and speak simple words like "talk, eat, wash, desk." 4) Short phrases: with the improvement of the patient's vocalization, increase the number of his vocabulary and expressions, ask him to speak aloud, slowly at first and then more quickly, phrases like "before the meal, wash your hands," and, "after the meal, rinse your mouth," etc. 5) Speak short sentences: if the patient can speak phrases clearly, let him articulate short sentences by combining phrases. 6) Speak long sentences: let the patient combine short sentences into long ones, such as "We should maintain good hygiene, wash the hands before a meal and rinse the mouth after a meal, otherwise we will suffer from disease."

(2) Language-connecting training: for instance, when the doctor speaks the first half of a sentence, the patient replies with the second half. For example, when the patient hears the expression of "before the meal", he should reply with, "wash your hands."

(3) Repetition exercises: repeat the words, phrases and sentences the doctor has said.

(4) Words of command exercises: the when doctor points to a picture or a word or a phrase, the patient should speak out and explains its meaning.

In general, the best time for a patient to practice language training is when he is in best condition and in a good mood. The practice should be done gradually: three to four hours a day. Such a training will be effective if it is continued every day.

4. HOW SHOULD THE PATIENTS TRAIN THEMSELVES IN DAILY LIFE?

The apoplectic patient can take advantage of daily activities to do rehabilitative exercises, which is beneficial to rehabilitation of affected limbs, others' understanding of the patient's mood and pathological condition as well as restoration of normal life and general rehabilitation.

(1) Face-washing exercise: The patient washes his face with the healthy hand first and then with the affected hand.

(2) Putting on and taking off clothes: When dressing, the patient puts clothes on the affected limbs first; when undressing, he takes the clothes off the healthy limbs first.

(3) Dining exercise: use chopsticks with the healthy hand and support the wrist with the affected hand in dining.

(4) Housework exercise: when the patient can take care of himself in daily life, he can use his affected hand to help the healthy hand open and close doors and windows, mop the floor, wash bowls, fold up a quilt, dry things outdoors, etc.

(5) Social training: The patient can walk, or take a bus in the company of family members.

5. WHAT PROBLEMS SHOULD THE PATIENTS TAKE INTO CONSIDERATION IN THE PROCESS OF REHABILITATION?

The rehabilitation of the patient needs the help of his relatives or friends. According to statistics, patients aged 70 or more can enjoy a period of normal life after rehabilitation, but begin to suffer from obvious retrogression five years later. So care should be taken to prevent retrogression.

(1) Be careful in terms of safety, avoid accidents such as bone fracture, dislocation and ecchymoma.

(2) Reinforce the functions of the healthy limbs and the compensatory functions of the affected limbs, strictly following the standards of rehabilitation exercise.

(3) Prevent disuse syndrome, adhesion of the shoulder joints, subluxation as well as contracture and deformity of the limbs.

(4) Use a walking stick. When the patient walks, he should carry a stick as long as the height from his feet to the top of his greater femoral trochanter.

(5) Take a small amount of exercise in the initial stage. Avoid doing hasty or excessive rehabilitation exercise.

6. HOW TO REASONABLY ARRANGE HOME-BASED REHABILITATION FOR THE PATIENTS?

The rehabilitation at home is very important. Since home-based rehabilitation is long-term work, it should be carried out with a proper plan and appropriate arrangement.

1) 8:00-9:00: Practice both passive and active functional exercises of the patient's upper and lower limbs slowly. Language training is done together with self-massage.

2) 9:00-10:00: Tuina therapy.

3) 10: 00-10:20: Full relaxation and language training with music.

4) 10:20-11:00: Language training.

5) 13:00-14:30: Midday nap.

6) 15:30-16:30: Practice both passive and active functional exercise of the patient's upper and lower limbs. Language training is done together with self-massage.

7) 16:30-17:30:Tuina therapy.

8) 18:00-19:00: Language training.

9) 20:00-21:00: Language training.

7. HOW SHOULD THE PATIENTS SCIENTIFICALLY ARRANGE THEIR HOME-BASED REHABILITATION?

Good daily living can help recover the functions of the patient's cerebral neural cells, which is vital to the recovery of the function of the limbs after apoplexy.

(1) The living room must face south with sufficient sunshine through its door and windows. Keep the temperature between 18⁰C and 22⁰C. The room should be bright, warm and dry.

(2) Keep the room well ventilated. Don't hang wet clothes indoors.

(3) Put some vases of flowers indoors, or plant some flowers and grass in the yard, so as to cultivate a good temperament, purify the air and eliminate mental stress and tiredness.

(4) Guarantee eight hours of sleep from ten o'clock in the evening to six o'clock the next morning. Have a nap for an hour and a half after lunch. Measures should be taken to ensure the quality of sleep. After waking up, the patient should feel refreshed and comfortable.

8. WHAT CARE SHOULD BE TAKEN WHEN HELPING THE PATIENTS IN THE TOILETS?

Only when the patient is in stable condition with keen consciousness and sound mentality can he or she enter a toilet. Performing toilet is also a kind of exercise, particularly good for exercising the functions of the heart and lungs and digestion, and also effective for restoring the ability of self-care and full recovery. The following points must be taken into account.

(1) The patient with cerebral hemorrhage can be allowed to enter a toilet three or four weeks after onset.

(2) A nurse must stand on the healthy side of the patient and the patient must support himself by holding the nurse with his healthy hand.

(3) Before entering a toilet, the patient must practice sitting and standing so as to prevent postural hypotension and urinating syncope.

(5) The floor in the toilet must be dry. The patient had better wear slip-free shoes and keep warm.

9. WHAT CARE SHOULD BE TAKEN WHEN HELPING THE PATIENTS TO BATHE?

A nurse should scrub the bed-ridden patient in time to maintain the physiological functions of skin, promote blood circulation lest skin infections and bedsores occur.

(1) Turn the body properly: Usually turn the healthy side.

(2) After the critical period, encourage the patient to scrub his body on his own. This is beneficial to activating joints and promoting blood circulation.

(3) Before scrubbing and bathing, the patient should first empty the bowels and urinate. The door and windows should be closed and the room temperature kept between 23⁰C and 30⁰C. Water about 50⁰C should be prepared for bathing.

(4) The scrubbing and bathing order is from the face to the neck, upper limbs, chest and abdomen, back and lower limbs. Soak the hands and feet in the water; carefully scrub the postauricular part, the neck, armpits and perineum; use clean water and a new towel when scrubbing the perineum and feet; keep the washed parts of the body covered and warm; after scrubbing, change to clean underwear and bed sheet.

(5) In the course of scrubbing, keep watch on the patient and check for the appearance of

petechia, eruption, edema, damage and infection. Timely treatment should be given if there is any.

10.WHAT CARE SHOULD BE TAKEN WHEN HELPING THE PATIENTS TO WASH?

During rehabilitation, the patient should make efforts to take a hot bath in the bathing-room. Hot bathing not only can wash away and get rid of bodily dirt, but also promote blood circulation, prevent skin infection and promote restoration of functions.

(1) The condition of the patient should be stabilized. Before bathing, the patient's blood pressure and pulse should be examined to see if there are any abnormal changes.

(2) Supply a handle or a chair for the patient and there should be one to two persons for aid and protection.

(3) Keep the room temperature between 23°C and 30°C and water temperature at 50°C. The door and windows should not be closed too tight. Take measures to prevent the patient from sweating too much. Ask the patient to drink 200 ml to 30 ml of light salty water after bathing.

(4) In the course of bathing, frequently ask the patient whether he is feeling dizzy, panicky or oppressed. Observe whether there are any signs of faintness, such as pale complexion and rapid beating of the pulse. If there is any, wrap the body with a towel, open the windows, and support the patient to stand for a while or lie down on the bed.

(5) Don't bathe within half an hour after meal or on an empty stomach.

11. HOW SHOULD THE PATIENTS SELECT FOOD?

The patient should have a diet with more vegetables, fruits and beans but less fat.

(1) Meat has to be well combined with vegetables. It is better for the patient to have food with higher protein such as bean products, eggs without yolk, lean meat and grain products. This kind of diet will prevent declination of memory, inertia, edema, anemia and lower resistance due to long-term intake of food with low protein.

(2) The patient should take less animal fat and internal organs such as heart, intestines, brains, yolks and fish eggs. It is better for the patient to have food with low fat and a diet with bean oil, peanut oil, sunflower seeds oil and sesame oil in order to reduce cholesterol, cirrhosis and arteriosclerosis.

(3) The patient should control the intake of sweet food and avoid overeating. Eating too much sugar leads to excessive neutral fat and arteriosclerosis. So, control of sweet food and sugar not only supplements the energy of the body, but also prevents the occurrence of other diseases.

(3) The patient should take various vitamins, minerals, and inorganic salt, calcium, compound vitamin B, vitamin E, etc.

12. WHAT MEDICINAL FOODS ARE SUITABLE FOR PATIENTS WITH PARALYSIS?

Abstinence from some foods is beneficial to the patient. The following medicinal foods are recommended.

(1) Meat and eggs: lean pork, egg without yolk, sheat-fish, and eel.

(2) Vegetables: potato, bean curd, bean sprout, pumpkin, cucumber, radish, celery, seaweed, black sesame, corn, mussel rape, soya bean, carrot, and black fungus.

(3) Fruits: hawthorn fruit, orange, pear, apple, date, and banana.

(4) Spices: onion, ginger, garlic, and vinegar.

(5) Fresh milk.

13. WHAT IS THE RELATIONSHIP BETWEEN PROTEIN AND WIND STROKE?

A common misconception prevails among apoplectic patients that they should rather not eat any meat, fish or egg, when they know they suffer from high blood fat and high cholesterol.

It is known to all that sheat-fish, eel, grass carp, lean pork, egg without yolk contain a large amount of protein that the human body needs. Protein is indispensable to the daily activities of the human body, ranging from composition of the cells to the structure of the human body, from growth and development of the body to repair of injured tissues, from metabolism to enzyme, from immune antibody to the composition of hormones, from preserving vital energy to delaying senility.

Research has revealed that the amino acid contained in protein can, through the central nerve system, reduce the morbidity of apoplexy and increase the rate of existence and rehabilitation by means of regulating blood pressure, reducing hypertension and improving the blood vessel elasticity. Besides, protein constitutes a material base for human memory and has great significance in preventing occurrence of senile dementia. So, having both meat and vegetable is the best for an apoplectic patient.

14. WHAT IS THE RELATIONSIIIP BETWEEN SMOKING AND DRINKING AND WIND STROKE?

Tobacco contains over 20 kinds of poisonous substances, among which nicotine can lead to spasms of the blood vessel, higher blood pressure, fast beating of the heart, acceleration of arteriosclerosis, promotion of platelet aggregation, increase of blood viscosity, and the slowed flow of the bloodstream. All these are etiological factors of apoplexy. According to statistics, the incidence of apoplexy among long-term heavy smokers is 3.5 times that of non-smokers.

Overdrinking or frequent drinking of strong liquor on an empty stomach will excite or inhibit the central nerves, causing high blood pressure and a rapid heart beat. Once the cerebral vessels disrupt, it is likely to cause hemorrhagic apoplexy. According to statistics, the incidence of apoplexy among long-term heavy drinkers is twice that of non-drinkers, although it is beneficial to the human body to drink in moderation low-alcohol drinks such as wine or medicinal wine according to a doctor's prescription.

15. CAN THE PATIENTS DRINK TEA?

Tea contains many vitamins such as Vitamin C and E and catechin, which can exert biological efficacy on metabolism. For example, Vitamin C can protect intact vascular walls and avoid vascular rupture; catechin can build up vascular elasticity and prevent sclerosis of blood vessels; Vitamins E and C and tea polyphenol can reduce blood fat; coffee alkali and tea alkali, which can excite the cerebral cortex and the respiratory and circulatory centers, help improve memory and eliminate tiredness. Furthermore, tea also contains trace elements that the human body needs such as cuprum, fluorine, magnesium and molybdenum. All in all, drinking tea properly, particularly green tea, helps the patient recover. But, for those who suffer from anemia, urinary stones, ulceration of the gastro enteric tract, habitual constipation, liver disease, malnutrition and neurasthenia, or those who have taken aspirin, ephedrine, and atropine medicine, and drinking tea is forbidden before sleep and immediately after meal.

16. HOW TO TREAT THE PATIENTS WITH PSYCHOLOGICAL THERAPY?

Patients with apoplexy usually suffer from psychological problems, such as anxiety of becoming disabled or dying soon. So, psychotherapy is very important.

(1) Doctors or nurses should pay attention to psychotherapy: They should frequently enter the ward to inquire about the condition of the patient, detect any problems and deal with them in a timely way. They should act not only as doctors or nurses, but also as relatives of the patient, trying to comprehend the patient's mental state, removing his or her psychic conflict, explaining the pathological condition to enable the patient to cooperate actively in the treatment.

(2) Self-mental adjustment of the patient: The patient should maintain a positive attitude toward disease, read more delightful books for the sake of his health, eliminate fear, stay happy and optimistic, free himeself from vexation and irritation, and avoid a pessimistic mood. Only by doing so, can the patient cooperate with the doctors. Besides, the patient should persist in doing active or passive functional training as far as health allows.

(4) The family members should cooperate in applying psychotherapy. In order to remove the patient's loneliness, they should talk with the patient, calming and encouraging him; in nursing, they should speak to him with a kind and pleasant countenance and affection, avoiding

hurting his feelings; during the course of feeding him with medicine and food, washing face, bathing, helping him go to toilet, turning the body and doing passive functional training or Tuina, they should never show any signs of impatience. This way of caring for the patient will be advantageous for quick recovery. As for the patient who is able to walk, the family members should accompany him; for the patient who has language problems, the family members should patiently help him do language training. This is very important for the patient to maintain a good mood and gain confidence in overcoming the disease.

17. CAN WIND STROKE OCCUR AMONG PATIENTS WITH CERVICAL VERTEBRAL DISORDER?

The patient with cervical artery syndrome is likely to develop apoplexy when he suddenly turns his head, leading to such symptoms as dizziness, nausea, vomiting, blurred sight, tinnitus, or even sudden falling down. These symptoms are caused by inflammatory edema of the tissues surrounding the cervical vertebrae due to osseous hyperplasia that results in the narrowing or spasm of the cervical artery and insufficient supply of blood to the brain. If cerebral arteriosclerosis is present, it will aggravate the insufficient supply of the blood for the brain and further slow blood circulation in the cerebral vessels and cause platelet aggregation, thereby bringing about thrombus and ischemic apoplexy. Therefore, the treatment of apoplectic patients of cervical vertebral syndrome should focus on both apoplexy and cervical vertebral syndrome.

18. WHY CAN HYPOTENSION LEAD TO WIND STROKE?

Cerebral vessels can regulate themselves within a certain range of blood pressure. When cerebral vessels are in disorder, their self-regulation function can only exert effect within a higher blood pressure. If the blood pressure is too low, spasms of the blood vessel may occur, resulting in ischemia, hypoxia and infarction of the cerebral tissues. At the same time, it may lead to a slow flow of the bloodstream and platelet aggregation that further results in an increase of blood viscosity and induces thrombus and apoplexy. So, the middle-aged and the aged with very low blood pressure should pay attention to treatment. For patients with high blood pressure, while using drugs for reducing it they should take care to prevent excessive decrease of blood pressure leading to apoplexy.

19. CAN THE VESSELS BE DREDGED AFTER THE TREATMENT OF CEREBRAL THROMBOSIS?

The pathological cause for cerebral thrombus is the athermanous sclerosis plaque of local cerebrovascular membrane that leads to coarse lumen of the blood vessel and platelet aggregation, making the lumen of blood vessels narrow. If the lumens of blood vessels are completely obstructed, they cannot be dredged no matter what therapies are used. However, therapies, such as promoting Qi flow, activating blood and resolving stasis in TCM as well as surgical bypass operation on the blood vessels, can start collateral circulation in the milieu of pathological changes, which can supply cerebral tissues with blood from bypass blood vessels and improve the symptoms of ischemia, thus reducing the damage of brain tissues and restoring the function of nerves.

20. WHY IS WIND STROKE HEREDITARY?

Clinical practice has shown that the genetic factor in apoplectic patients is comparatively obvious. Those who have a constitution of hereditary factors for apoplexy, such as hypertension, disturbance in the metabolism of fat and protein, tend to be victims of apoplexy. The death of their parents due to apoplexy is five times that of the general people.

Investigation has discovered that the incidence of hypercholesterolemia and high blood coagulation state is comparatively higher among the family members of the patients with ischemic apoplexy; while the family members of the patients with hemorrhagic apoplexy, apart from hypercholesterolemia, tend to have low blood coagulation. It is thus evident that in some patients apoplexy is hereditary. Apoplexy, like hypertension, is obviously hereditary. For this reason, family members must take measures to prevent apoplexy. To maintain stability of blood pressure and to reduce weakening of the elasticity of the blood vessels wall are very important steps in preventing hereditary apoplexy.

Appendix 1

FIGURES INDICATING THE MUSCLES THAT DOMINATE THE MOVEMENT OF THE MAIN JOINTS IN THE HUMAN BODY

Table 1 Atlantooccipital joint flexor

Name	Location and form	Starting point	Ending point
Sternocleidomastoid muscle	Located obliquely at both sides of the neck and streaky in form	Anterior to the manubrium of the sternum and the sternum end of the clavicle	Mastoid process of the temporal bone
Anterior scalene muscle	At both sides of the cervical section of the spinal column	Transverse process of the cervical vertebra	First rib
Medial scalene muscle			
Posterior scalene muscle			Second rib

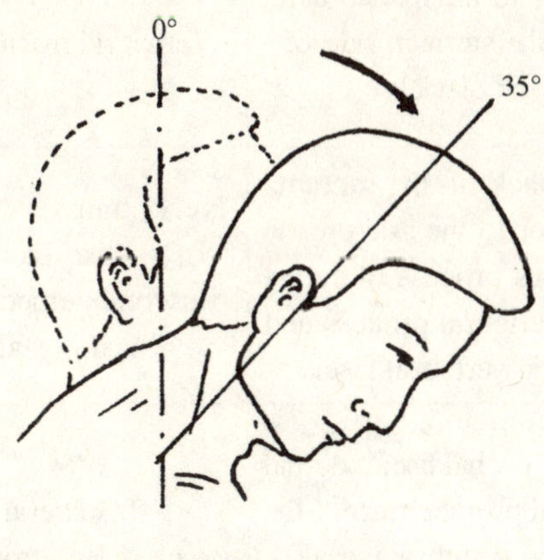

Fig. 1-l Atlantooccipital joint flexion (anterior flexion of the head)

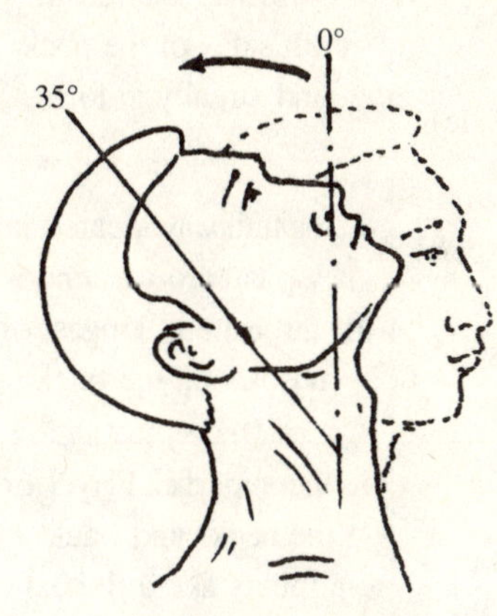

Fig.1-2 Extension of the atlantooccipital joint (posterior flexion of the head)

Table 2 Atlantooccipital joint extensor

Name	Location and form	Starting point	Ending point
Sternocleido-mastoid muscle	Obliquely located at both sides of the neck and streaky in form	Anterior to the manubrium of the sternum and at the sternum side of the clavicle	Temporal mastoid process
Erector spinal muscle	Longitudinally located in the spinal groove, and is the largest and longest of muscles on the back	At the back of the sacrum posterior to the iliac crest, spinous process of the lumbar vertebral process and thoracic vertebral fascia	Neck, transverse process of the thoracic vertebrae, temporal mastoid, and costal angle
Trapezius muscle	In the superficial layer of the neck and back, appears like a deltoid broad muscle and combines both sides into trapezius muscle	Superior nuchal line, external occipital protuberance, 7th cervical vertebra and all spinous processes of the horacic vertebrae	1/3 lateral to the clavicle, acromion and scapular spine

Table 3 Atlantooccipital joint lateral flexor

Name	Location and form	Starting point	Ending point
Sternocleido-mastoid muscle (same side)	Obliquely located at both sides of the neck and streaky in form	Anterior to the manubrium and at the sternum side of the clavicle	Temporal mastoid process
erector spinal muscle (same side)	Longitudinally located in the spinal groove, and is the largest and longest of muscles on the back	At the back of the sacrum, posterior to the iliac crest spinous process of the lumbar vertebral process and thoracic vertebral fascia	Neck, transverse process of the thoracic vertebrae,temporal mastoid, and costal angle
Trapezius muscle (same side)	In the superficial layer of the neck and back, appears like a deltoid broad muscle and combines both sides into trapezius muscle	Superior nuchal line, external occipital protuberance, 7th cervical vertebra and all spinous processes of the thoracic vertebrae	1/3 lateral to the clavicle, acromion and scapular spine

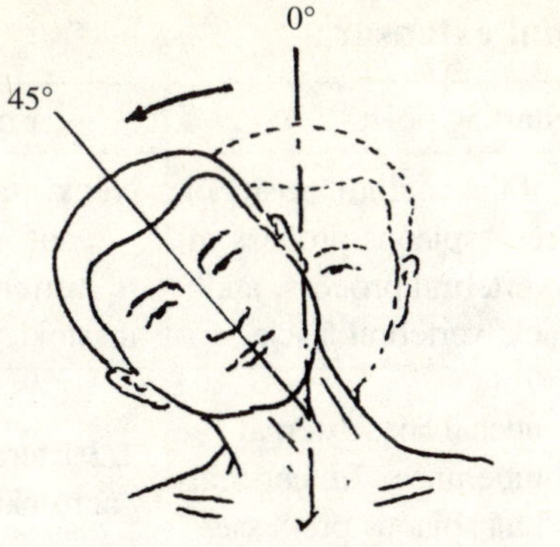

Fig. 1-3 Lateral flexion of the atlantooccipital joint (lateral flexion of the head)

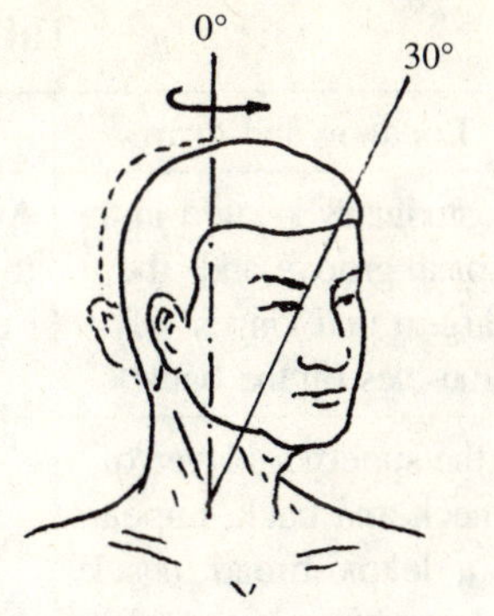

Fig. 1-4 Rotation of the atlantooccipital joint (rotation of the head)

Table 4 Atlantooccipital joint rotator

Name	Location and form	Starting point	Ending point
Sternocleidomastoid muscle (same side)	Obliquely located at both sides of the neck and streaky in form	Anterior to the manubrium of the sternum and at the sternum side of the clavicle	Temporal mastoid process
Trapezius muscle (opposite side)	In the superficial layer of the neck and back, appears like a deltoid broad muscle and combines both sides into trapezius muscle	Superior nuchal line, external occipital protuberance, 7th cervical vertebra and all spinous processes of the thoracic vertebrae	1/3 lateral to the clavicle, acromion and scapular spine

Table 5 Spinal flexor

Name	Location and form	Starting point	Ending point
Rectal abdominal muscle	At both sides of the anterior midline along the abdomen, in the sheath of the rectal abdominal muscle, broad in the upper part and narrow in the lower part	Pubic symphysis and pubic crest	Xiphoid process and anterior to the 5th and 7th costal cartilages
External oblique muscle of the abdomen	Anterior and lateral to the superficial layer of the abdomen, and a broad muscle	Lateral to the inferior position of eight ribs	Posterior fibers: the anterior fibers of the iliac crest changing into aponeurosis
Internal oblique muscle of the abdomen	In the deep layer of the external oblique muscle of the abdomen, and fan-shaped	1/3 lateral to the thoracolumbar fasciailiac crest and inguinal ligament	Posterior part of the muscle bundle: lower border of three inferior ribs. Most of the muscle bundle: white line

Table 6 Spinal extensor

Name	Location and form	Starting point	Ending point
Erector spinal muscle	Longitudinally located in the spinal groove and the largest and longest of muscles on the back	At the back of the sacrum, posterior to the iliac crest, spinous process of the lumbar vertebral process, and the thoracic vertebral fascia	Neck, transverse process of the thoracic vertebrae,temporal mastoid, and costal angle
Trapezius muscle	In the superficial layer of the neck and back, appears like a deltoid broad muscle and combines both sides into trapezius muscle	Superior nuchal line, external occipital protuberance, 7th cervical vertebra and all spinous processes of the thoracic vertebrae	1/3 lateral to the clavicle, acromion and scapular spine

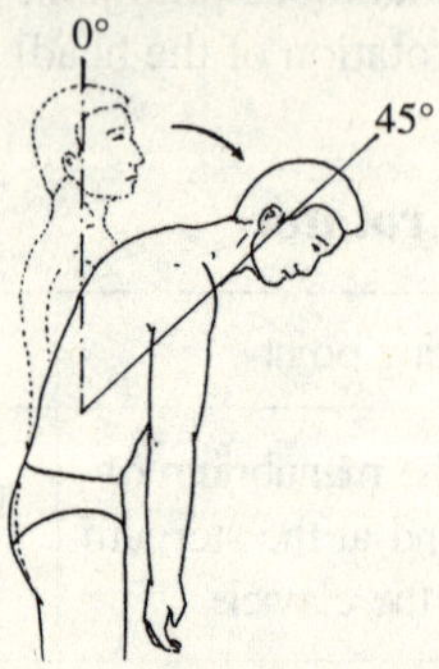

Fig. 1-5 Flexion of the spinal column (anterior flexion of the waist)

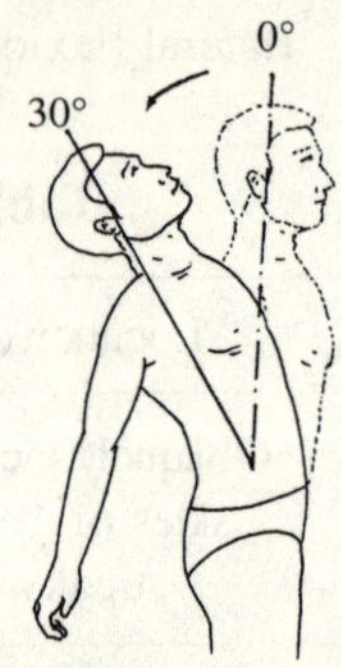

Fig. 1-6 Extension of the spinal column (posterior flexion of the waist)

Table 7 Lateral flexor of the spinal column

Name	Location and form	Starting point	Ending point
Quadrate muscle of the loins (same side)	Lateral to the posterior wall of the abdomen and both sides of the spinal column, and is a rectanglular flat muscle	Posterior to the iliac crest	12th rib and the 1st-4th transverse processes of the lumbar vertebrae
Erector spinal muscle (same side)	Longitudinally located in the spinal groove, and is the largest and longest of muscles on the back	At the back of the sacrum, posterior to the iliac crest, spinous process of the lumbar vertebral process and thoracic vertebral fascia	Neck, transverse process of the thoracic vertebrae, temporal mastoid, and costal angle
Rectal abdominal muscle (same side)	At both sides of the anterior midline along the abdomen, in the sheath of rectus abdominis, broad in the upper part and narrow in the lower part	Pubic symphysis and pubic crest	Xiphoid process and anterior to the 5th and 7th costal cartilages
External oblique muscle of the abdomen (same side)	Anterior and lateral to the superficial layer of the abdomen, and is a broad muscle	Lateral to the inferior position of eight ribs	Posterior fibers: the anterior fibers of the iliac crest changing into aponeurosis

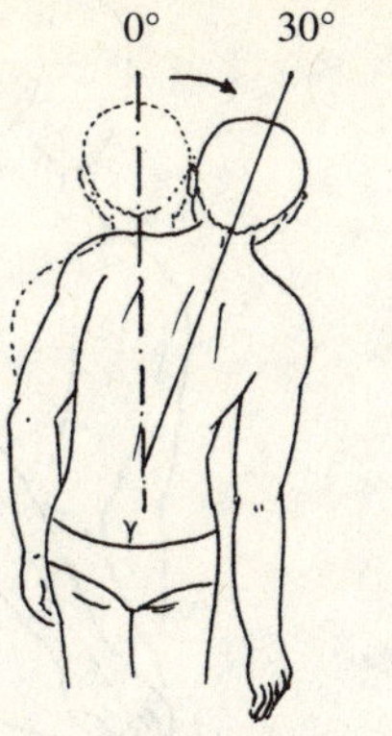

Fig. 1-7 Lateral flexion of the spine (lateral flexion of the waist)

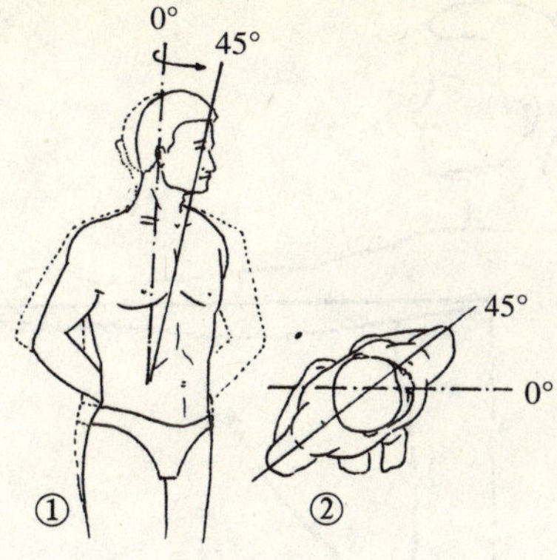

Fig. 1-8 Rotation of the spine(rotation of the waist)

Table 8 Rotator of the spinal column

Name	Location and form	Starting point	Ending point
External oblique muscle of the abdomen (opposite side)	Anterior and lateral to the superficial layer of the abdomen, and is a broad muscle	Lateral to the inferior position of eight ribs	Posterior fibers: the anterior fibers of the iliac crest changing into aponeurosis
Internal oblique muscle of the abdomen	In the deep layer of the external oblique muscle of the abdomen and fan-shaped	1/3 lateral to the thoracolumbar fascia, iliac crest and inguinal ligament	Posterior part of the muscle bundle: lower border of three inferior ribs.Most of the muscle bundle: white line

Table 9 Flexor of the shoulder joint

Name	Location and form	Starting point	Ending point
deltoid muscle (anterior part of the muscle bundle)	In the shoulder, and triangular in form	Anterior part of the muscle bundle: acromion	Tuberosity of the humeral deltoid muscle
Biceps muscle of the arm	At the anterior part of the upper arm, and fusiform in shape	Long head: supraglenoid tubercle of the scapula. Short head: coracoid process of the scapula	Radial tuberosity
Coracobrachial muscle	Thin and long, located deep in the biceps muscl of the arm	Coracoid process of the scapula	Medial side of the middle part of the humerus
Greater pectoral muscle	Broad, thick and flat, covering most part of the anterior wall of the thorax, and flat-shaped	Half of the medial side of the clavicle, sternum and 1st-6th costal cartilages	Greater tubercle crest of the humerus

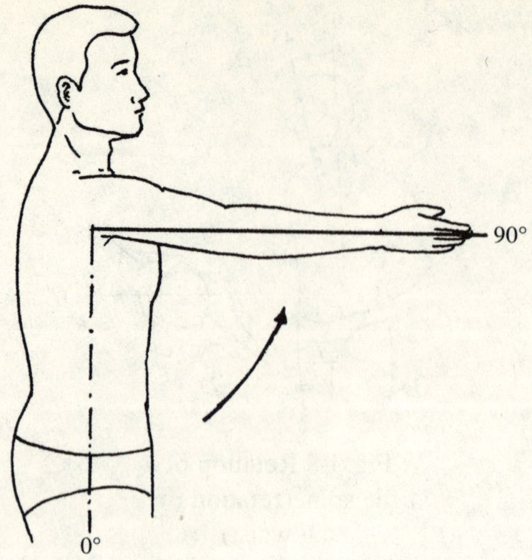

Fig. l-9 Flexion of the shoulder joint

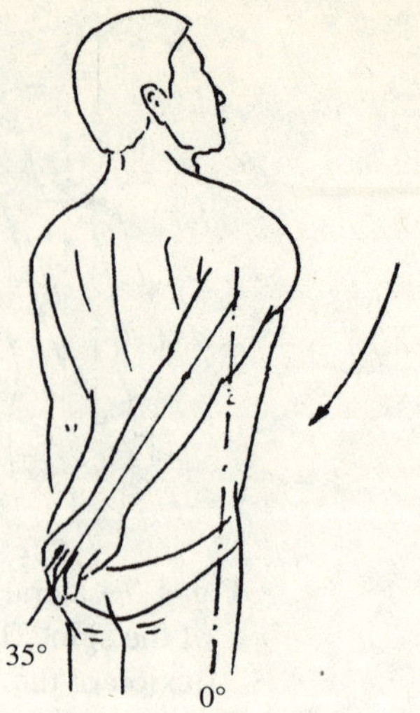

Fig. l-10 Extension of the shoulder joint

Table 10 Extensor of the shoulder joint

Name	Location and form	Starting point	Ending point
Deltoid muscle (posterior part of the muscle bundle)	Located in the shoulder and triangular in form	Posterior part of the muscle bundle: scapular spine	Tuberosity of the humeral deltoid muscle
Teres major muscle	Inferior to the lower fossa of the scapular spine	Dorsal part of the inferior angle of the scapular spine	crest of the small humeral tubercle
Broad muscle of the back	At the lower part of the back and inferior and lateral to the thorax, appears like a broad triangular muscle, and is the largest muscle in the human body	6 inferior spinous processes of the thoracic vertebrae, all the spinous processes of the lumbar vertebrae, median sacral crest, posterior part of the iliac crest	Near the small tubercle of the humerus

Table 11 Abductor of the shoulder joint

Name	Location and form	Starting point	Ending point
Deltoid muscle	In the shoulder and triangular in form	Lateral to the clavicle, acromion and scapular spine	Tuberosity of the humeral deltoid muscle
Supraspinous muscle	Inside the supraspinous fossa of the scapula, and oval in shape	Supraspinous fossa	Superior part of the greater tubercle of the humerus

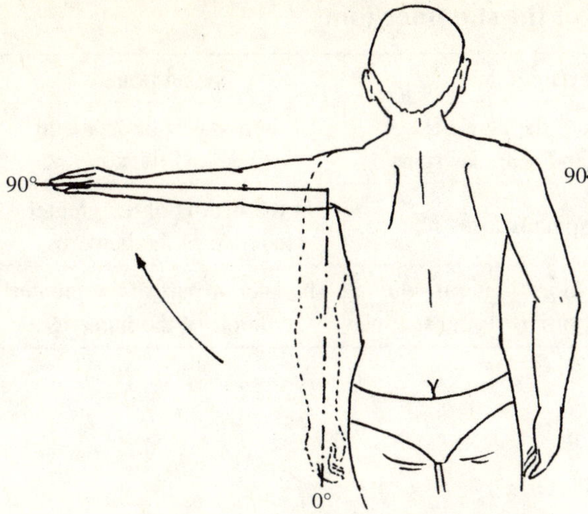

Fig. 1-11 Abduction of the shoulder joint

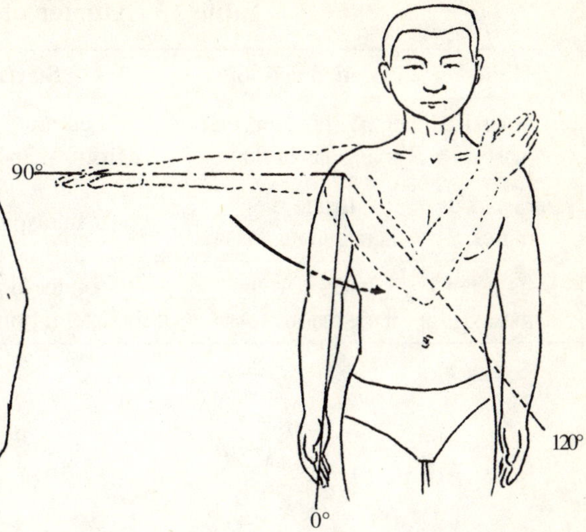

Fig. 1-12 Adduction of the shoulder joint

Table 12 Adductor of the shoulder joint

Name	Location and form	Starting point	Ending point
Teres major muscle	Inferior to the infraspinous fossa	Dorsal part of the inferior angle of the scapular spine	crest of the small humeral tubercle
Subscapular muscle	At the lateral wall of the thorax; a flat and wide multi-pennate muscle	subscapular fossa	Small humeral tubercle
Coracobrachial muscle	At the medial and anterior side of the upper arm	Coracoid process of the scapula	Small tubercle crest of the humerus
Brachial triceps (long head)	Posterior to the upper arm	Long head: infraglenoid tubercle of the scapula	Ulna olecranon
Greater pectoral muscle	Broad, thick and flat, covering most part of the anterior wall of the thorax, shaped like a fan	Half of the medial side of the clavicle, sternum and 1st-6th costal cartilages	greater tubercle crest of the humerus
Broad muscle of the back	At the lower part of the back and inferior and lateral to the thorax; shaped like a broad triangular muscle; the largest muscle in the human body	6 inferior spinous processes of the thoracic vertebrae, all the spinous processes of the lumbar vertebrae, median sacral crest, posterior part of the iliac crest	Near the small tubercle of the humerus

Table 13 Extorter of the shoulder joint

Name	Location and form	Starting point	Ending point
Deltoid muscle	In the shoulder, and triangular in shape	Lateral to the clavicle, acromion and scapular spine	Tuberosity of the humeral deltoid muscle
Infraspinous muscle	Inside the infraspinous fossa	Infraspinous fossa	In the middle of the greater tubercle of the humerus
teres minor muscle	Inferior to the infraspinous fossa	2/3 on the dorsal-lateral side of the lateral border of the scapula	The inferior part of the greater tubercle of the humerus

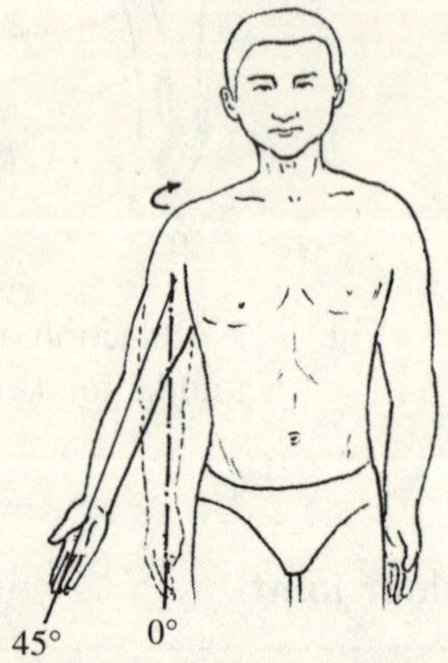

Fig. 1-13 Extorsion of the shoulder joint

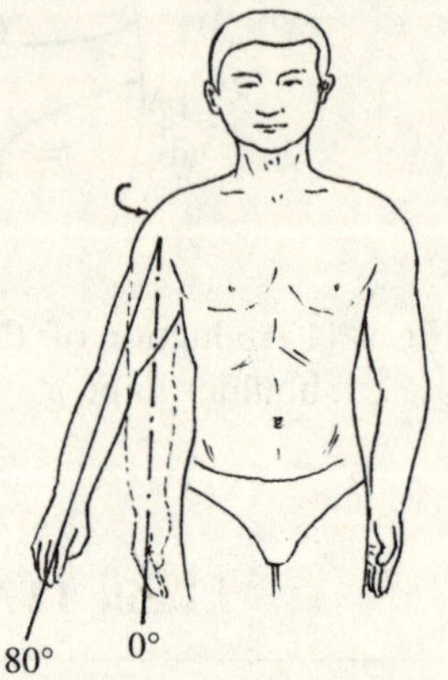

Fig. 1-14 Intorsion of the shoulder joint

Table 14 Intorter of the shoulder joint

Name	Location and form	Starting point	Ending point
Deltoid muscle (anterior muscle bundle)	In the shoulder, and triangular in shape	Anterior part of the muscle bundle: acromion	Tuberosity of the humeral deltoid muscle
Teres major muscle	Inferior to the lower fossa of the scapular spine	Dorsal part of the inferior angle of the scapular spine	Crest of the small humeral tubercle
Subscapular muscle	At the lateral wall of the thorax; a flat and wide multi-pennate muscle	Subscapular fossa	Small humeral tubercle
Greater pectoral muscle	Broad, thick and flat, covering most part of the anterior wall of the thorax, and shaped like a fan	Half of the medial side of the clavicle, sternum and 1st-6th costal cartilages	Greater tuber clecrest of the humerus
Broad muscle of the back	At the lower part of the back and posterior and lateral to the thorax.; shaped like a broad triangular muscle; the largest muscle in the human body	6 inferior spinous processes of the thoracic vertebrae, all the spinous processes of the lumbar vertebrae, median sacral crest, posterior part of the iliac crest	Near the small tubercle of the humerus

Table 15 Flexor of the elbow joint

Name	Location and form	Starting point	Ending point
Biceps muscle of the arm	At the anterior part of the upper arm, and fusiform in shape	Long head: supraglenoid tubercle of the scapula. Short head: coracoid process of the scapula	Radial tuberosity
Brachial muscle	Inferior to the anterior part of the upper arm	Anterior to the lower part of the humerus	Ulna tuberosity
Brachioradial muscle	Located lateral and anterior to the forearm	Superior to the lateral epicondyle of the humerus	Radial styloid process
Round pronator muscle	Anterior to the upper and middle sections of the forearm	Humeral epicondyle and deep fascia of the forearm	Middle part lateral to the humerus
Radial flexor muscle of the wrist	Located anterior to the forearm		Base of the second metacarpal bone

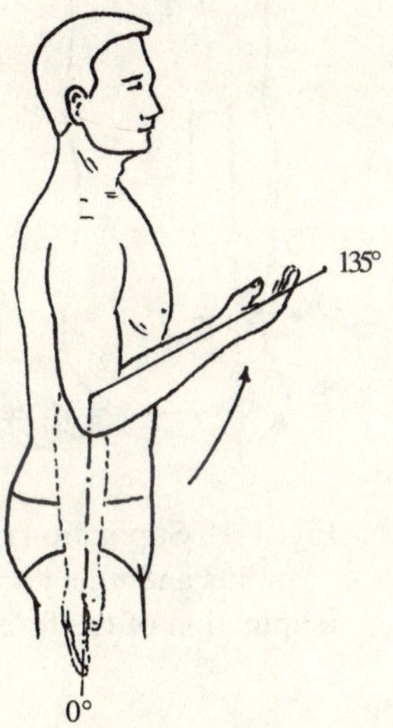

Fig. 1-15 Flexion of the elbow joint

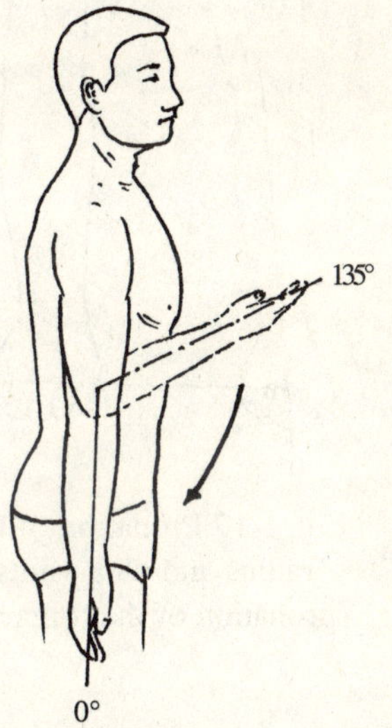

Fig. 1-16 Extension of the elbow joint

Table 16 Extensor of the elbow joint

Name	Location and form	Starting point	Ending point
Brachial triceps	Posterior to the upper arm	Long head: infraglenoid tubercle of the scapula.Lateral head: at the osseous surface lateral and superior to the sulcus of the radial nerve posterior to the humerus.Medial head: at the osseous surface inferior to the sulcus of the radial nerve	Ulna olecranon

Table 17 Pronators of the radial and ulna joints

Name	Location and form	Starting point	Ending point
Round pronator muscle	Anterior to the upper and middle sections of the forearm	Medial epicondyle of the humerus and deep fascia of the forearm	Middle part lateral to the humerus
Quadrate pronator muscle	In the deep layer of the distal end anterior to the forearm; flat and square in shape	Anterior to 1/4 part inferior to the ulna	Anterior to 1/4 part inferior to the radius

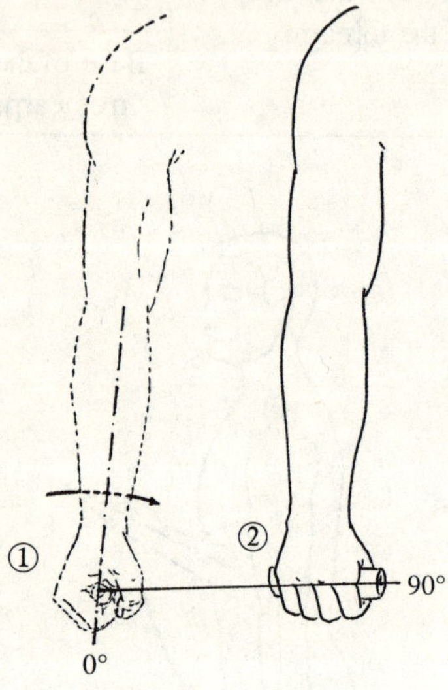

Fig. 1-17 Pronation of the radius and ulna joints (pronation of the forearm)

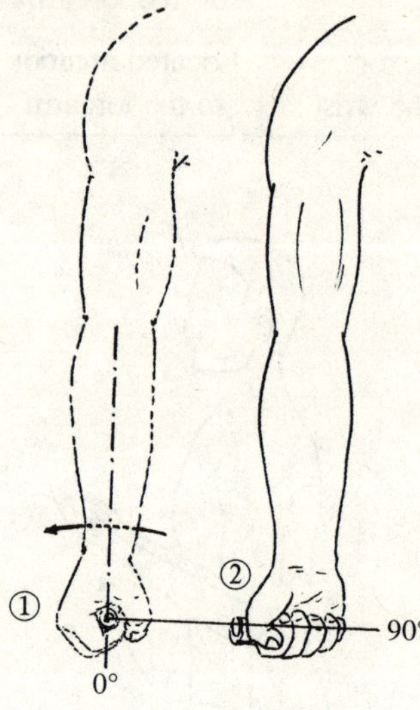

Fig. 1-18 Supination of the radius and ulna joints (supination of the forearm)

Table 18 Supinators of the radius and ulna joints

Name	Location and form	Starting point	Ending point
Biceps muscle of the arm	At the anterior part of the upper arm and fusiform in shape	Long head: upraglenoid tubercle of the scapula. Short head: coracoid process of the scapula	radial tuberosity
supinator	Near the posterior part of the forearm	At the external epicondyle of the humerus and the upper part of the lateral border of the ulna	The upper part of the anterior surface of the radius

Table 19 Flexor of the radiocarpal joint

Name	Location and form	Starting point	Ending point
Radial flexor muscle of the wrist	At the medial side of the forearm	Medial epicondyle of the humerus and deep fascia of the forearm	Base of the 2nd metacarpal bone
ulnar flexor muscle of the wrist	At the medial side anterior to the forearm	Medial epicondyle of the humerus and deep fascia of the forearm	pisiform bone
Long palmar muscle	Between the radial flexor muscle and ulnar flexor muscle of the wrist; the belly is small and the tendon slender and long	Medial epicondyle of the humerus and deep fascia of the forearm	Palmar aponeurosis
Superficial flexor muscle of the fingers	In the deep layer of the long palmar muscle	Medial epicondyle of the humerus and anterior to the ulna and radius	Lateral to both sides of the body of the middle sections of 2nd-5th fingers
Long flexor muscle of the thumb	At the radial side in the deep layer anterior to the forearm	Anterior to the upper part of the radius and ulna and the interosseous membrane	Base of the distal section of the thumb
Deep flexor muscle of the fingers	In the deep layer of the superficial flexor muscle of the fingers	Anterior to the upper part of the radius and ulna and the interosseous membrane	Base of the distal sections of 2nd-5th fingers

Table 20 Extensor of the radiocarpal joint

Name	Location and form	Starting point	Ending point
Long radial extensor muscle of the wrist	In the superficial layer posterior to the forearm, arrayed from the radius to the ulna	Lateral epicondyle of the humerus	Base of the 2nd metacarpal bone
Short radial extensor muscle of the wrist	In the superficial layer posterior to the forearm, arrayed from the radius to the ulna	Lateral epicondyle of the humerus	Base of the 2nd metacarpal bone
Extensor muscle of the fingers	In the superficial layer posterior to the forearm, arrayed from the radius to the ulna	Lateral epicondyle of the humerus	The middle sections and the base of the distal sections of 2nd-5th fingers
extensor muscle of the little finger	In the superficial layer posterior to the forearm, arrayed from the radius to the ulna	Lateral epicondyle of the humerus	Aponeurosis on the back of the little finger
Ulnar and carpal extensor muscle	In the superficial layer posterior to the forearm, arrayed from the radius to the ulna	Lateral epicondyle of the humerus	Base of the 5th metacarpal bone
Short extensor muscle of the thumb	In the deep layer posterior to the forearm, arrayed from the radius to the ulna	posterior to the humerus and ulna, and the interosseous membrane	base of the proximal section of the thumb
Long extensor of the thumb	In the deep layer posterior to the forearm, arrayed from the radius to the ulna	posterior to the humerus and ulna, and the interosseous membrane	Base of the distal section of the thumb
Extensor muscle of the index finger	In the deep layer posterior to the forearm, arrayed from the radius to the ulna	posterior to the humerus and ulna, and the interosseous membrane	Dorsal aponeurosis of the index finger

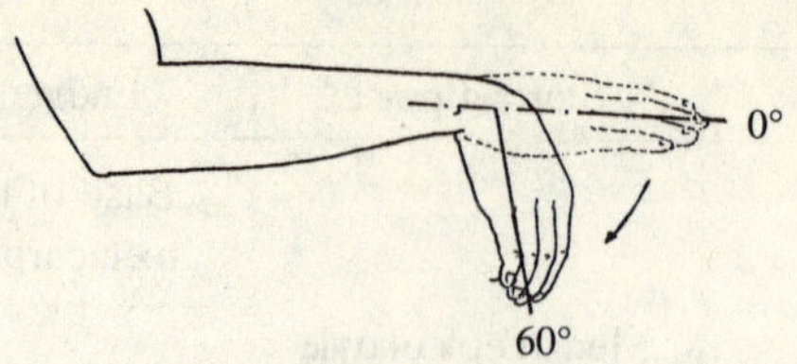

Fig. 1-19 Flexion of the radiocarpal joint (wrist flexion)

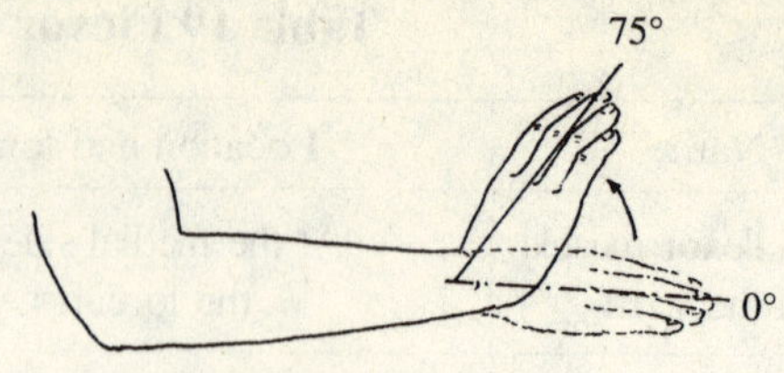

Fig. 1-20 Extension of the radiocarpal joint (wrist extension)

Table 21 Abductor of the radiocarpal joint

Name	Location and form	Starting point	Ending point
Radial flexor muscle of the wrist	Anterior to the medial side of the forearm	Medial epicondyle of the humerus and the deep fascia of the forearm	Middle section lateral to the radius
Long radial extensor muscle of the wrist	On the lateral side of the superficial layer posterior to the forearm	Lateral epicondyle of the humerus	Base of the 2nd metacarpal bone
short radial extensor muscle of the wrist			Base of the 3rd metacarpal bone

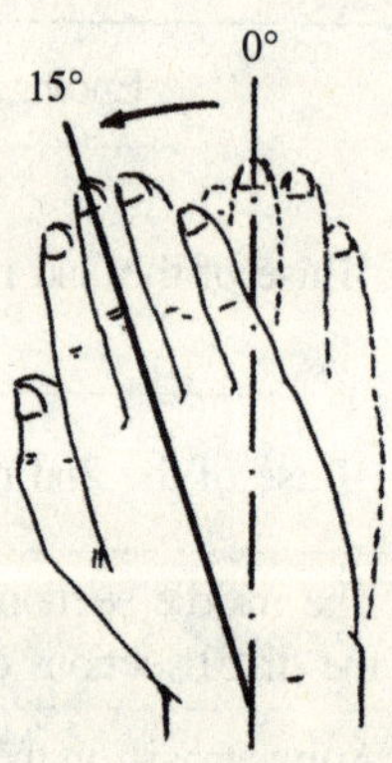

Fig. 1-21 Abduction of the radiocarpal joint

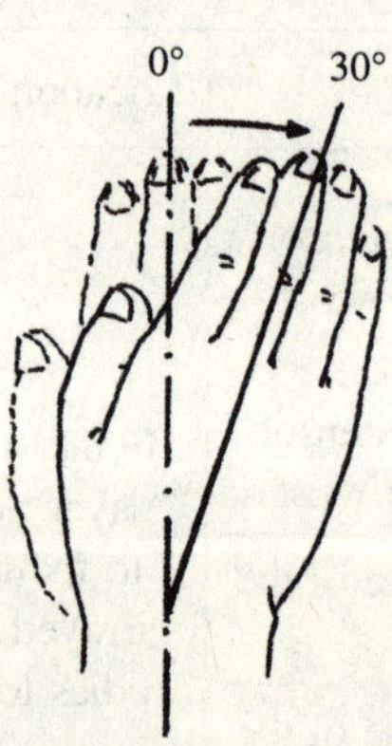

Fig. 1-22 Adduction of the radiocarpal joint

Table 22 Adductor of the radiocarpal joint

Name	Location and form	Starting point	Ending point
Ulnar flexor muscle of the wrist	Located the most medial to the forearm	Medial epicondyle of the humerus and deep fascia of the forearm	Pisiform bone
Ulnar extensor muscle of the wrist	In the superficial layer at the ulnar side posterior to the forearm	Lateral epicondyle of the humerus	Base of the 5th metacarpal bone

Table 23 Flexor of the thumb joint

Name	Location and form	Starting point	Ending point
Long flexor of the thumb	In the deep layer at the radial side anterior to the forearm	Anterior to the radius and ulna and the interosseous membrane	Base of the distal section of the thumb
Short flexor of the thumb	In the superficial layer at the medial side of the thenar prominence	Flexor retinaculum and trapezium bone	Base of the proximal section of the thumb

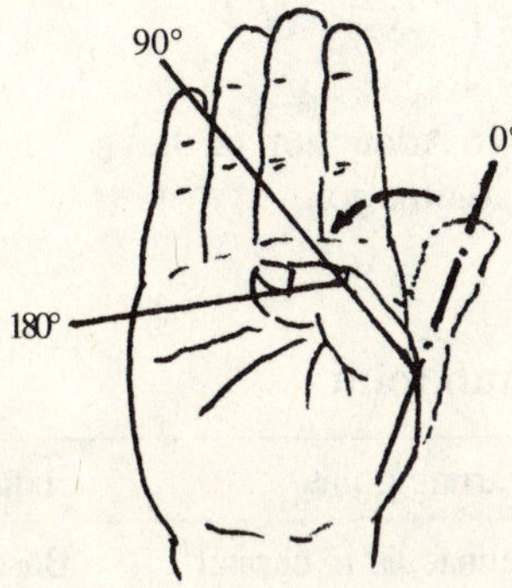

Fig. 1-23 Flexion of the thumb joint

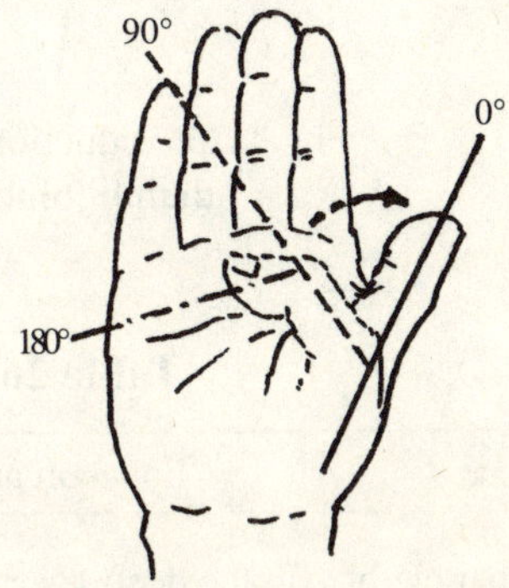

Fig. 1-24 Extension of the thumb joint

Table 24 Extensor of the thumb joint

Name	Location and form	Starting point	Ending point
Short extensor muscle of the thumb	In the deep layer near the lateral part posterior to the forearm	Posterior to the radius and ulna and the interosseous membrane	Base of the proximal section of the thumb
Long extensor muscle of the thumb			Base of the distal section of the thumb

Table 25 Abductor of the thumb joint

Name	Location and form	Starting point	Ending point
Long abductor muscle of the thumb	In the deep layer at the radial side posterior to the forearm	Posterior to the radius and ulna and the interosseous membrane	Base of the 1st metacarpal bone
Short abductor muscle of the thumb	In the superficial layer lateral to the thenar prominence	Flexor retinaculum and scaphoid bone	Base of the proximal section of the thumb

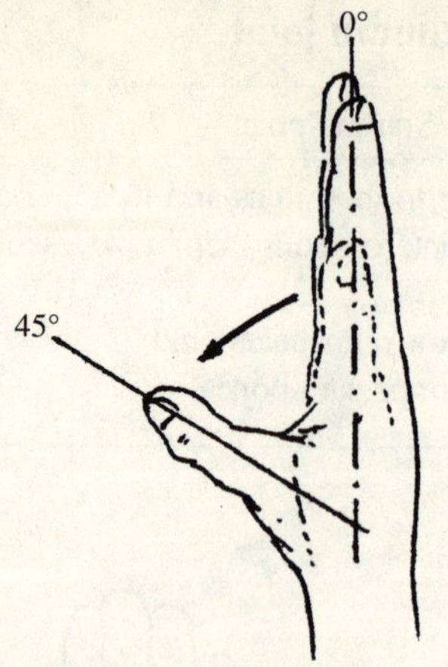

Fig. 1-25 Abduction of the thumb joint

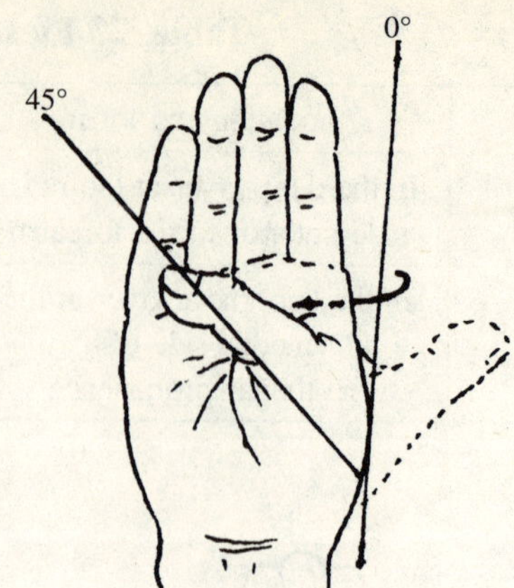

Fig. 1-26 Adduction of the thumb joint

Table 26 Adductor of the thumb joint

Name	Location and form	Starting point	Ending point
Adductor muscle of the thumb	In the deep layer at the medial side of the thenar prominence	Flexor retinaculum, capital bone, the 2nd and 3rd metacarpal bones	Base of the proximal section of the thumb

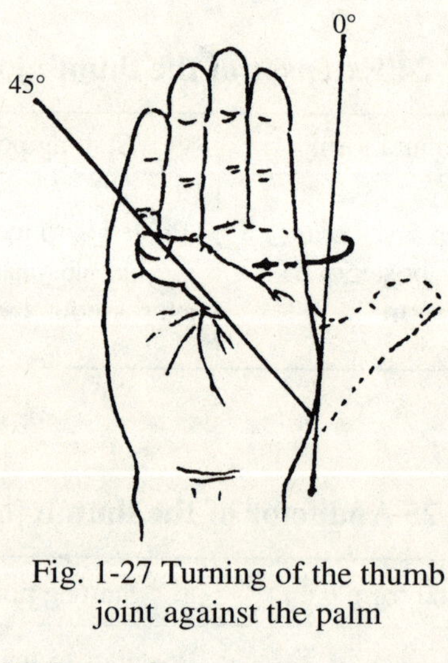

Fig. 1-27 Turning of the thumb joint against the palm

Table 27 Opposing muscle of the thumb joint

Name	Location and form	Starting point	Ending point
Opposing muscle of the thumb	In the deep layer of the thenar prominence near the medial side	Flexor retinaculum and trapezium bone	Lateral part of the palmar side of the 1st metacarpal bone

Table 28 Flexors of the joints of the 2nd-5th fingers

Name	Location and form	Starting point	Ending point
Superficial flexor muscle of the finger	Anterior and medial to the forearm and in the deep layer of the long palmar muscle	Medial epicondyle of the humerus, anterior to the ulna and radius	Lateral to both sides of the middle section of the 2nd-5th fingers
Deep flexor muscle of the finger	In the deep layer of the superficial flexor muscle of the finger	The upper part of the ulna and radius and the interosseous membrane	Base of the distal section of the 2nd-5th fingers
Lumbricus muscles	On the center of the palm in thin streaky form	Radial side of the deep flexor muscle of each finger	Dorsal aponeurosis of the 2nd-5th fingers
Volar interosseous muscles	In the intermetacarpal spaces	Medial surface of the 2nd metacarpal bone, lateral surface of the 4th and 5th metacarpal bone	Base of the proximal section and dorsal aponeurosis of the 2nd, 4th and 5th fingers
Dorsal interosseous muscles		All intermetacarpal spaces, their both heads starting from the opposite side of the metacarpal bone	Base of the proximal section and dorsal aponeurosis of the 2nd-5th fingers

Table 29 Abductors of the joints of the 2nd-5th fingers

Name	Location and form	Starting point	Ending point
Extensor muscle of the finger	In the superficial layer of the forearm near the ulnar side	Base of the middle and distal sections of the 2nd-5th fingers	Base of the middle and distal sections of the 2nd-5th fingers
Extensor muscle of the small finger			Dorsal aponeurosis of the small finger
extensor muscle of the index finger	In the deep layer of the forearm near the ulnar side	Posterior to the ulna and radius and the interosseous membrane	Dorsal aponeurosis of the index finger
Lumbricus muscles	On the center of the palm in thin streak form	Radial side of the deep flexor muscle of each finger	Dorsal aponeurosis of the 2nd-5th fingers
Volar interosseous muscle	In the intermetacarpal spaces	Medial surface of the 2nd metacarpal bone, lateral surface of the 4th and 5th metacarpal bone	Base of the proximal section and dorsal aponeurosis of the 2nd, 4th and 5th fingers
Dorsal interosseous muscles	In the intermetacarpal spaces	All intermetacarpal spaces, their both heads starting from the opposite side of the metacarpal bone	Base of the proximal section and dorsal aponeurosis of the 2nd-5th fingers

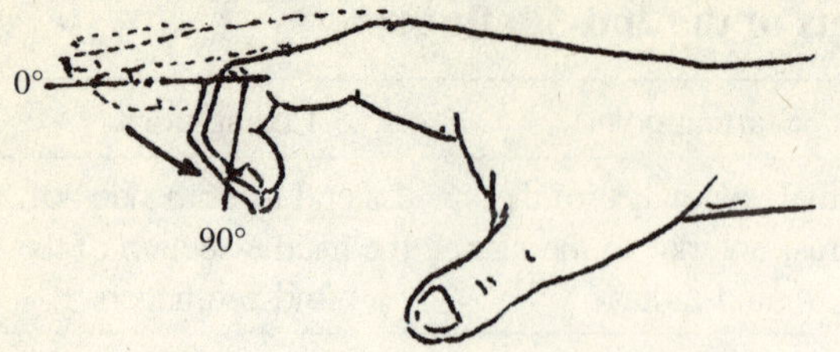

Fig. 1-28 Flexion of the joints of the 2nd-5th fingers

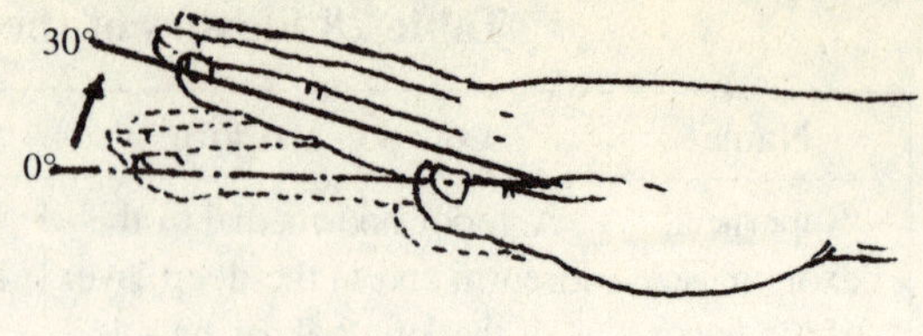

Fig. 1-29 Extension of the joints of the 2nd-5th fingers

Table 30 Abductors of the joints of the 2nd-5th finger

Name	Location and form	Starting point	Ending point
Abductor muscle of the small finger	In the superficial layer medial to the hypothenar prominence	Pisiform bone and flexor retinacula	Base of the proximal section of the little finger
Dorsal interosseous muscles	In the intermeta-carpal spaces	All intermetacarpal spaces, their both heads starting from the opposite side of the metacarpal bone	Base of the proximal section and dorsal aponeurosis of the 2nd-5th fingers

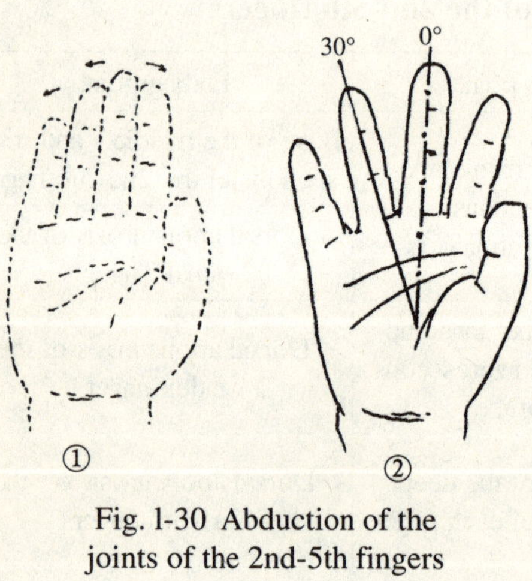

Fig. 1-30 Abduction of the joints of the 2nd-5th fingers

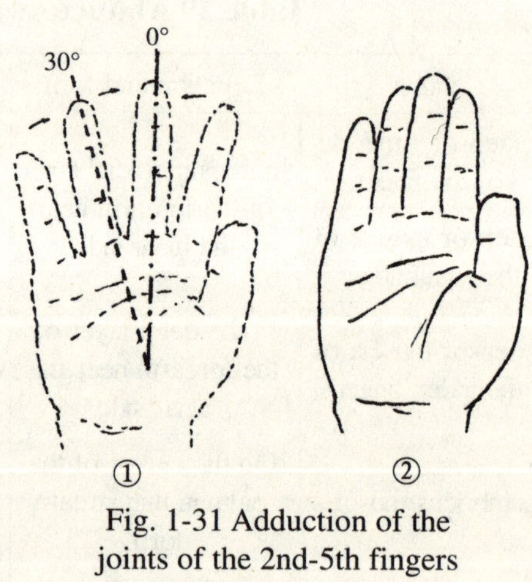

Fig. 1-31 Adduction of the joints of the 2nd-5th fingers

Table 31 Adductors of the joints of the 2nd-5th fingers

Name	Location and form	Starting point	Ending point
Volar interos-seous muscle	In the intermet-acarpal spaces	Medial surface of the 2nd metacarpal bone, lateral surface of the 4th and 5th metacarpal bone	Base of the proximal section and dorsal aponeurosis of the 2nd, 4th and 5th fingers

Table 32 Flexor muscles of the hip joint

Name	Location and form	Starting point	Ending point
Musculus rectus femoris	Located right anterior to the thigh	Anterior inferior iliac spine	Tuberosity of the tibia
Sartorius muscle	Located obliquely at the medial side of the thigh, teniform in shape and the longest muscle in the body	Anterior superior iliac spine	Medial surface of the upper part of the tibia
Greater psoas muscle	Anterior and medial to the pelvis	Lateral side and transverse process of the lumbar vertebral body	Lesser trochanter of the femur
Iliac muscle	Anterior and lateral to the pelvis, flat in form	Iliac fossa	
Tensor muscle of the fascia lata	Anterior and lateral to the upper part of the thigh	Anterior superior iliac spine	Lateral condyle of the tibia

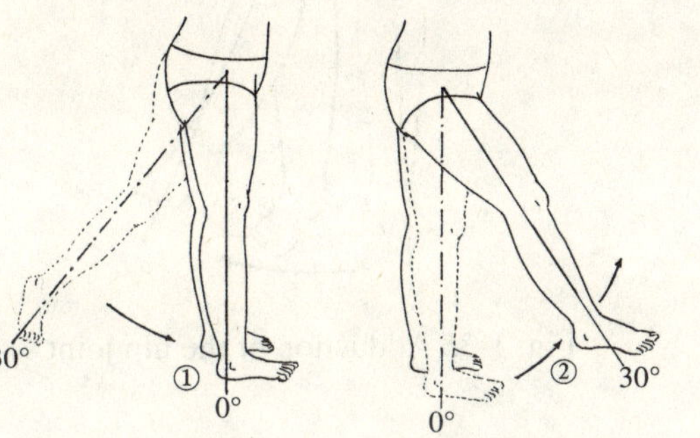

Fig. 1-32 Flexion of the hip joint

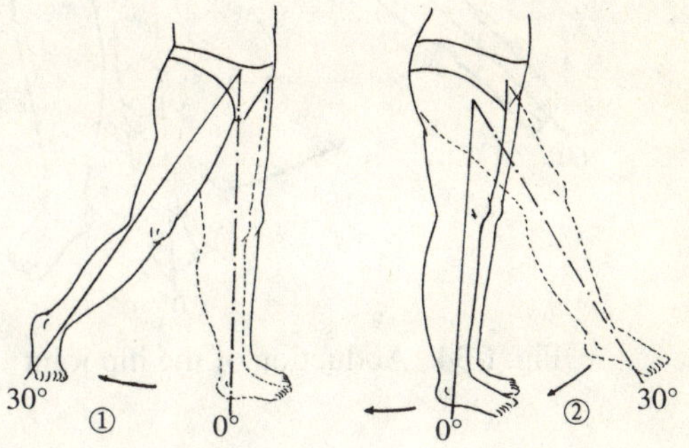

Fig. 1-33 Extension of the hip joint

Table 33 Extensor of the hip joint

Name	Location and form	Starting point	Ending point
Biceps muscle of the thigh	Lateral to the thigh	Long head: ischial tuberosity. Short head: flinea aspera femoris	Fibula head
Semitendinos-us muscle	At the medial side of the thigh; half of it long and thin tendon	Ischial tuberosity	Medial side of the upper part of the tibia
Semimembra-nosus muscle	In the deep and medial layer posterior to the thigh; half of it flat thin aponeurosis		Posterior to the medial condyle of the tibia
Greater gluteal muscle	Beneath the skin over the buttocks, and large and thick	On the external surface of the wing of the ileum and the dorsal side of the sacrum	Iliotibial tract and gluteal muscle tuberosity on the femur

Table 34 Abductor of the hip joint

Name	Location and form	Starting point	Ending point
Middle gluteal muscle	In the deep layer of the large gluteal muscle and shaped like a fan	On the lateral side of the iliac wing	Greater trochanter of the femur
Lesser gluteal muscle	In the deep layer of the middle gluteal muscle and shaped like a fan		

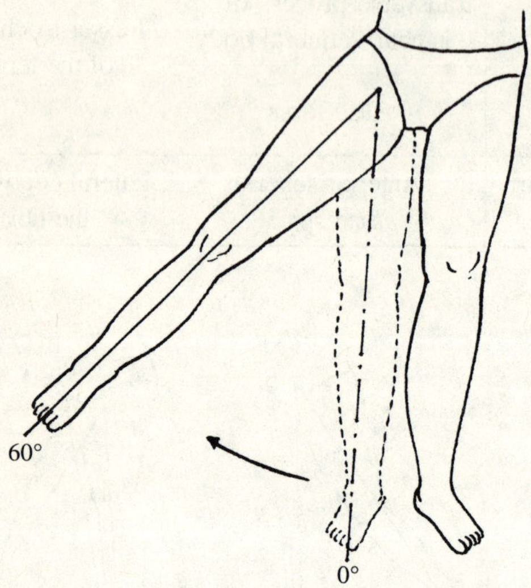

Fig. 1-34 Abduction of the hip joint

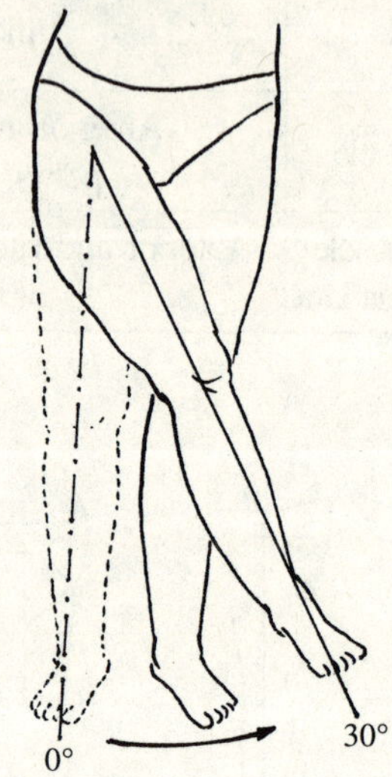

Fig. 1-35 Adduction of the hip joint

Table 35 Adductor muscle of the hip joint

Name	Location and form	Starting point	Ending point
Pubic muscle	In the superficial layer of the thigh, arranged from the lateral to the medial side	Osseous facet of the pubic branch, ischial ramus and ischial tuberosity	Linea aspera femoris
Long adductor muscle			
Gracilis muscle			Medial to the upper part of the femur
Short adductor muscle			Linea aspera femoris
Great adductor muscle	In the deep layer at the medial side of the thigh and triangular in shape		Linea aspera femoris and tuberosity of the femoral adductor muscle

Table 36 Lateral rotator of the hip joint

Name	Location and form	Starting point	Ending point
Middle gluteal muscle (posterior part of the muscle bundle)	Below the buttocks, in the deep layer of the great gluteal muscle, and fan-shaped	External facet of the iliac wing	Greater trochanter of the femur
Small gluteal muscle (posterior part of the muscle bundle)	Below the buttocks, in the deep layer of the middle gluteal muscle, and fan-shaped		
Piriformis muscle	Below the buttocks, inferior to the small gluteal muscle, and pear-shaped	In the pelvis, anterior to the sacrum and lateral to the anterior sacral foramina	
Internal obturator muscle	Below the buttocks, inferior to the piriformis muscle	On the medial side of the obturator membrane and the osseous facets around it	Trochanteric fossa
Quadrate muscle of the thigh	Below the buttocks and the internal obturator muscle	Ischial tuberosity	Intertrochanteric crest
External obturator muscle	Below the buttocks and deep in the internal obturator muscle	On the lateral side of the obturator membrane and the osseous facets around it	Trochanteric fossa
Greater psoas muscle	Anterior and medial to the pelvis	On the lateral side and the transverse process of the lumbar vertebral body	Lesser trochanter of the femur
Iliac muscle	Anterior and lateral to the pelvis, and fan-shaped	Iliac fossa	

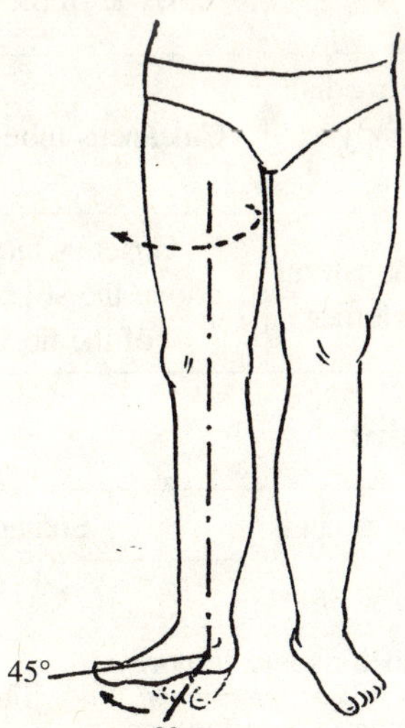

Fig. 1-36 Lateral rotation of the hip joint

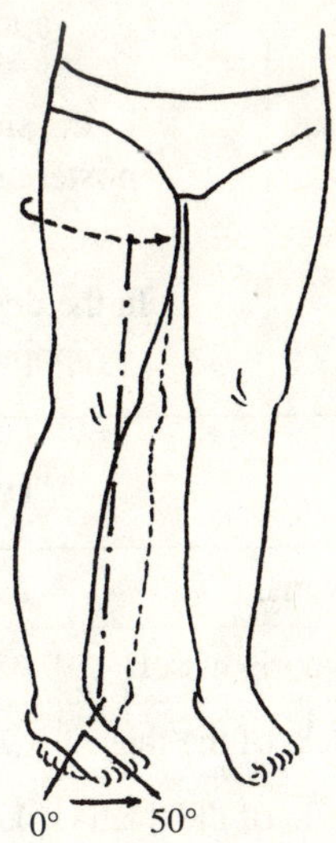

Fig. 1-37 Medial rotation of the hip joint

Table 37 Medial rotator of the hip joint

<table>
<tr><th>Name</th><th>Location and form</th><th>Starting point</th><th>Ending point</th></tr>
<tr><td>Middle gluteal muscle (posterior part of the muscle bundle)</td><td>Below the buttocks, in the deep layer of the great gluteal muscle, and fan-shaped</td><td rowspan="2">External facet of the iliac wing</td><td rowspan="2">Greater trochanter of the femur</td></tr>
<tr><td>Small gluteal muscle(posterior part of the muscle bundle)</td><td>Below the buttocks, in the deep layer of the middle gluteal muscle, and fan-shaped</td></tr>
</table>

Table 38 Flexor muscle of the knee joint

<table>
<tr><th>Name</th><th>Location and form</th><th>Starting point</th><th>Ending point</th></tr>
<tr><td>Sartorius muscle</td><td>Located obliquely at the medial side of the thigh, teniform in shape; the longest muscle in the body</td><td>Anterior to the superior iliac spine</td><td>On the medial surface of the upper part of the tibia</td></tr>
<tr><td>Biceps muscle of the thigh</td><td>On the lateral side posterior to the thigh</td><td>Long head: ischial tuberosity. Short head: flinea aspera femoris</td><td>Fibula head</td></tr>
<tr><td>Gracilis muscle</td><td>In the superficial layer on the medial side of the thigh</td><td>Pubic branch, ramus of the ischiu,surface of the ischial tuberosity</td><td rowspan="2">Medial to the upper part of the tibia</td></tr>
<tr><td>Semitendinosus muscle</td><td>Located at the medial side of the thigh, half of it appearing like a thin tendon</td><td rowspan="2">Ischial tuberosity</td></tr>
<tr><td>Semimembran-osus muscle</td><td>In the deep layer posterior to the thigh, half of it in flat and thin aponeurosis</td><td>Posterior to the medial condyle of the tibia</td></tr>
<tr><td>Gastrocnemius muscle</td><td>In the superficial layer posterior to the shank</td><td>Posterior to the medial and lateral condyle of the femur</td><td>Calcaneus tuberosity</td></tr>
<tr><td>Popliteal muscle</td><td>In the deep layer of the popliteal fossa</td><td>Lateral part of the lateral condyle of the femur</td><td>Osseous facet above the soleal line of the tibia</td></tr>
</table>

Table 39 Extensors of the knee joint

<table>
<tr><th>Name</th><th>Location and form</th><th>Starting point</th><th>Ending point</th></tr>
<tr><td>Rectus femoris muscle</td><td>Anterior to the thigh</td><td>Inferior iliac spine</td><td rowspan="4">Tibial tuberosity</td></tr>
<tr><td>Medial muscle of the thigh</td><td>Medial to the thigh</td><td>Medial lip of the linea aspera femoris</td></tr>
<tr><td>Lateral muscle of the thigh</td><td>Lateral to the thigh</td><td>Lateral lip of the linea aspera femoris</td></tr>
<tr><td>Middle muscle of the thigh</td><td>Deep in the rectus femoris muscle</td><td>Anterior to the femur</td></tr>
</table>

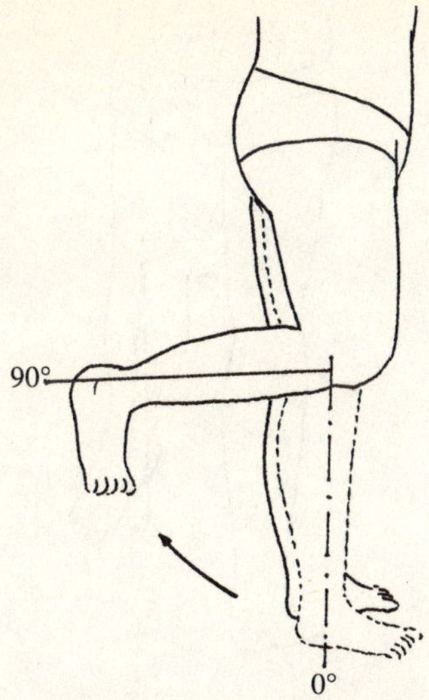

Fig. 1-38 Flexion of the knee joint

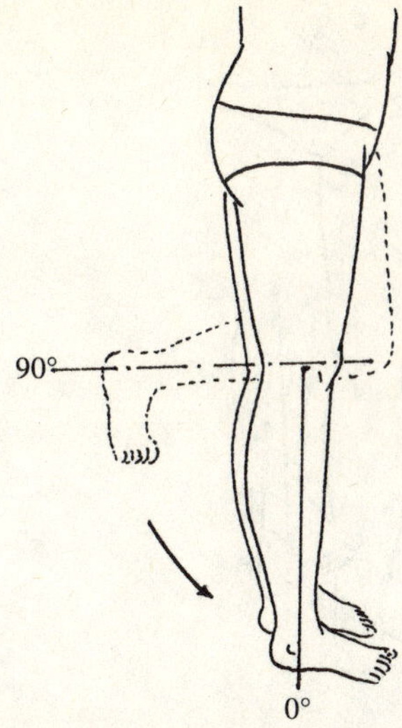

Fig. 1-39 Extension of the knee joint

Table 40 Lateral rotators of the knee joint

Name	Location and form	Starting point	Ending point
Biceps muscle of the thigh	Posterior to the lateral side of the thigh	Long head: ischial tuberosity. Short head: flinea aspera femoris	Fibula head

Table 41 Medial rotators of the knee joint

Name	Location and form	Starting point	Ending point
Sartorius muscle	Located obliquely at the medial side of the thigh, and teniform in shape; the longest muscle in the body	Anterior to the superior iliac spine	Medial surface of the upper part of the tibia
Biceps muscle of the thigh	In the superficial layer medial to the thigh	Pubic branch, ramus of the ischium, surface of the ischial tuberosity	
Semitendinosus muscle	Located at the medial side of the thigh, half of it appearing like a thin tendon	Ischial tuberosity	
Semimembranosus muscle	In the deep layer posterior to the thigh, half of it in flat and thin aponeurosis		Posterior to the medial condyle of the tibia
Popliteal muscle	In the deep layer of the popliteal fossa	Lateral part of the lateral condyle of the femur	Osseous facet above the soleal line of the tibia

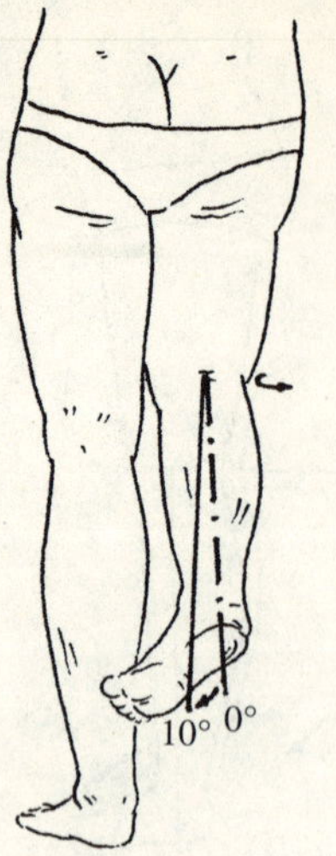

Fig. 1-40 Lateral rotation of the knee joint

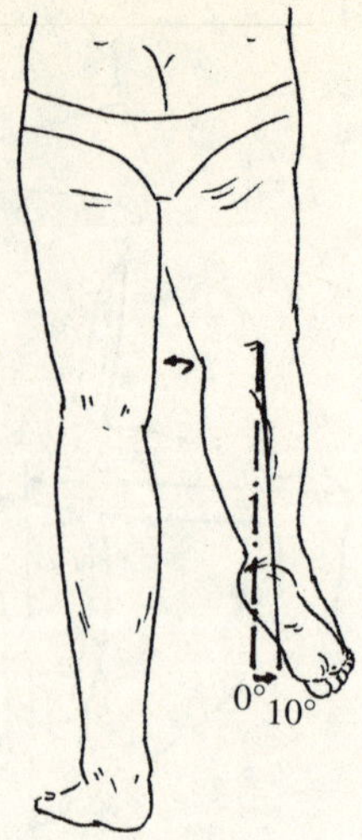

Fig. 1-41 Medial rotation of the knee joint

Table 42 Flexors of the ankle joint

Name	Location and form	Starting point	Ending point
Gastrocnemius muscle	In the superficial layer posterior to the shank	Posterior to the medial and lateral condyle of the femur	Calcaneus tuberosity
Soleus muscle	In the interior layer of the gastrocnemius muscle, and flatfish-shaped	Superior to the posterior part of the fibia and the soleal line of the tibia	
Long muscle of the fibia	In the superficial layer lateral to the fibula	Lateral surface of the fibula	Medial side of the cuneiform bone and base of the 1st metatarsal bone
Short muscle of the fibia	In the deep layer lateral to the fibula		Tuberosity of the 5th metatarsal bone
Long flexor muscle of the toe	In the deep layer posterior to the fibula in the shank	Posterior surface of the fibula	Base of the distal section of the 2nd-5th toes
Long flexor muscle of the big toe	In the deep layer posterior to the fibula in the shank	Posterior surface of the fibula	Base of the distal section of the big toe
Posterior muscle of the tibia	Between the long flexor muscle of the toe and the long flexor muscle of the big toe	Posterior to the tibia, fibia and periosteum of the shank	Tuberosity of the navicular bone and medial, intermediate and lateral to the cuneiform bone

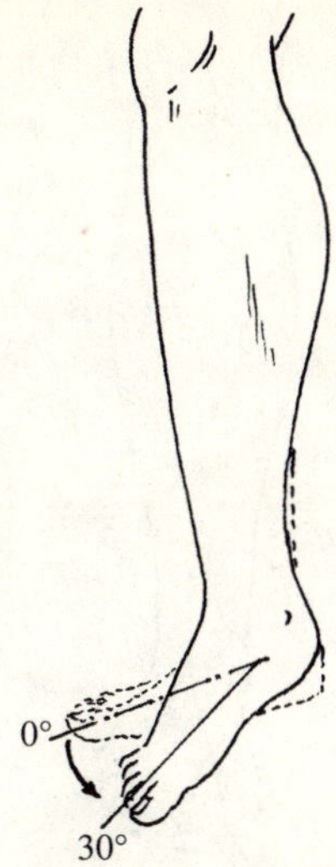

Fig. 1-42 Flexion of the ankle joint

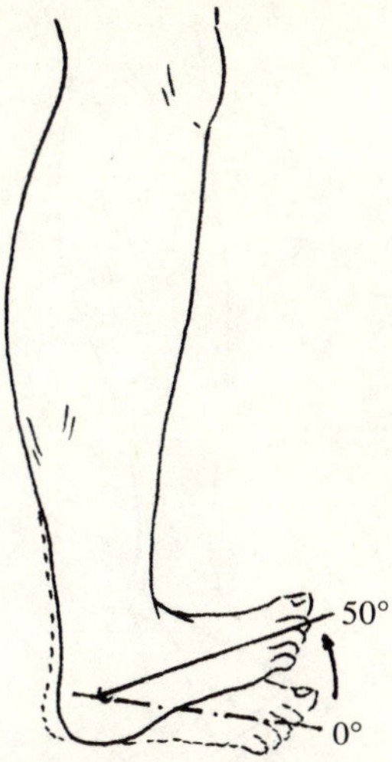

Fig. 1-43 Extension of the ankle joint

Table 43 Extensors of the ankle joint

Name	Location and form	Starting point	Ending point
Anterior muscle of the tibia	Anterior to the interosseous membrane of the shank, arranged from the medial to the lateral side	Lateral side of the tibia	Medial side of the cuneiform bone and the sole surface of the 1st metatarsal bone
Long extensor of the toe		Anterior to the fibula	Base of the middle and distal sections of the 2nd-5th toes
Long extensor of the big toe		Medial side of the fibula and the interosseous membrane	Digital base of the distal section of the big toe
The third fibial muscle		Frontal of the fibula	Base of the 5th metatarsal bone

Table 44 Eversion muscles of the ankle joint

Name	Location and form	Starting point	Ending point
Long muscle of the fibia	In the superficial layer lateral to the fibula	Lateral surface of the fibula	Medial side of the cuneiform bone and base of the 1st metatarsal bone
Short muscle of the fibia	In the deep layer lateral to the fibula		Tuberosity of the 5th metatarsal bone
The third muscle of the fibia	Most lateral to the interosseous membrane of the shank	Anterior to the fibia	Base of the 5th metatarsal bone

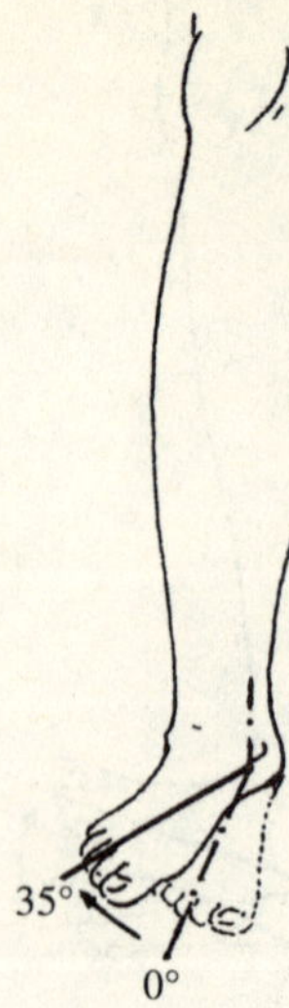

Fig. 1-44 Eversion of the ankle joint

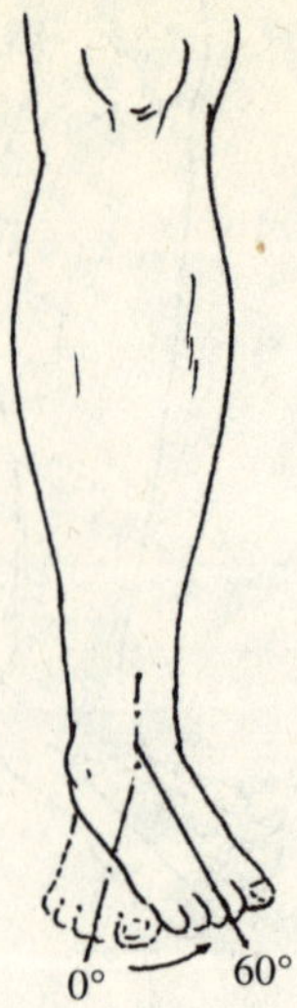

Fig. 1-45 Inversion of the ankle joint

Table 45 Inversion muscles of the ankle joint

Name	Location and form	Starting point	Ending point
Anterior muscle of the tibia	Anterior to the medial side of the interosseous membrane of the shank	Lateral to the tibia	Medial cuneiform bone and the base of the 1st metatarsal bone
Long flexor muscle of the toe	In the deep layer posterior to the shank	Posterior to the tibia	Base of the distal section of the 2nd-5th metatarsal bones
Long flexor muscle of the big toe	In the deep layer of the fibial side posterior to the shank	Posterior to the fibula	Base of the distal section of the big toe
Posterior muscle of the tibia	Between the long flexor muscle of the toe and the long flexor muscle of the big toe	Posterior to the tibia, fibia and the periosteum of the shank	Tuberosity of the navicular bone and medial, intermediate and lateral to the cuneiform bone

Table 46 Flexor muscle of the big toe

Name	Location and form	Starting point	Ending point
Long flexor muscle of the big toe	In the deep layer posterior to the shank	Posterior to the fibula	Base of the distal section of the big toe
Short flexor muscle of the big toe	Medial to the foot sole	Medial side of the cuneiform bone	Base of the proximal section of the big toe

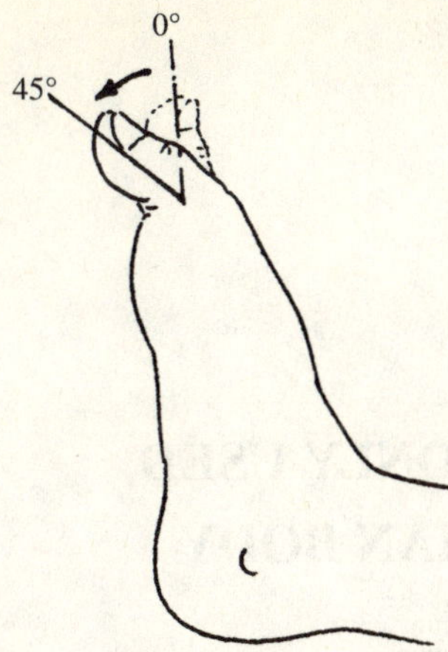

Fig. 1-46 Flexion of the big toe joints

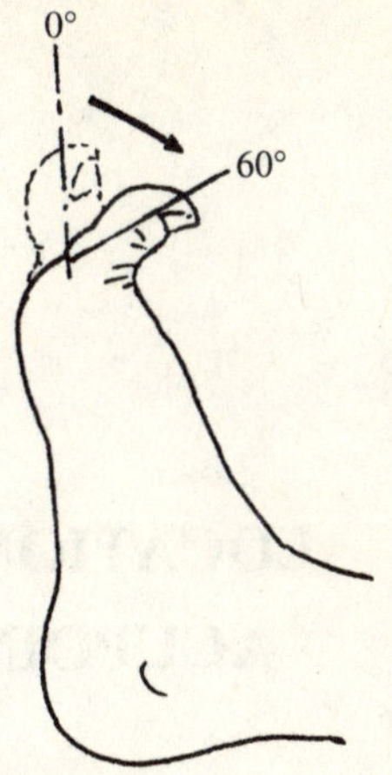

Fig. 1-47 Extension of the big toe joints

Table 47 Extensors of the big toe joints

Name	Location and form	Starting point	Ending point
Long extensor muscle of the big toe	Anterior and lateral to the interosseous membrane of the shank	Medial side of the fibia and interosseous membrane	Base of the distal section of the big toe
Short extensor muscle of the big toe	Mdial to the dorsum of the foot	Anterior to the upper and lateral parts of the calcaneus	Base of the proximal section of the big toe

Table 48 Flexors of the joints of the 2nd-5th toes

Name	Location and form	Starting point	Ending point
Long flexor muscle of the toe	In the deep layer at the tibial side posterior to the shank	Posterior to the fibula	Base of the distal section of the 2nd-5th toes
Short flexor muscle of the toe	In the middle part of the foot dorsum	Anterior to the upper and lateral parts of the calcaneus	Base of the middle section of the 2nd-5th toes

Table 49 Extensors of the joints of the 2nd-5th toes

Name	Location and form	Starting point	Ending point
Long extensor muscle of the toe	Anterior and medial to the interosseous membrane of the shank	Anterior to the fibula	Base of the middle and distal sections of the 2nd-5th toes
Short extensor muscle of the toe	Middle and lateral sections of the foot dorsum	Anterior to the upper and lateral parts of the calcaneus	Base of the proximal section of the 2nd-5th toes

Appendix 2
LOCATION OF THE COMMONLY USED ACUPOINTS ON THE HUMAN BODY

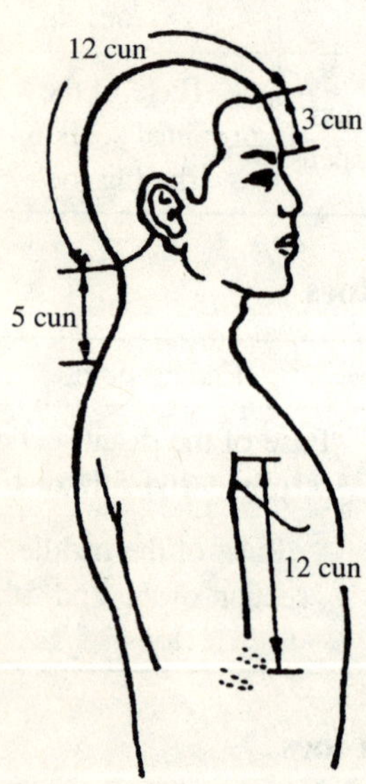

Fig. 2-1 Perpendicular *cun* measurement of the head (lateral side)

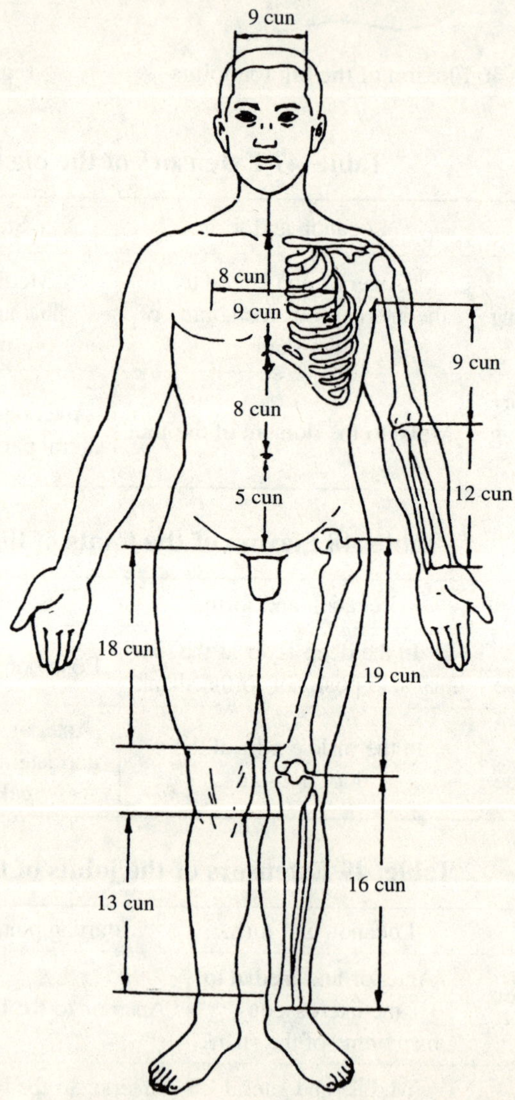

Fig. 2-2 Proportional *cun* measurement of bones (frontal)

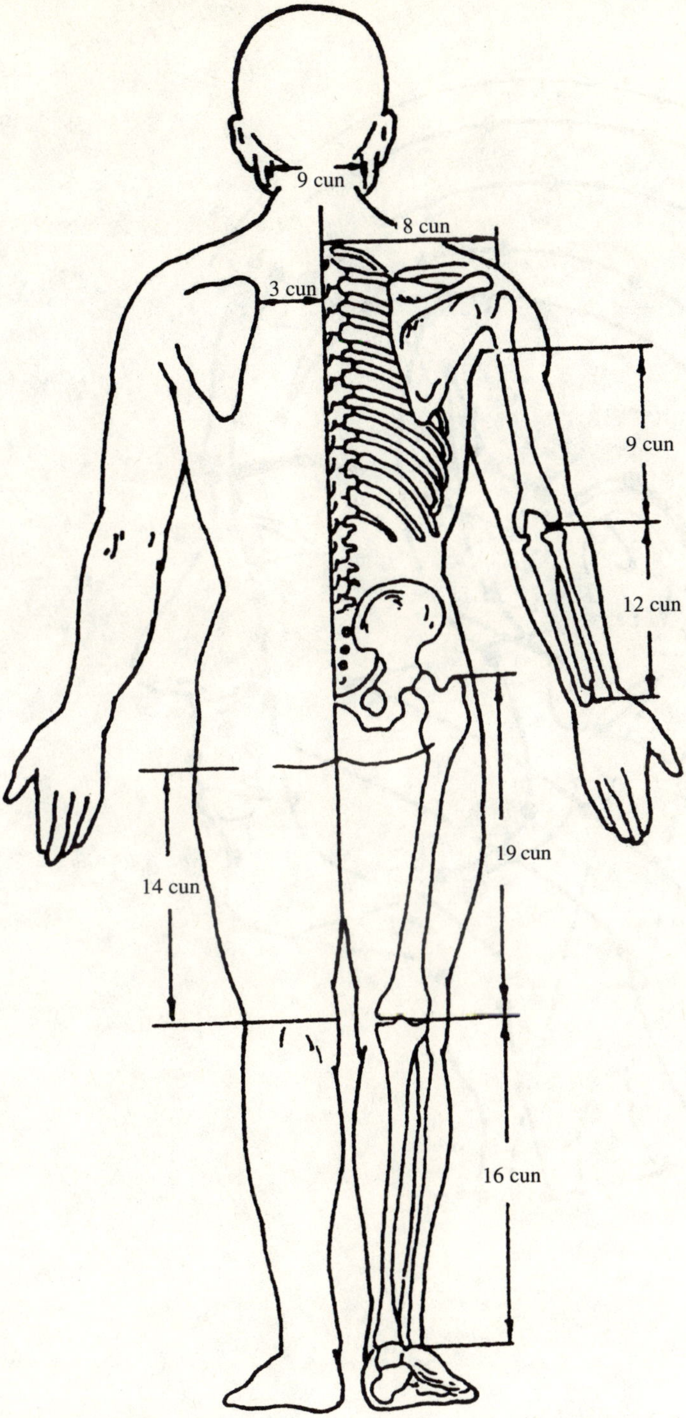

Fig. 2-3 Proportional *cun* measurement of bones (back)

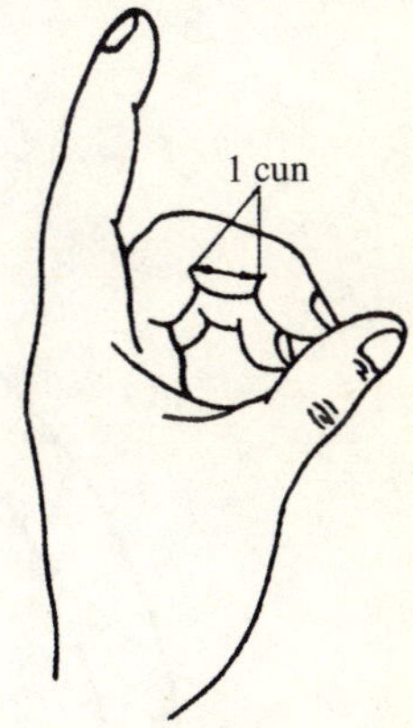

Fig. 2-4 Middle finger *cun*

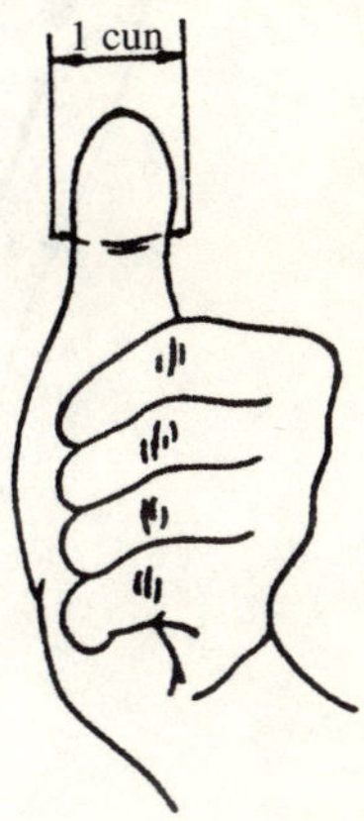

Fig. 2-5 Transverse finger *cun*

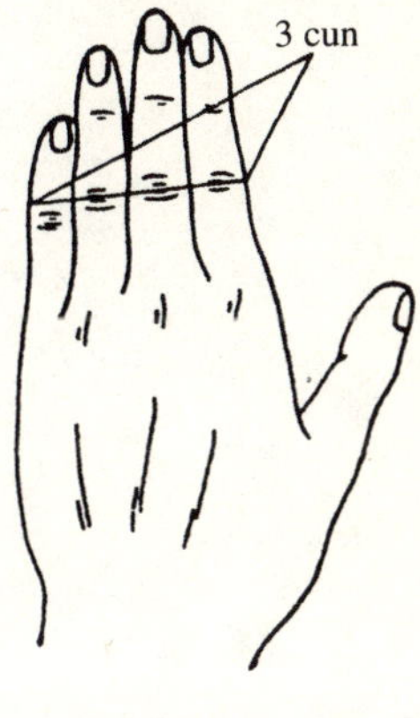

Fig. 2-6 Thumb *cun*

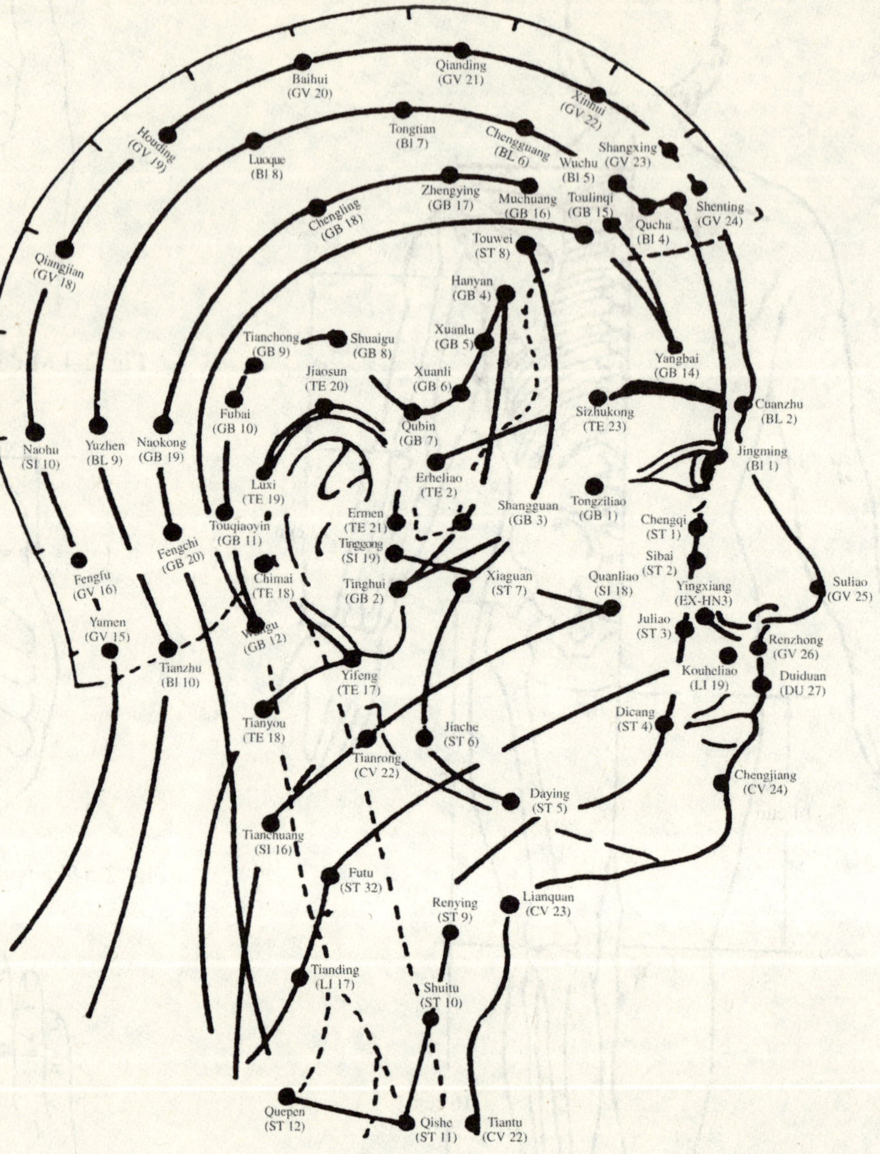

Fig. 2-7 Acupoints located on the face and head (lateral)

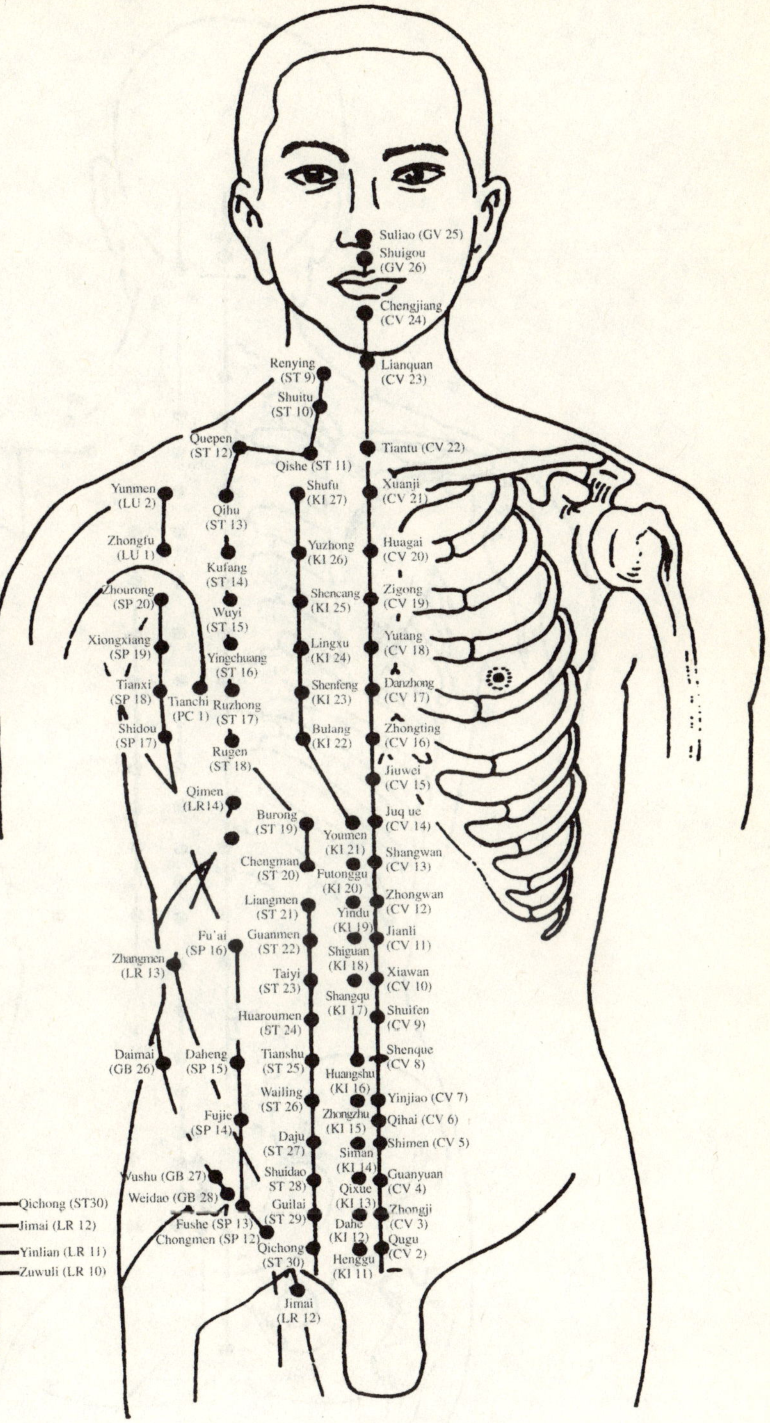

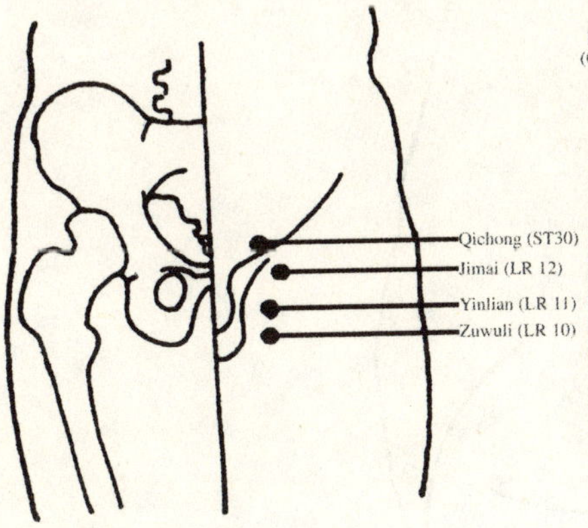

Fig. 2-8 Zuwuli (LR 10), Yinlian (LR 11) and Jimai (LR 12) acupoints

Fig. 2-9 Acupoints located on the chest and abdomen

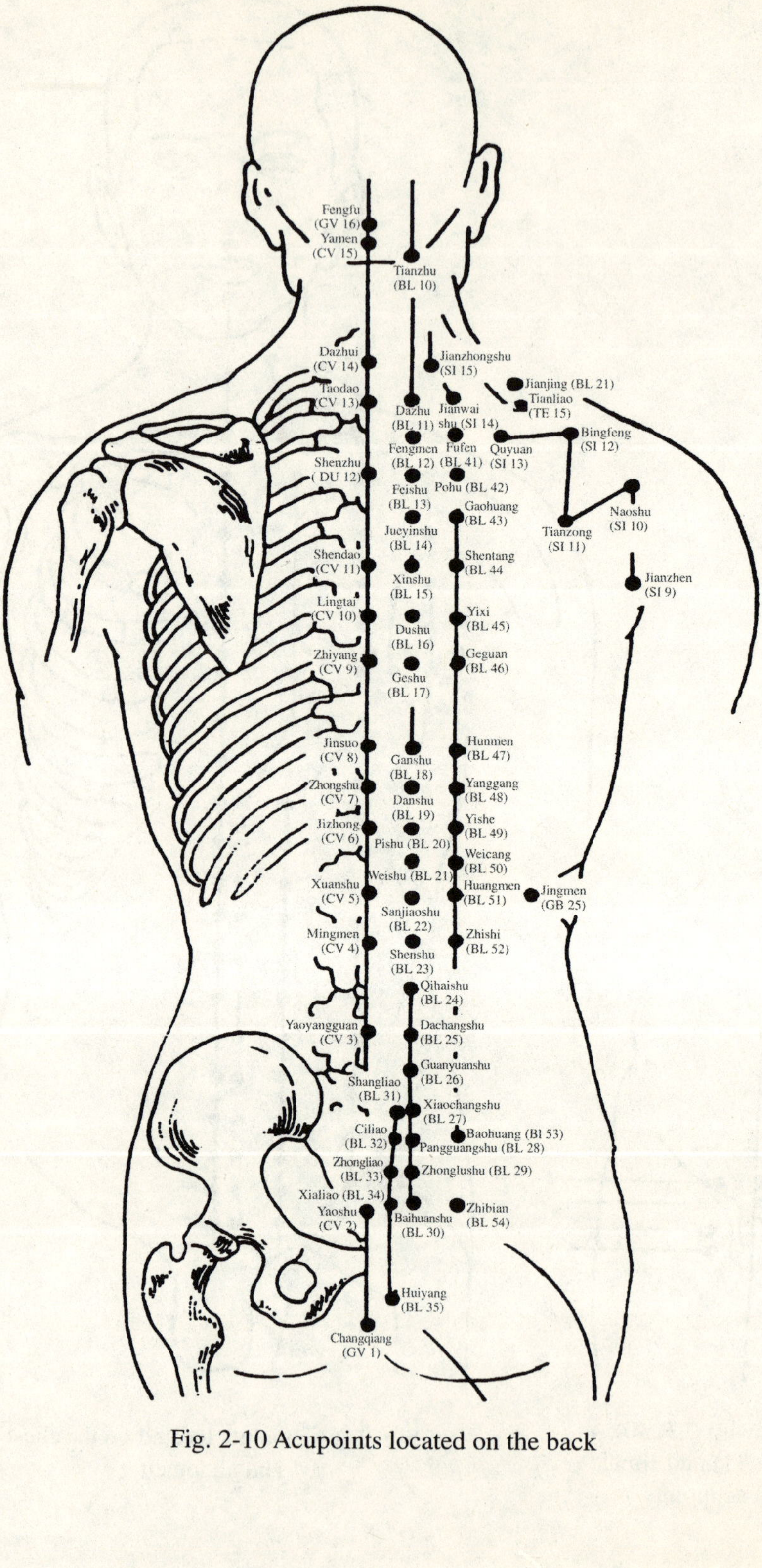

Fig. 2-10 Acupoints located on the back

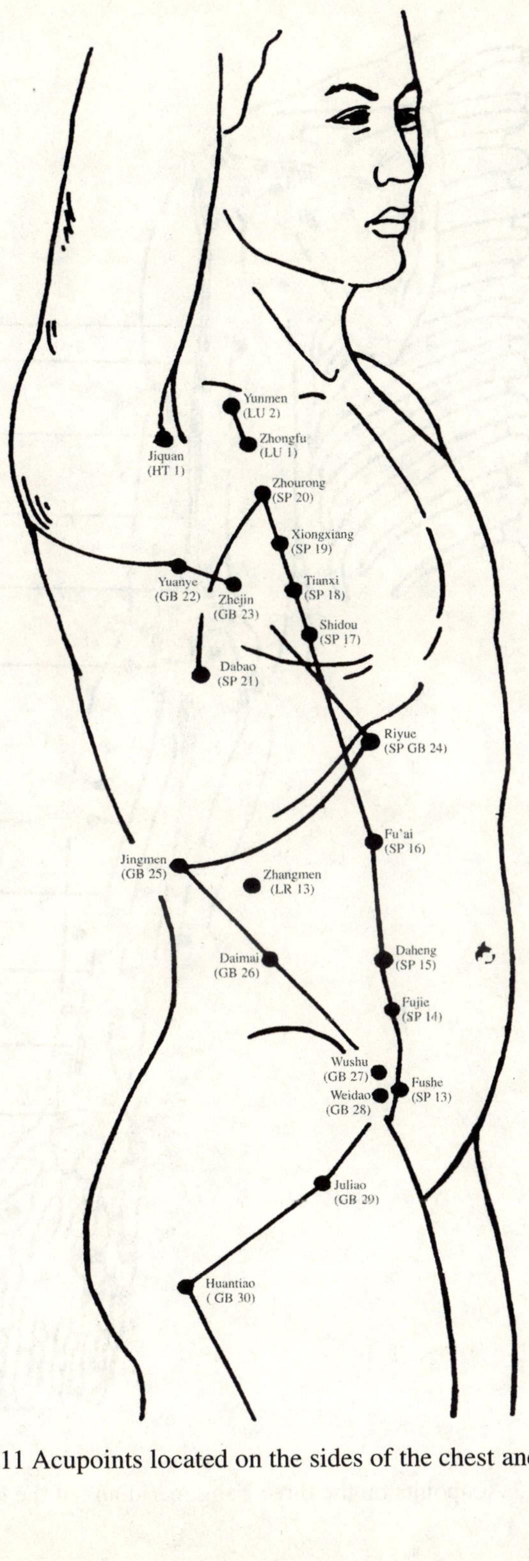

Fig. 2-11 Acupoints located on the sides of the chest and abdomen

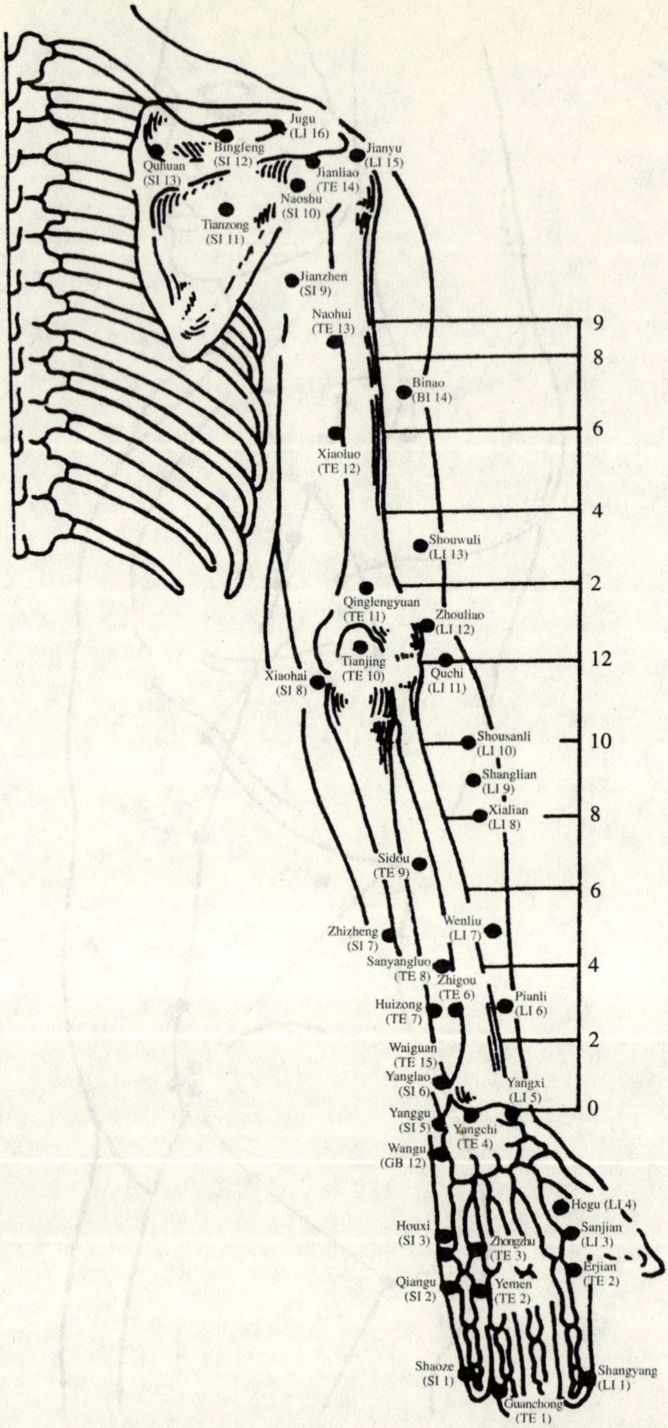

Fig. 2-12 Acupoints on the three Yang meridians of the hand

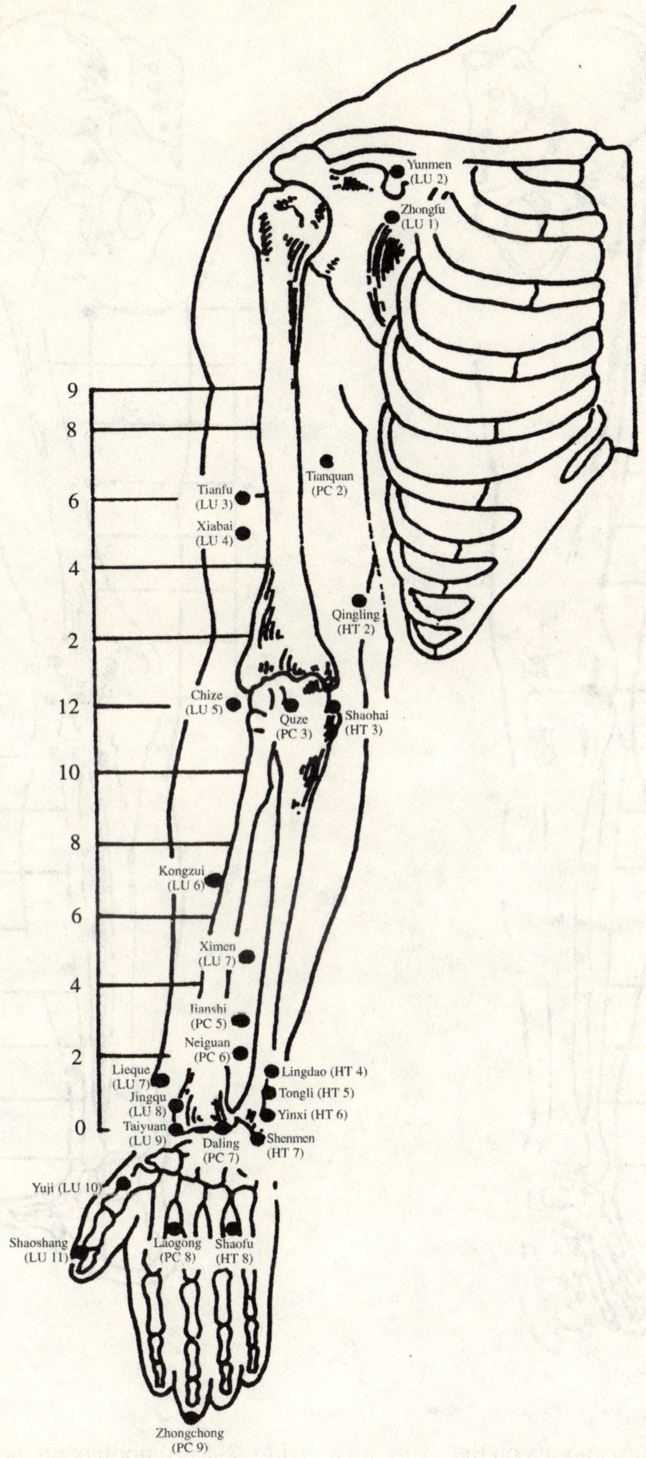

Fig. 2-13 Acupoints on the three Yin meridians of the hand

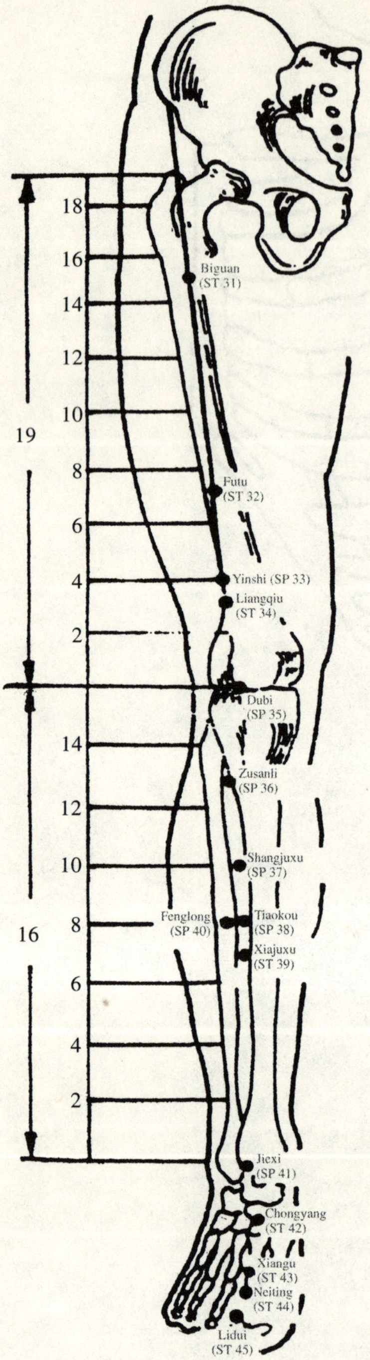

Fig. 2-14 Acupoints on the stomach meridian (lower limb)

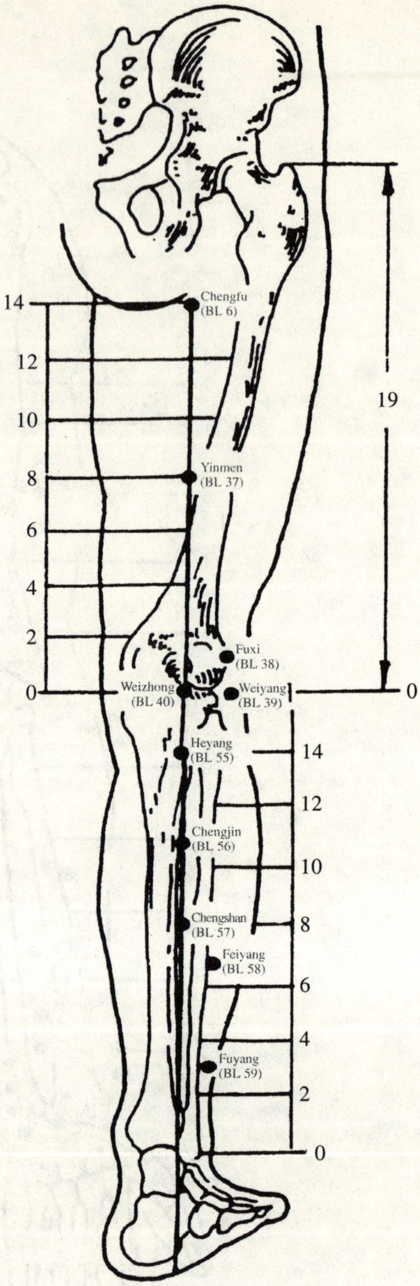

Fig. 2-15 Acupoints on the bladder meridian (lower limb)

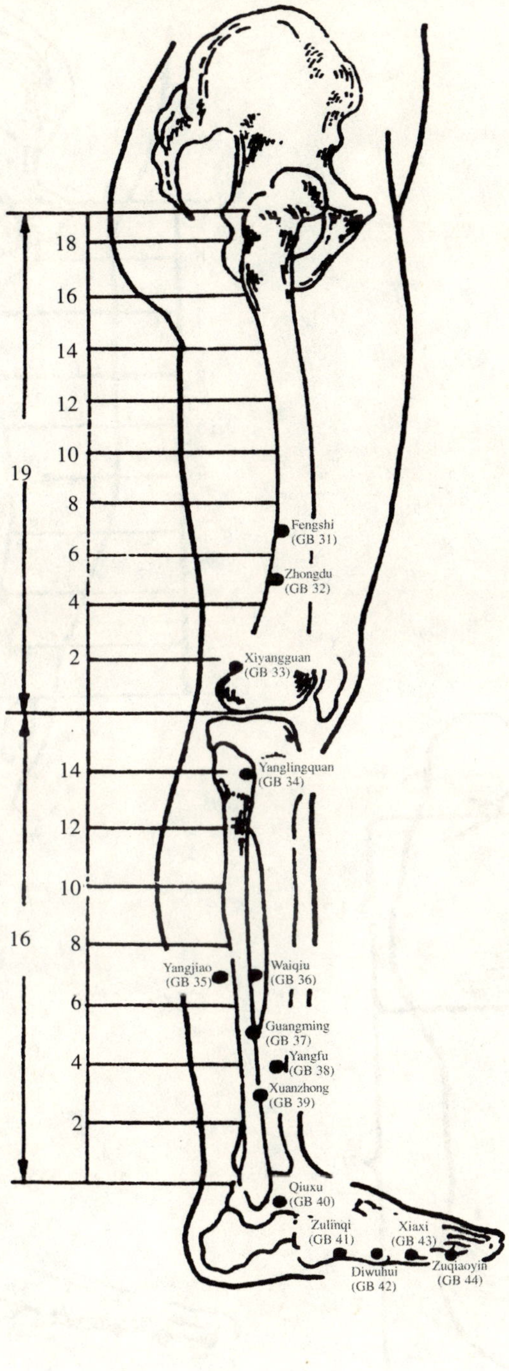

Fig. 2-16 Acupoints on the gallbladder meridian (lower limb)

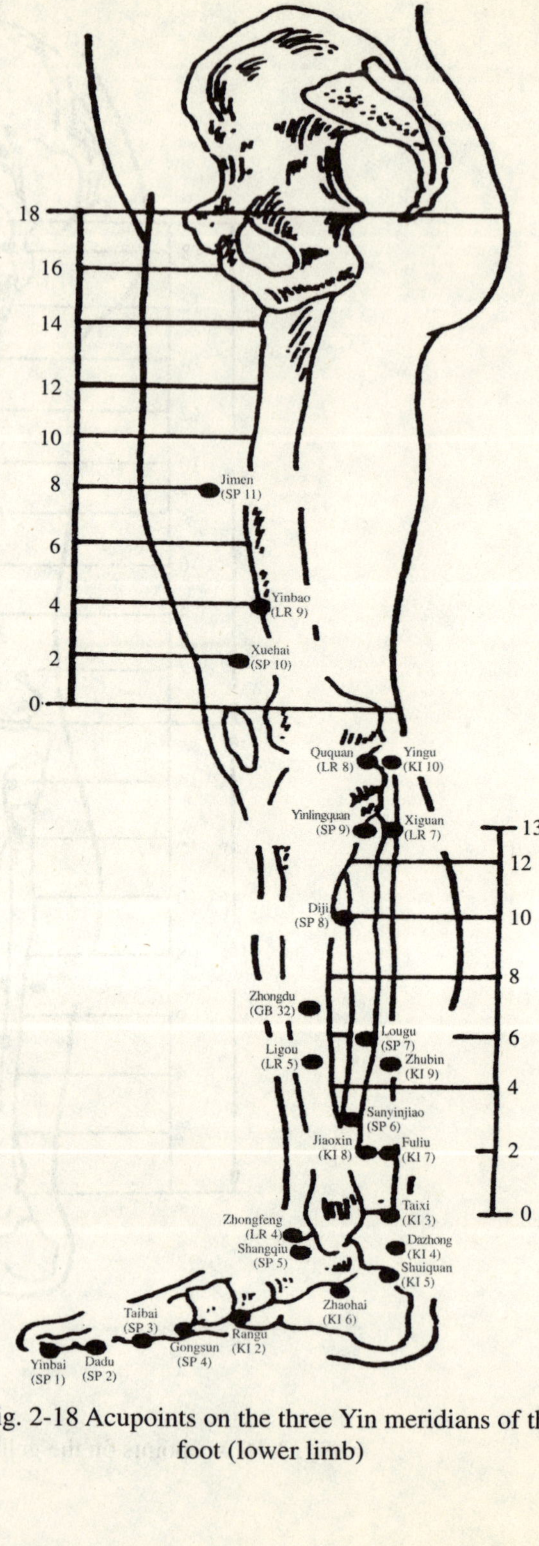

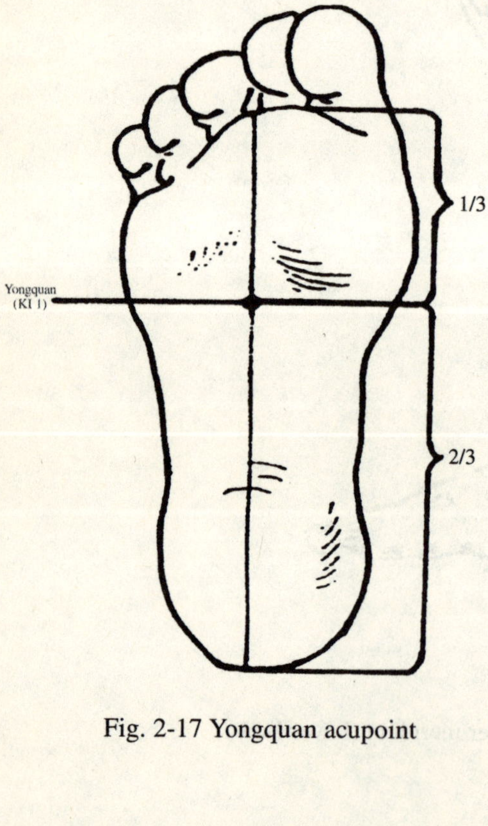

Fig. 2-17 Yongquan acupoint

Fig. 2-18 Acupoints on the three Yin meridians of the foot (lower limb)

图书在版编目（CIP）数据

中风偏瘫中医康复术详图解/潘畅 著.
一北京：外文出版社，2004
ISBN 7-119-03192-9

I. 中… II. 潘… III. 中风一中医学：康复医学一图解
IV. R255.2-64

中国版本图书馆 CIP 数据核字（2002）第 082087 号

英文翻译 李照国等 **英文审定** 梁良兴
责任编辑 胡开敏 **插图绘制** 徐 麟
封面设计 蔡 荣 **印刷监制** 张国祥

中风偏瘫中医康复术详图解
潘 畅著
*

外文出版社出版
（中国北京百万庄大街 24 号）
邮政编码 100037
外文出版社网址:
http://www.flp.com.cn
外文出版社电子信箱:
info@flp.com.cn
sales@flp.com.cn

中国国际图书贸易总公司发行
(中国北京车公庄西路 35 号)
北京邮政信箱第 399 号 邮政编码 100044
2004 年(16 开)第 1 版
2004 年第 1 版 第 1 次印刷
(英)
ISBN 7-119-03192-9/R·187(外)
08000（精）
14-E-3386S